A COMPANION TO SPECIALIST SURGICAL PRACTICE

Breast and Endocrine Surgery

A COMPANION TO SPECIALIST SURGICAL PRACTICE

Series editors

Sir David C. Carter
O. James Garden
Simon Paterson-Brown

Breast and Endocrine Surgery

Edited by

John R. Farndon

Professor and Head of Department
University Department of Surgery
Bristol Royal Infirmary
Bristol

W B Saunders Company Limited
London · Philadelphia · Toronto · Sydney · Tokyo

W. B. Saunders Company Ltd 24–28 Oval Road
London NW1 7DX

The Curtis Center
Independence Square West
Philadelphia, PA 19106-3399, USA

Harcourt Brace & Company
55 Horner Avenue
Toronto, Ontario M8Z 4X6, Canada

Harcourt Brace & Company, Australia
30–52 Smidmore Street
Marrickville, NSW 2204, Australia

Harcourt Brace & Company, Japan
Ichibancho Central Building, 22-1 Ichibancho
Chiyoda-ku, Tokyo 102, Japan

A catalogue record for this book is available from the British Library

ISBN 0-7020-2144-X

Typeset by Florencetype Ltd, Stoodleigh, Devon
Printed in Great Britain by The Bath Press, Bath

Contents

Contributors

Nigel D. S. Bax *PhD FRCP (Lon) FRCP (Ed)*
Academic Dean of Medicine, South East Asia, University of Sheffield;
Dean, Asean Sheffield Medical College, Ipoh, Perak, Malaysia;
Honorary Consultant Physician, Royal Hallamshire Hospital, Central
Sheffield University Hospital Trust, Sheffield, UK

J. Michael Dixon *BSc(Hons) MBChB MB FRCS (Ed) FRCS (Eng)*
Honorary Senior Lecturer in Surgery, Department of Surgery, Royal
Infirmary; Consultant Surgeon, Edinburgh Breast Unit, Western
General Hospital, Edinburgh, UK

John R. Farndon *BSc MD FRCS*
Professor and Head of Department, University Department of
Surgery, Bristol Royal Infirmary, Bristol, UK

Janet Hardy *MB ChB FRACP MD*
Consultant Physician, Department of Palliative Medicine, Royal
Marsden Hospital, Surrey, UK

Mark W. Kissin *MChir FRCS*
Consultant Breast Surgeon & Quality Assurance Co-ordinator for
Breast Screening in South West Thames Region, Royal Surrey
County & St Luke's Hospital Trust, Surrey, UK

Robert C. F. Leonard *BSc MBBS MD FRCP FRCPE*
Consultant Medical Oncologist, Edinburgh Breast Unit, Western
General Hospital, Edinburgh, UK

Robert E. Mansel *MS FRCS*
Professor of Surgery, University of Wales College of Medicine,
Cardiff, UK

Radu Mihai *MD*
Research Fellow, University Department of Surgery, Bristol Royal
Infirmary, Bristol; University Assistant, Department of
Endocrinology, Carol Davila University, Bucharest, Romania

Jeffrey A. Norton *MD*
Professor of Surgery, Chief of Endocrine & Oncologic Surgery,
Washington University School of Medicine, St Louis, Missouri, USA

Gary R. Peplinski *MD*
General Surgery Resident, Department of Surgery, Washington
University School of Medicine, St Louis, Missouri, USA

Hemant Singhal *MBBS FRCS*
University of Wales College of Medicine, Cardiff, UK

Richard Sainsbury *MD FRCS*
Consultant Surgeon, Breast Clinic, The Royal Infirmary, Lindley, Huddersfield, UK

W. James B. Smellie *MB BChir FRCS*
Directorate of Surgery, St Thomas' Hospital, London, UK

Malcolm H. Wheeler *MD FRCS*
Consultant Surgeon, University Hospital of Wales, Cardiff, UK

H. Frank Woods *DPhil FRCP (Lon) FRCP (Ed)*
Sir George Franklin Professor of Medicine, University of Sheffield; Honorary Consultant Physician, Royal Hallamshire Hospital, Central Sheffield University Hospital Trust, Sheffield, UK

Anthony E. Young *MChir FRCS*
Consultant Surgeon, Directorate of Surgery, St Thomas' Hospital, London, UK

Foreword

General surgery defies easy definition. Indeed, there are those who claim that it is dying, if not yet dead – a corpse being picked clean by the vulturine proclivities of the other specialties of surgery. Unfortunately for those who subscribe to this view, general surgery is not lying down, indeed it is rejoicing in a new enhanced vigour, as this new series demonstrates.

The general surgeon is the specialist who, along with his other colleagues, provides a 24-hour, 7-day, emergency surgical cover for his, or her, hospital. Also it is to general surgical clinics that patients are referred, unless their condition is manifestly related to one of the other surgical specialties e.g. urology, cardiothoracic services, etc. Moreover trainees in these specialities must, during their training, receive experience in general surgery, whose techniques underpin the whole of surgery. General surgery occupies a pivotal position in surgical training. The number of general surgeons required to serve a community, outstrips that required by any other surgical specialty.

General surgery is a specialty in its own right. Inevitably, there are those who wish to practice exclusively one of the sub-specialties of general surgery, e.g. vascular or colorectal surgery. This arrangement may be possible in a few large tertiary referral centres. Although the contribution of these surgeons to patient care and to advances in their discipline will be significant, their numbers are necessarily low. The bulk of surgical practice will be undertaken by the general surgeon who has developed a sub-specialty interest, so that, with his other colleagues in the hospital, comprehensive surgery services can be provided.

There is therefore a great need for a text which will provide comprehensively the theoretical knowledge of the entire specialty and act as a guide for the acquisition of the diagnostic and therapeutic skills required by the general surgeon. The unique contribution of this companion is that it comes as a series, each chapter fresh from the pen of a practising clinician and active surgeon. Each volume is right up to date and this is evidenced by the fact that the first volumes of the series are being published within 12 months from the start of the project. This is a series which has been tightly edited by a team from one of the foremost teaching hospitals in the United Kingdom.

Quite properly the series begins with a volume on emergency surgery and critical care – two of the greatest challenges confronting the practising surgeon. These are the areas that the examination candidate finds the greatest difficulty in acquiring theoretical knowledge and practical experience. Moreover, these are the areas in which advances are at present so rapid that they constantly test the experienced consultant surgeon.

This series not only provides both types of reader with the necessary up-to-date detail but also demonstrates that general surgery remains as challenging and vigorous as it ever has been.

Sir Robert Shields *DL, MD, DSc, FRCS(Ed, Eng, Glas, Ire),*
FRCPEd, FACS
President, Royal College of Surgeons of Edinburgh

Preface

A Companion to Specialist Surgical Practice was designed to meet the needs of the higher surgeon in training and busy practising surgeon who need access to up-to-date information on recent developments, research and data in the context of accepted surgical practice.

Many of the major surgery text books either cover the whole of what is termed 'general surgery' and therefore contain much which is not of interest to the specialist surgeon, or are very high level specialist texts which are outwith the reach of the trainee's finances, and though comprehensive are often out of date due to the lengthy writing and production times of such major works.

Each volume in this series therefore provides succinct summaries of all key topics within a specialty and concentrates on the most recent developments and current data. They are carefully constructed to be easily readable and provide key references.

A specialist surgeon, whether in training or in practice, need only purchase the volume relevant to his or her chosen specialist field plus the emergency surgery and critical care volume, if involved in emergency care.

The volumes have been written in a very short time frame, and produced equally quickly so that information is as up to date as possible. Each volume will be updated and published as a new edition at frequent intervals, to ensure that current information is always available.

We hope that our aim – of providing affordable up-to-date specialist texts – has been met and that all surgeons, in training or in practice will find the volumes to be a valuable resource.

Sir David C. Carter *MD, FRCS(Ed), FRCS(Glas), FRCS(Eng), Hon FRCS(Ire), Hon FACS, FRCP(Ed), FRS(Ed)*
Chief Medical Officer in Scotland
Formerly Regius Professor of Clinical Surgery, University Department of Surgery, Royal Infirmary, Edinburgh

O. James Garden *BSc, MB, ChB, MD, FRCS(Glas), FRCS(Ed)*
Professor of Hepatobiliary Surgery of the Royal Infirmary; Director of Organ Transplantation, University Department of Surgery, Royal Infirmary, Edinburgh

Simon Paterson-Brown *MS, MPhil, FRCS(Ed), FRCS(Eng), FCSHK*
Consultant General and Upper Gastrointestinal Surgeon, University Department of Surgery, Royal Infirmary, Edinburgh

Acknowledgements

I am indebted to all the authors who have contributed to this volume for their perseverance and expertise. I am grateful to my fellow editors for assistance and advice in the initial planning of this book. The series editors give special thanks to Rachael Stock and Linda Clark from W. B. Saunders for their initial persuasion, continuing enthusiasm and ongoing support. I am grateful to my secretaries Alison Foxwell and Carol Bond, for their expert help with the preparation and editing of the manuscripts. Finally, as always, I am indebted to my wife, Chris, for her never-ending support in yet another academic venture.

J. R. FARNDON

1 Parathyroids – primary and secondary disease

Radu Mihai
John R. Farndon

Primary hyperparathyroidism

Primary hyperparathyroidism (1°HPT) is a common endocrine disorder, occurring as frequently as diabetes mellitus and hyperthyroidism. Because many patients remain asymptomatic, the reported incidence varies according to the means of diagnosis and the population studied and has increased significantly since the use of multichannel biochemical analysers. In the UK the incidence was estimated to be 25 per 100 000 general population[1] but it may be 1 in 1000 of a blood donor panel, 1 in 680 in a hospital population and 1 in 500 in women older than 45 years. The prevalence in older women might be up to 1%.

Aetiology

Monoclonality

Monoclonality has been demonstrated using X chromosome inactivation analysis in parathyroid adenomas,[2,3] in parathyroid hyperplasia in patients with familial multiple endocrine neoplasia (MEN) type 1[4,5] and in sporadic multigland 1°HPT.[6]

The molecular events associated with the development of parathyroid neoplasia have not been entirely characterised but at least three tumour-specific molecular genetic defects have been implicated.

1. Cyclin D_1 overexpression has been demonstrated in some parathyroid adenomas. It is due to a clonal chromosomal inversion by which the 5′-regulatory region of the parathyroid hormone (PTH) gene on chromosome 11 is juxtaposed to the *PRAD1* (parathyroid adenoma 1) gene[7,8] leading to expression of cyclin D_1 oncogene – a cell cycle regulator of G1/S transition.[9]
2. Retinoblastoma (*RB*) gene deletion has been found in some aggressive and malignant parathyroid tumours.[10] *RB* is a growth suppressor gene acting as a negative regulator of the G1/S transition

in normal cells.[11] The simultaneous deregulation of the RB and cyclin D pathways also described in several other tissues suggest a multicomponent model of tumorigenesis.

3. Loss of a tumour suppressor gene is suggested by the loss of heterezygosity in more than 25% of parathyroid adenomas on chromosome arms 11q, 1p,[12] 6q, and 15q[13] but no such genes have been identified or cloned. Analysis of *p53*, a well-studied tumour suppressor gene, shows that none of its characteristic mutations appear in either parathyroid adenomas or carcinomas[14] and allelic loss of p53 gene appears in only a minority of carcinomas.[15]

One or more such chromosomal abnormalities are present in most parathyroid tumours studied, suggesting that parathyroid cells, like many other cell types, require the accumulation of multiple genetic lesions. Mechanisms involved in parathyroid tumorigenesis in familial syndromes are discussed in Chapter 4.

Genetic defects might explain the abnormal growth or proliferation of parathyroid cells but do not account for or correlate with the loss of sensitivity to extracellular calcium concentration – the biochemical hallmark of 1°HPT. The recent cloning of a calcium-sensing receptor (CaR) from parathyroid cells[16] raises the hypothesis that dysfunction of this CaR might explain the abnormal Ca^{2+}-regulated PTH secretion in hyperparathyroidism. It is known that inactivating mutations of CaR cause autosomal dominant hypercalcaemic disorders (i.e. familial hypocalciuric hypercalcaemia and neonatal severe hyperparathyroidism[17]) but no such mutations have been identified in parathyroid tumours[18] and allelic losses on chromosome 3 at the CaR locus appear in less that 10% of tumours.[19] A substantial reduction in the intensity of CaR immunostaining has been described in parathyroid adenomas[20] and this decreased expression of CaR would be compatible with the functional abnormalities. In addition, a member of the low density lipoprotein receptor superfamily was reported to be another putative Ca^{2+} sensor on parathyroid cells[21] with reduced expression in 1°HPT.[22]

Radiation-associated HPT

In some series, 15–20% of patients give a history of prior irradiation but radiation-associated disease rather than radiation-induced is preferred, because an aetiological link cannot be established. A dose–response relationship exists, with an excess relative risk increased significantly by 0.11/cGy and this is not influenced by gender or age at first presentation.[23]

Mechanisms

In 1°HPT, the frequency and length of pulses of PTH secretion are not abnormal but patients have an increased basal secretion and increased amplitude of PTH pulses.[24]

Although PTH secretion is still modulated by plasma calcium levels, a decreased sensitivity of parathyroid cells to extracellular calcium has been demonstrated by studies *in vivo* and *in vitro*. This induces an increased set-point (defined as calcium level at which PTH secretion is inhibited by 50%) and a shift to the right of the inverse sigmoidal relationship between PTH secretion and calcium concentration. These functional abnormalities explain the maintenance of high plasma PTH levels in the face of hypercalcaemia.

PTH binds to specific receptors on the membrane of target cells and induces activation of several intracellular second messengers (cAMP, IP_3, Ca^{2+}). PTH receptors are widely distributed in a variety of cells other than the 'traditional' renal and bone target cells, including fibroblasts, chondrocytes, vascular smooth muscle, fat cells and placental trophoblasts.[25]

An important regulator of parathyroid cell growth is active vitamin D_3 ($1,25(OH)_2D_3$), which also inhibits PTH gene transcription by binding to its receptor (VDR) in specific regions of the PTH gene promoter. It is assumed that impaired effects of vitamin D_3 may contribute to the enhanced secretion and proliferation seen in 1°HPT. The VDR genotype *bb* is found in 60% of postmenopausal women with 1°HPT[26] and since this genotype is linked to decreased transcriptional activity or messenger RNA stability, it will account for reduced VDR expression and impeded regulatory actions of vitamin D.

Current data suggest that the biochemical severity of 1°HPT is determined by a combination of parameters, such as Ca-receptor content, set-point, gland size and secretory output per cell. It remains to be determined whether the pathogenesis of 1°HPT represents a primary abnormality in the control of cell growth with a secondary change in Ca-receptor expression and function, a primary alteration in Ca-sensing pathways predisposing to somatic mutations in genes controlling growth or a combination of these two mechanisms.

Presentation

Asymptomatic disease

Asymptomatic disease may be found in up to 50% of patients, although definition criteria differ between centres. Such a high prevalence of asymptomatic patients contrasts markedly with earlier studies in which less than 1% of diagnosed patients were considered without identifiable symptoms. If followed for up to 10 years most asymptomatic patients deteriorate and might require surgery. Even patients with mild asymptomatic 1°HPT already have significant bone loss at diagnosis and parathyroidectomy has only an initial positive effect on bone mineralisation but no long-term advantage.[27]

Renal manifestations

Renal manifestations have decreased from 60–70% to 10–20% over the last decades. It is unclear what constitutional or environmental factors affect this incidence since many patients now lack renal manifestations despite having had the disease for many years. Polyuria, back pain, colic and haematuria are possible symptoms and signs.

There are two broad categories of kidney lesions: anatomical (nephrolithiasis and nephrocalcinosis) and functional (a spectrum of tubular and glomerular disorders). Functional changes occur in the absence of any demonstrable renal calcification. Reductions in glomerular filtration rate determine elevations of blood urea nitrogen and creatinine. Impairment of bicarbonate transport in the proximal tubule causes renal proximal tubular acidosis type II. This hyperchloraemic acidosis due to excess PTH contrasts with mild alkalosis accompanying hypercalcaemia of other causes (as in malignancy and vitamin D intoxication). Aminoaciduria, glycosuria and a decreased capacity to concentrate urine (nephrogenous diabetes insipidus) are reported. The pathogenesis of nephrolithiasis still remains unclear and there is no correlation with hypercalciuria. The propensity for crystallisation and crystal growth of stone-forming constituents of urine is increased by the urinary acidosis and excess of vitamin D and/or calcium in the diet provides a positive risk factor.

Skeletal involvement
Osteitis fibrosa cystica has decreased in incidence from more than 50% in 1930–1950 to 9% in the 1970s and nearly zero in recent series. Excess PTH initiates bone remodeling and increased bone resorption is associated with enhanced bone formation. There are region-specific differences in bone mass, with low values in areas with cortical bone (e.g. radius) and normal/high values in vertebrae and iliac crest (trabecular bone).

Histological bone markers of excess PTH include reduction in the number of trabeculae, increase in multinucleated osteoclasts, Howship's lacunae on the surface of the bone and replacement of normal cellular and marrow elements by fibrovascular tissue. Fractures are rarely seen today (Figure 1.1).

Articular manifestations
Chondrocalcinosis with attacks of pseudogout, juxta-articular erosions, traumatic synovitis and periarthritis are recognised complications of 1°HPT.

Neuromuscular and neuropsychiatric manifestations
The real incidence of these is difficult to evaluate because some of the symptoms may be non-specific or reflect degenerative or ageing features. Extreme weakness and fatigue, particularly involving proximal musculature of the lower extremities can be present and improves after surgery. Many patients with 1°HPT are asymptomatic. Some, however, have severe muscular weakness which may be confused with amyotrophic lateral sclerosis or muscular dystrophy. Gross atrophy of the muscles involved can be detectable on clinical examination.

Figure 1.1
Brown tumour of the mandibula in a patient with primary hyperparathyroidism

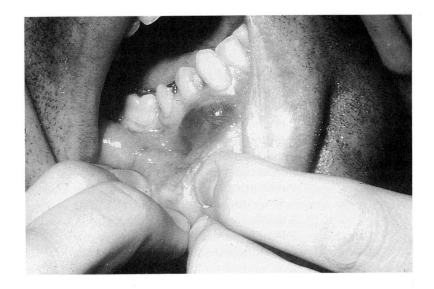

A loss of 'well-being' is frequently encounted. Depression, apathy, lethargy, confusion, personality changes, memory impairment and occasionally overt psychosis are the effect of hypercalcaemia and excess PTH.

Gastrointestinal involvement

Anorexia, nausea, dyspepsia, constipation and abdominal pain are frequent symptoms. Peptic ulcer disease appears to be a true manifestation of symptomatic 1°HPT and not just a coincidental relationship. In a minority of patients, ulcers are part of the Zollinger–Ellison syndrome or MEN 1 with gastrin-producing tumours.

Pancreatitis may occur but a cause–effect relationship is uncertain. In acute 1°HPT, 25% of patients may have pancreatitis. Normocalcaemia in a patient with severe acute pancreatitis should raise the question of 1°HPT as an aetiological factor, saponification calcium absorption giving a spurious normal calcium level.

Hypertension

High blood pressure is often present at the time of diagnosis but a specific correlation is not easily identified. Plasma renin activity, plasma aldosterone and whole-body exchangeable sodium do not differ between normotensive and hypertensive patients with 1°HPT and are unchanged after surgery. A role of impaired renal function is supported by the inverse relationship between mean arterial pressure and glomerular filtration rate before and after parathyroidectomy. Recently a parathyroid hypertensive factor (PHF) has been purified from plasma of spontaneously hypertensive rats (SHRs) and culture medium from organ culture of SHR parathyroid glands.[28] It was reported that in patients with 1°HPT, the presence of PHF is linked with hypertension and postparathyroidectomy blood pressure falls in parallel with PHF levels.[29]

Increased risk of premature death

Although an overall cure rate of 97% is achieved in patients undergoing surgery, a study of 896 patients revealed an increased risk of premature death, better survival being reported for patients who underwent parathyroidectomy at an early stage of disease.[30] Additional mortality due mainly to cardiovascular disease was also reported for mild and non-progressive forms of disease. The death rate attributable to 1°HPT in the USA in 1986, however, was only 57 for the entire population and an additional 157 deaths were attributable to hypercalcaemic complications.[31] These officially reported figures may underestimate the real mortality and a prospective study of sufficient size and design is needed to answer this question.

Other clinical manifestations

Rickets in children with 1°HPT is explained by enhanced bone resorption/turnover and limited dietary calcium intake due to anorexia. Neonatal tetany in children of mothers with HPT occurs because chronic hypercalcaemia during gestation inhibits the function of the newborn parathyroids.

Normocalcaemic hyperparathyroidism is defined as completely normal total serum calcium in the presence of symptoms or complications of 1°HPT. Factors known to decrease calcium levels (such as decreased serum albumin levels, vitamin D deficiency, severe pancreatitis, increased phosphate intake and hypomagnesiaemia) should be eliminated during the diagnostic work-up.

Most patients are identified because of a renal calculus and most of them have hypercalciuria.[32] They present a diagnostic challenge to differentiate from idiopathic hypercalciuria (assumed to be due to increased intestinal absorption, diminished tubular resorption of calcium resulting in a renal leak or a primary urinary phosphate leak). A failure to distinguish these two possibilities may lead to inappropriate neck exploration in patients with idiopathic hypercalciuria or to an overlooked diagnosis in those with 1°HPT.

Hypercalcaemic crisis

Hypercalcaemia is a common metabolic emergency, occurring in 0.5% of hospitalised patients. The severity of clinical manifestations often correlates with the degree of hypercalcaemia. Neuromuscular, renal and gastrointestinal manifestations are influenced by the time course of developing hypercalcaemia and the intercurrent medical conditions.

Hypercalcaemia associated with malignancy is the most common cause. Generally, the higher the levels of plasma calcium, the more likely that malignancy is the underlying cause. Acute 1°HPT is more frequent in patients with long-standing hypercalcaemia, very large parathyroid adenomas, radiographic evidence of osteitis fibrosa cystica (50%) and a history of nephrolithiasis (60%).[33] Sarcoidosis, milk-alkali syndrome and adrenal insufficiency are very rare causes of hypercalcaemic crisis. For a biochemical diagnosis it is important to use calcium values corrected for albumin (since it may be reduced in anorexic patients and catabolic status associated with neoplasia) or ionised calcium measurements.

Marked dehydration due to anorexia, nausea or vomiting leads to more severe hypercalcaemia. Weakness and lethargy lead to immobilisation, which accentuates bone resorption. Confusion and frequent and significant cognitive impairment and coma are possible. If untreated, the condition will proceed to oliguric renal failure, cardiac arhythmia and death.

Familial hyperparathyroidism is presented in Chapter 4.

Differential diagnosis of hypercalcaemia includes several important conditions (Table 1.1) but more than 80% of patients with persistent hypercalcaemia will have either HPT or malignancy.

Table 1.1 *Other causes of hypercalcaemia*

Malignancy	Multiple myeloma Skeletal metastasis from breast, lung or other cancers Skeletal carcinomatosis
Iatrogenic	Treatment with thiazide diuretics Excess intake of vitamin D and/or calcium Treatment with Lithium
Immobilisation	
Familial diseases familial hypocalciuric hypercalcaemia	Abnormality of the calcium receptor (see text): must be checked by 24-hour urinary calcium excretion
metaphyseal chondrodysplasia Jansen	Constitutive activity of PTH/PTHRP receptor (very rare)
Granulomatous diseases	Sarcoidosis Tuberculosis
Endocrine diseases	Thyrotoxicosis Phaeochromocytoma Adrenal crisis
Renal failure	
Milk-alkali syndrome	

Breast and lung cancer account for 60% of hypercalcaemia of malignancy; renal cell cancer for 10–15%, head and neck carcinomas 10%, and haematological malignancies 10%. Many neoplastic tissues express high levels of PTH-related peptide (PTH-RP), a hormone with possible paracrine/autocrine functions in multiple adult and fetal tissues. Although its coding genes and chemical structure differ from PTH[34] the two peptides act on similar/identical receptors (see reviews in reference 25).

The history should include a careful drug history (to uncover the use of diuretics or antacids), a positive family history of hypercalcaemia (the possibility of familial hypocalciuric hypercalcaemia) or other endocrine tumours (the possibility of MEN syndromes).

Familial hypocalciuric hypercalcaemia (FHH) is an autosomal dominant disorder associating hypercalcaemia, low urinary calcium excretion and very few symptoms. PTH levels are usually within the normal range but are considered inappropriately elevated considering the calcium level. Several mutations in the calcium receptor gene can induce its low affinity for Ca^{2+} and a single defective allele causes FHH whereas two defective alleles cause neonatal severe hyperparathyroidism.

If referral occurs through physician colleagues it is hoped that sarcoidosis, thyrotoxicosis, tuberculosis and Addison's disease will have been excluded. Milk-alkali syndrome is now very rare, since H_2-blockers and proton-pump inhibitors make the use of high doses of alkaline compounds unnecessary.

Investigative techniques

Laboratory tests

Plasma and urine electrolytes

1. High total calcium/ionised calcium. Determination of total calcium continues to be used as a screening tool since it is widely available, inexpensive and has a low experimental error. Because it is generally accepted that most protein-bound calcium is in the form of calcium albuminate, corrected values for plasma albumin levels offer more reliability. When an abnormality of calcium metabolism is suspected, however, the direct measurement of the ionised fraction is the investigation of choice.[35] An increased plasma ionised calcium should raise the suspicion of 1°HPT in patients with minimal, intermittent or no elevation of the total calcium levels. The diagnosis is then supported by non-suppressed intact PTH levels (see reference 6)
2. Hypophosphataemia and phosphaturia
3. Hyperchloraemia and increased chloride to phosphate ratio (values > 33 confirm 1°HPT, whereas ratios of 17–32 are obtained in other clinical situations)

4. Hypercalciuria (> 10 mmol day^{-1}) is present in 75% of hypercalcaemic patients. Excess calcium spillage supports the diagnosis of 1°HPT but, more importantly, loss of less than 2 mmol of calcium per day must alert the clinician to the diagnosis of familial hypercalcaemic hypocalciuria. This condition may mimic 1°HPT very closely, with normal/high levels of parathyroid hormone inappropriate in the face of hypercalcaemia. Repeated urinary calcium determination, enquiry into family history and measurement of the serum calcium in first-degree siblings (being an autosomal dominant disorder) will confirm the correct diagnosis and save the patient an unnecessary neck exploration.

PTH level

Increased intact PTH level is essential for diagnosis. The initial pitfalls generated by measuring the biologically inactive C-terminal fragments of PTH are overcome by the new assay using two antibodies to identify only intact PTH. More recently, rapid PTH immunoradiometric and immunochemiluminometric assays have been described, which recognise the intact PTH molecule and can be used intraoperatively to confirm removal of all overactive parathyroid tissue. A similar method has been proposed for lateralisation of parathyroid adenomas by PTH estimation in left versus right internal jugular veins at the beginning of surgery.[36]

Serum alkaline phosphatase

An increased serum alkaline phosphatase is not usually seen since bone involvement is decreasing in severity.

Cyclic adenosine monophosphate and hydroxyproline

Increased urinary excretion of nephrogenous cyclic adenosine monophosphate (marker of PTH action of renal tubules) and hydroxyproline (marker of bone breakdown) are useful but not essential for diagnosis. Intraoperative measurement of nephrogenous cAMP can be used to prove the adequacy of resection, because its short half-life (2–4 min) allows detection of a quick decline following removal of hyperfunctional parathyroid tissue.

EDTA infusion test

The differential diagnosis of hypercalcaemia can be difficult, and this has led to the development of a hypocalcaemic stimulation test using an infusion of disodium EDTA or an intramuscular injection of salmon calcitonin. In 1°HPT EDTA always, and calcitonin usually (80%), induces an increase in PTH levels. No such rise is demonstrated in patients with other causes of hypercalcaemia.

Calcium infusion test

An intravenous calcium infusion test is used to demonstrate reduced suppressibility of PTH levels (the set-point abnormality). Patients with

1°HPT do not have a significant PTH response, while in normal individuals intact PTH suppress below 70% of baseline at 60 min after a 1000 mg calcium load. Simultaneous abnormal suppression of nephrogenous cAMP with oral calcium loading has also been used as a diagnostic test.

MEN syndromes

Since 1°HPT is the commonest component of the MEN syndromes it might be assumed that patients presenting with 1°HPT represent a population at increased risk for either of the two syndromes. However, serum gastrin, prolactin and calcitonin are needless determinations in patients without any clinical indication of MEN syndromes.[37]

Radiological studies

Parathyroid imaging is not needed before initial surgery because failure to localise will not influence the biochemically confirmed diagnosis and because a unilateral positive image will not obviate the need for bilateral neck exploration. All the imaging techniques available have insufficient sensitivity and specificity and none is adequate alone.

Ultrasonography is easily available but ineffective in localising small adenomas (weighing less than 500 mg). It produces satisfactory results in localising adenomas weighing more than 1 g, but these adenomas should not present a problem to an experienced endocrine surgeon. Intraoperative ultrasonography with 10 MHz probe is useful in locating intrathyroidal adenomas and during surgical re-exploration of the neck.

Subtraction scanning using technetium–thallium relies on the fact that thallium (^{201}Tl-chloride) is trapped in both thyroid and parathyroid tissue whereas technetium (^{99m}Tc-pertechnetate) is trapped only in thyroid (Fig 1.2). It seems that the uptake of thallium by parathyroids relates to mitotic activity (DNA profile) rather than gland weight.[38] Sensitivity up to 85% and specificity of about 90% have been reported.

The more recent technique of technetium–sestamibi scanning is becoming the initial investigation of choice.[39] Sestamibi accumulates into mitochondria of parathyroid cells in a manner similar to that described for thallium but its emission spectrum enhances the sensitivity for both smaller and deeper lesions. In addition, sestamibi scanning permits single photon emission computed tomography (SPECT) imaging, with a tridimensional data display and markedly improved spatial resolution.[40]

Computed tomography localises ectopic and mediastinal glands, but can be limited by artefacts from metallic clips from previous surgery. **Magnetic resonance imaging** (MRI) is best suited for locating ectopic glands, because the signal intensity of parathyroid adenomas is similar to that of thyroid gland and fat and MRI will therefore miss adenomas in close vicinity of thyroid. Comparison of the STIR (short tau inversion recovery) sequence images (which differentiate from fat tissue) with concomitant T1 images (which have better image detail) provides improved anatomical localisation.[41] In some centres MRI is the most accurate non-invasive localisation study, especially when gadolinium enhancement is used.

Positron emission tomography with [11C]methionine or glucose analogues is still experimental.[42]

The advantage and cost-effectiveness of preoperative localisation and unilateral neck exploration in 1°HPT are controversial issues. Some say preoperative localisation of a solitary parathyroid adenoma (eventually coupled with confirmation of excision of all hyperfunctional tissue by quick PTH assay) may optimise operative time with unilateral neck exploration.[43,44] Others report unacceptably high surgical failure rates for unilateral neck exploration guided by preoperative localising studies compared with a bilateral neck exploration by an experienced endocrine surgeon.[45]

Tests for localisation after operative failure

1. Venous sampling for PTH levels can be done before following neck exploration. A significant gradient between neck and peripheral blood will exclude the mediastinal parathyroid as the cause of 1°HPT and 'mapping' of the neck is helpful during the second exploration.
2. Measuring PTH by immunoradiometric assay in percutaneous needle aspirates of cervical masses was proposed as a method to confirm parathyroid adenomas[46] but the small size and profound position of most parathyroid tumours make this method difficult to apply.
3. Methylene blue is currently used by a few surgeons.
4. Limited arteriography is possible but rarely used in current practice.
5. Combined use of Tc-sestamibi and a hand-held gamma-detecting probe may prove feasible for intraoperative localisation of abnormal parathyroid tissue but the technique is still experimental.

Bone lesions

The earliest changes are seen on radiographs of the hands where subperiosteal erosions can be detected in the phalanges (especially the radial aspect of the middle phalanges) and terminal tufts. The skull demonstrates a mottled appearance with lucent cystic areas ('pepperpot skull' in its most florid form; Fig. 1.3) and any bone may demonstrate cystic lesions due to osteoclastomas or brown tumours. These lesions may lead to pathological fractures. Subtle bone changes are rarely detected on skeletal surveys and there is little justification for this investigation unless there are specific symptoms.

Abnormal bone density can be demonstrated by ^{125}I bone densitometry, X-ray spectrophotometry or single-photon absorptiometry. The densitometric site at which evidence of PTH-mediated bone

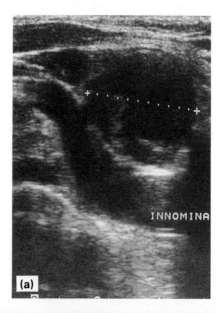

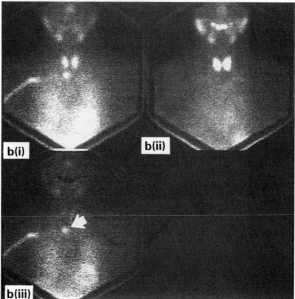

Figure 1.2 *Parathyroid imaging. (a) Ultrasound image of a parathyroid adenoma in close vicinity with the inominate artery. (b) Technetium-thalium subtraction scan: (i) thallium uptake by both thyroid and parathyroid; (ii) technetium uptake by the thyroid; (iii) the subtracted image, demonstrating an area of increased uptake on the left side of the neck, corresponding to left lower parathyroid.*

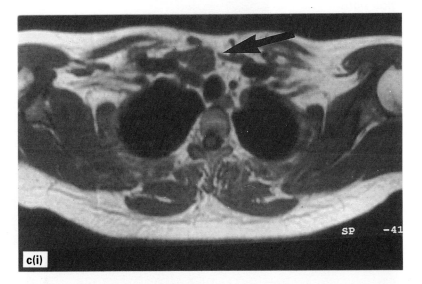

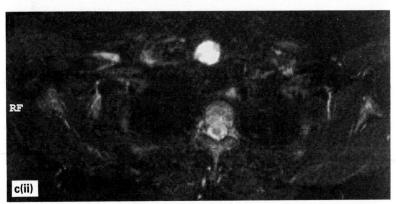

Figure 1.2 *(continued)   (c) Magnetic resonance image of the same adenoma in T2 (i) and STIR sequence (ii). (Courtesy of Dr J Caballa, Department of Radiology, Bristol Royal Infirmary, Bristol, UK)*

resorption is greatest is the cortical distal third of the radius. Bone mass can be evaluated by single- and dual-photon absorptiometry, quantitative CT and dual-energy X-ray absorptiometry (DEXA scan). In many patients there is an initial rapid loss in bone mass followed by a period of stable disease with little progression at the time of diagnosis of 1°HPT.

Pathological basis for primary hyperparathyroidism

Adenomas are found in 80% of patients. Chief cells, oxyphil cells and water clear cells are present in differing proportions in parathyroid

Figure 1.3
Radiological signs of primary hyper-parathyroidism: salt and pepper aspect of the skull.

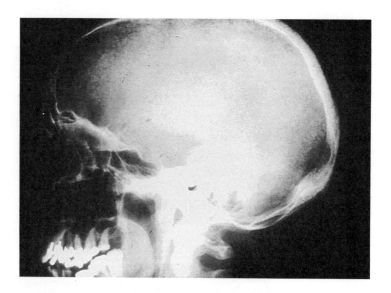

adenomas. An acinar pattern can be observed in some tumours. The presence of a rim of compressed normal tissue will support the diagnosis of an adenoma. Their weight ranges from 70 mg to 20 g.

Double adenomas are probably a distinct entity. Patients with persistent or recurrent 1°HPT caused by missed/not recognised double adenomas are older, nephrolithiasis is less common and muscle weakness, neuropsychiatric disorders, constipation and weight loss are more severe than in patients with persistent or recurrent 1°HPT caused by hyperplasia.[47]

Hyperplasia can be found in as many as 15–20% of patients. It can occur alone or in association with certain familial endocrinopathies. The first intimation of hyperplasia might be the uncovering of multiple-gland disease in a patient presenting in a conventional way. Intraoperative assessment is not always easy, even with the help of frozen sections and a skilled pathologist. Four gland enlargement is unusual in the hyperplasia of sporadic 1°HPT and as normal-sized glands frequently coexist with enlarged ones, the histological diagnosis may be difficult.

Carcinomas occur in about 1% of all patients with an equal male/female incidence at a mean age of 50 years. There are no obvious clinical or biochemical markers to distinguish patients with carcinoma and histological studies do not always help because they lack diagnostic predictability. Carcinoma is often confirmed only when the patient subsequently develops local recurrence or metastases.

The accurate diagnosis of malignancy is very difficult. Vascular and capsular invasion, the presence of fibrous bands, trabecular or rosette-like cellular architecture, the presence of mitotic figures have all been used to help distinguish carcinoma from adenoma, but the specificity of these criteria is low.

Chief cells predominate in carcinomas but oxyphil and transitional oxyphil cells may also be found. The architecture varies from a more solid to a trabecular pattern but there are no great differences between adenoma and carcinoma. Oxyphil cell carcinoma is often only recognised when metastases develop, 5–8 years after the initial surgery.

Parathyroid carcinomas usually continue to function and troublesome hypercalcaemia adds considerably to the patient's suffering. Occasionally they are non-secretory although they have consistent light and electron microscopic features and parathyroid hormone immunoreactivity is demonstrable.

Flow cytometry analysis of DNA content in parathyroid lesions does little to enhance the distinction between benign and malignant lesions. In patients with clinically or pathologically demonstrated parathyroid cancer, however, flow cytometry may differentiate the likely indolent disease (diploid tumours) from tumours more likely to behave aggressively (aneuploid).[48] Mitotic activity constitutes a prognostic risk factor but is of limited diagnostic significance. In half the carcinomas, the frequency of mitoses does not exceed values recorded in benign parathyroid lesions.[49]

Ectopic PTH secretion is extremely rare, quoted only as case reports of small cell lung cancer[50] and ovarian carcinoma, where DNA rearrangement and amplification in the regulatory region of one PTH gene allele have been demonstrated.[51]

Neonatal HPT is a genetically transmitted autosomal dominant disease characterised by life-threatening marked hypercalcaemia and intense parathyroid hyperplasia and hypercellularity. The disease is due to a mutation in the calcium receptor gene which induces chief cells hyperplasia leading to severe hypercalcaemia which is fatal if not recognised and treated early. Patients appear to be homozygous for CaR mutations which determine familial benign hypocalciuric hypercalcaemia in heterozygotes (for a review see reference 52). Near-total parathyroidectomy controls the disease.

HPT in familial syndromes is presented in Chapter 4.

Management options

Treatment should be adapted to the severity of 1°HPT (Table 1.2).

Medical treatment

All HPT patients should be advised to avoid prolonged bed rest or dehydration and to ask medical advice if persistent vomiting or diarrhoea develop (since it can trigger a hypercalcaemic crisis).

A moderate dietary calcium intake is advisable because low intake further stimulates the parathyroids and high intake accentuates hypercalcaemia. However, a high calcium intake (up to 60 mmol/day vs. the currently recommended 20 mmol/day) over a 3-year period is

Table 1.2 *Therapeutic options adapted to the severity of disease[56]*

Mild hypercalcaemia (2.6–2.9 mmol l^{-1})	Moderate hypercalcaemia (2.9–3.3 mmol l^{-1})	Severe hypercalcaemia (over 3.4 mmol l^{-1})
50% symptomatic patients – surgery	Surgical treatment	Emergency treatment (see Table 7.3)

50% asymptomatic patients
  Mobilise
  Keep well hydrated
  Diet with moderate calcium
  Oestrogens to menopausal women
  Clodronate orally
		Surgical treatment on equilibrate patient

reported to reverse the degree of age-dependent hyperparathyroidism in postmenopausal women.[53]

No satisfactory medical therapy exists for the treatment of 1°HPT. Calcitonin and diphosphonates do not give good long-term control. The efficacy of the somatostatin analogue **octreotide** in the management of 1°HPT is low. It produces a significant decrease in urinary calcium but reductions in serum calcium and PTH levels are not significant[54] because parathyroid tissue is usually negative for somatostatin receptor expression.[55]

HRT in postmenopausal women may offer the advantage of oestrogenic effects on the bone.

Emergency treatment of hypercalcaemic crisis

Rehydration   It often takes 4–6 litres to restore the volume status in the first 24 h. This will increase calcium excretion by 100–300 mg day^{-1}, but rarely normalises serum calcium if used alone.

Forced saline diuresis   Loop antidiuretics depress the proximal tubular reabsorptive mechanisms for calcium and increase urinary calcium excretion by 800–1000 mg day^{-1}. Frusemide, ethacrynic acid or bumetamide are used, but should not be initiated until volume repletion has been achieved. The risks of forced diuresis include: cardiac decompensation (need central venous pressure monitoring), hypophosphataemia, hypokalaemia, hypomagnesaemia.

Antiresorptive agents   **Bisphosphonates** are effective osteoclast inhibitors and have become one of the mainstays of therapy for severe hypercalcaemia. The most potent is pamidronate, which is widely used in the treatment of acute hypercalcaemia. Details about each of the three main agents are presented in Table 1.3. For moderate hypercalcaemia, oral formulations should be available but oral pamidronate is unlikely to become available and oral etidronate is not very effective. Oral clodronate is effective and induces a significant fall in serum calcium in patients with 1°HPT and 3°HPT. The resulting decrease in bone turnover could potentially reduce the severity and magnitude of the 'hungry bone syndrome' post-parathyroidectomy.[57] The calcium-lowering effect is, however, incomplete and ill-sustained due to the unopposed effect of PTH on renal tubular reabsorption of calcium. It may be exploited in assessing the beneficial effects of parathyroidectomy on renal function and thus help identify patients who would benefit from surgery.

Gallium nitrate is an antiresorptive drug which did not prove as clinically efficient as initially hoped.

Calcitonin   This is a non-toxic therapy with a very rapid onset of action (within minutes) but limited usefulness. Its main indication remains the first 24–48 h of treatment of acute severe hypercalcaemia, in conjunction with more potent but slower acting therapies (as bisphosphonates).

Glucocorticoids   These may be useful in treating patients with other causes of hypercalcaemia, i.e. myeloma/lymphoma, granulomatous diseases (it decreases vitamin D production by activated macrophages in granulomas) and vitamin D intoxication.

Dialysis   This is reserved for patients with renal failure. Peritoneal dialysis can remove 500–2000 mg of calcium in 24 h, whereas haemodialysis clears 250 mg h^{-1}.

Intravenous phosphate therapy   This is dramatically effective but has serious potential hazards, such as precipitation of calcium phosphate in the skeleton, kidney, soft tissues and heart. With the availability of potent and hazard-free drugs, phosphates are rarely indicated.

Mithramycin (Plicamycin)   This was one of the first-line drugs especially for hypercalcaemia of malignancy despite its potentially disturbing side effects (Table 1.3). Its use is much reduced since the availability of bisphosphonates.

Asymptomatic HPT

The debate about the optimum treatment of asymptomatic 1°HPT continues. Some advocate parathyroidectomy for all patients with symptomless mild 1°HPT because:

1. Subtle physical and psychological changes are only appreciated on restoration of biochemical normality;
2. There is a risk of developing renal failure in the long term;
3. There is a risk of bone loss – this is especially important in elderly females;
4. Hypercalcaemia may contribute to confusion in the elderly;

Table 1.3 *Treatment of acute hypercalcaemia*

Treatment	Dose	Onset of action	Duration of action	Advantages	Disadvantages
Saline	4–6 l	Hours	During infusion	Rehydration	Cardiac overload, electrolyte disturbances (K, Mg, phosphates)
Loop diuretics	Frusemide 40 mg i.v. every 1–2 h	Hours	During infusion	Enhanced renal calcium excretion	Cardiac overload, electrolyte disturbances (K, Mg, phosphates)
Calcitonin	2–8 U kg^{-1} i.v., s.c. or i.m.	Hours	2–3 days	Rapid onset of action	Only modest reduction of plasma calcium levels, for only few days
Etidronate	25 mg/kg (single i.v. dose) or 7.5 mg/kg over few days	24–48 h	5–7 days	33–80% of patients are normocalcaemic by 7 days	Hyperphosphataemia
Pamidronate	30–90 mg (single i.v. or infusion over 24 h)	24–48 h	10–14 days	Potency: 70–100% of patients become normocalcaemic Immediate onset Prolonged duration of action	Adverse effects (1/3 patients) Limited/transient fever (20%), myalgias, hypophosphataemia, hypomagnesaemia
Clodronate	4–6 mg kg^{-1} in 2–4 h			Well tolerated	Potential nephrotoxicity
Galium nitrate		48–72 h	10–14 days	High potency	Contraindicated if renal impairment
Mithramycin	15–25 μg kg^{-1} over 4 h	6–12 h	Not sustained		Local/soft tissue irritation if extravasation occurs Increases in hepatic transaminases Nephrotoxicity, thrombocytopenia

5. There is a risk of hypercalcaemic crisis in the elderly, especially if an intercurrent illness produces dehydration;
6. The incidence and mortality from cardiovascular disease may be increased.

The workload of adopting such a policy would be considerable and it should be kept in mind that the preoperative risk factor profile is altered. Impairments in cardiovascular, respiratory and kidney functions and abnormal glucose control are frequent in these patients and they appear more likely to have a history of congestive heart disease, thromboembolic diseases, stroke or diabetes mellitus.[58]

Surgical treatment

Once the biochemical diagnosis of 1°HPT is confirmed there is no need to proceed to localisation procedures and neck exploration can be undertaken forthwith. Over 40 years ago Albright and Reifenstein[59] wrote: 'much mischief has been done by the "let's have a look" approach to the problem', 'a good thyroid surgeon is not enough' and 'there is no time like the first operation to uncover a small adenoma'. The identification of all glands is important as the search for a specific missing gland can then proceed logically based on anatomical and embryological knowledge.

Excellent monographs exist which describe the technical details of neck exploration and those by Gunn[60] and Wells et al.[61] are recommended.

The strap muscles are separated in the midline and elevated from the underlying thyroid. They need never be divided. There may be a need to divide the middle thyroid vein or the inferior thyroid veins but this should be avoided if possible. Preservation of the veins may be important if the exploration is unsuccessful and selective venous sampling is subsequently required.

The thyroid lobe is gently retracted toward the midline to allow examination of those areas where the glands are most likely to be found – just above the inferior artery and around the lower thyroid pole. The recurrent nerve must be protected; undue dissection or palpation near or directly on the nerve may interfere with its function. The nerve is sometimes closely applied to an abnormal parathyroid and it must be carefully dissected free. Diathermy should not be used in the vicinity of the nerve.

The glands are often enclosed within a fat pad beneath fascia and this has to be opened before the gland 'pops out'. This is particularly the case for glands within the thyrothymic ligament or thymus.

The vessels supplying a normal gland can be seen coursing into its substance and care must be taken not to devascularise these structures unwittingly. If a biopsy is taken it should be a sliver from the distal pole of the gland away from the feeding vessels. A silver clip placed across the distal third of a gland will both mark the gland and allow a bloodless biopsy.

All four glands should be visualised before a policy of resection and biopsy is decided. Too aggressive a biopsy policy will lead to an unacceptably high incidence of hypoparathyroidism.

By concentrating on the likely sites of the parathyroids a competent surgeon can successfully identify and remove abnormal tissue in 95% of patients. The presence of four normal glands will probably mean the wrong diagnosis since a fifth ectopic and abnormal gland is rare. The exploration must be carried superiorly above the upper thyroid pole and behind the pharynx and oesophagus. A full exploration and excision of the thymic upper poles should be performed, opening the carotid sheath and examining the lower thyroid poles. Intrathyroidal adenomas may be detected by intraoperative ultrasonography. In any event a careful description with a map should be kept with the location of all glands, with a notation whether biopsy was proven or not, and the presence of identifying landmarks, e.g. non-absorbable sutures or clips which might mark retained glands or biopsy sites.

Drains need not be placed. Most surgeons reapproximate the strap muscles and platysma and close the skin with clips or staples. No dressing is required.

Parathyroid adenomas

Unilateral parathyroidectomy without exploration of the contralateral side is claimed to eliminate the risk of persisting hypocalcaemia but may not uncover double adenomas. Methods proposed to ensure complete excision of sources of the excess PTH include urinary cAMP and intraoperative PTH levels.[62] PTH levels are reduced to half base line values within 10–15 min after successful parathyroidectomy whereas calcium levels fall to the normal range within 24–36 h. Hypocalcaemic symptoms and the need for supplements in the early postoperative period are not predicted by determination of an early plasma calcium level.[63]

Sporadic multiple gland hyperplasia

Excision of the enlarged glands, leaving normal 'sized' glands intact is adopted by some surgeons,[64] whereas others recommend 3 and 3½ glands excision.[65]

MEN syndromes

Treatment of HPT in patients with MEN syndromes is described in Chapter 4.

Parathyroid carcinoma

If the condition is recognised preoperatively (perhaps by suggestive features on computed tomography scan or palpable lymphadenopathy) en bloc resection offers the best results with central compartment dissection when there is evidence of regional node metastases.

Serum calcium and parathyroid hormone measurements are post-operative markers of tumour recurrence. Recurrence in the neck or lungs can often be treated surgically with en bloc radical dissection, mediastinal lymph node clearance and limited pulmonary resections. Palliation is obtained by reducing hypercalcaemia with mithramycin or disodium clodronate. Radiotherapy is of little use.

Multiple resections for local recurrence or metastases in patients with recurrent or distant disease appear to prolong survival and palliate the symptoms of hypercalcaemia.[66] The outlook is variable and, as with many endocrine tumours, some patients survive for many years with known indolent metastatic disease.

Overall results

The increased set point seen in $1°$HPT is normalised on the first post-operative day and baseline serum PTH levels are within the normal range 24–48 h after excision of the adenoma. The suppression of PTH levels during an oral calcium load is already normalised on the second postoperative day. A given decrease in extracellular calcium concentration is counteracted by a progressively larger increase in serum levels of intact PTH after parathyroid surgery; the reason for this increase in the 'secretory reserve' is not well understood.[67]

Persistent hyperparathyroidism is the commonest cause of postoperative hypercalcaemia, which is defined as continued hypercalcaemia in the immediate postoperative period or occurring within 1 year of surgery.

Recurrent hyperparathyroidism can be strictly defined as hypercalcaemia occurring after the following criteria have been met:

1. Identification and biopsy proof of all four parathyroids at the initial operation;
2. Complete removal of all abnormal tissue;
3. A normocalcaemic phase of 1 year or longer;
4. Abnormal tissue uncovered at re-exploration at a site of a previously normal gland.

These extremely rigorous criteria[68] are not usually fulfilled in today's surgical practice, when it is unusual to biopsy all glands.

True recurrent disease might account for 1% of persistent hypercalcaemia. If persistent disease is suspected the diagnosis must be checked and confirmed. If hyperparathyroidism is present the next steps require careful thought. There is no virtue in attempting to localize the abnormal tissue if the patient's general condition would not withstand re-exploration and its associated morbidity. If the diagnosis is confirmed and a decision is made to offer re-exploration then most surgeons would use localization procedures preoperatively. This would be carried out while consulting previous operation notes, operative maps and histology reports as these often indicate the likely site of abnormality. If, for example, all glands had been identified and biopsied as normal except the left lower parathyroid then techniques which look specifically in this area would be used to detect intrathyroid masses or mediastinal adenomas.

Reoperative surgery

Failure of the surgeon to locate the abnormal parathyroid tissue is a rare but important event. After unsuccessful surgery, the diagnosis of 1°HPT must be reconfirmed and the severity of the condition assessed because, even when successful, reoperation is associated with some increased morbidity. Operative and pathology reports are reviewed to assess the adequacy or extent of the previous operation. Localisation studies have a major influence on planning subsequent reoperation.

Current areas of research

Although major insights into the management and pathophysiology of primary hyperparathyroidism have been gained since Mandl performed the first parathyroidectomy in 1924, primary hyperparathyroidism remains an area with many unsolved questions. Genetic alterations and molecular pathways involved in parathyroid gland physiology and pathology and the relationship between abnormal parathyroid cell growth and hormone secretion in 1°HPT are not yet integrated into a simple model. The appropriate aggressiveness of treatment for patients with mild symptomatic disease is still not agreed. There is continued controversy concerning the advantages of unilateral exploration vs bilateral neck dissection in patients with positive imaging of one parathyroid adenoma. After identification of the plasma membrane calcium-receptor the development of pharmacological control of PTH secretion by interfering with the function of this receptor is an exciting prospect.

Secondary hyperparathyroidism

Introduction

Secondary HPT (2°HPT) is the condition in which PTH is secreted to compensate for a chronic calcium and/or phosphate imbalance. There is presumably no initial abnormality inherent within the parathyroid glands. Possible causes for 2°HPT are presented in Table 1.4.

Overall incidence

Some of the conditions listed are very rare and this section concentrates on renal 2°HPT. Nearly all patients with chronic renal failure develop some degree of 2°HPT, with a wide variation in the extent of disease. The prevalence of 2°HPT has been assessed at 67% using a bone biopsy technique[69] but improved and early medical treatment means that less then 5% of these patients will require parathyroidectomy.[70]

Table 1.4 *Possible causes for 2°HPT*

Chronic renal failure

Rickets
  vitamin D deficiency
  vitamin D resistance syndromes
  renal tubular phosphate-wasting disorders

Osteomalacia

Malabsorption

Pseudohypoparathyroidism

Complication of high-dose phosphate therapy in patients with X-linked
hypophosphataemia

Mechanisms

In most patients on long-term haemodialysis an increase in parathyroid size is noted, progressing from diffuse to nodular hyperplasia
and possible adenoma formation. A deficit of calcitriol synthesis is an
important factor for inducing 2°HPT and is aggravated by a reduced
expression of vitamin D receptors. With advanced chronic renal
failure, hyperphosphataemia is an additional important factor in
worsening HPT. A low calcium intake and the use of dialysate
containing low calcium levels may put the patients to a higher risk
for developing 2°HPT. These metabolic abnormalities are amplified
by the decreased expression of the calcium sensor receptor in the parathyroid cells.

Although the process starts as a four gland response to a metabolic
drive, worsening 2°HPT involves monoclonal recruitment of cell
subpopulation.[6] The higher proliferation rate of cells within areas of
nodular hyperplasia[71] and their higher set-point for Ca^{2+}-controlled
PTH secretion than in the cells obtained from diffuse hyperplasia[72]
suggest a more aggressive response of some cell subpopulations.

In vivo dynamic tests of parathyroid gland function suggest that
calcium-regulated PTH secretion does not differ with the degree of
2°HPT. Set point values in patients with 2°HPT do not correspond to
basal serum PTH levels, to the maximum serum PTH in response
to hypocalcaemia or to the minimum serum PTH level during hypercalcaemia. Some propose that variations in parathyroid gland size are
the major contributor to excessive PTH secretion in patients with
chronic renal failure[73] and not a functional abnormality.

Increased plasma levels of PTH have extensive metabolic influence.
The effects on bone are discussed in a later section. Detrimental
effects on remnant nephrons and a suppressive effect on tubular
proteinase activities have been described in an experimental model.[74]

The severity of 2°HPT seems to accentuate the resistance to erythropoietin (in addition to iron deficiency, aluminium toxicity and marrow
dysfunction) and most patients need a higher dose to achieve an
adequate haematocrit.[75]

Presentation

The frequency and severity of symptoms of 2°HPT are highly variable.

Bone disease
Patients with chronic renal failure present with osteitis fibrosa cystica
(OFC) or less frequently with osteomalacia, which may eventually lead
to skeletal deformities or fractures. OFC occurs to some degree in up
to 95% of these patients. Physical findings may include a funnel chest
deformity and sternal bowing due to rib deformities, height reduction
from kyphosis and vertebral crush fractures. Bone pain occurs
primarily in the thoracolumbar spine and lower extremity and it is
exacerbated by weight bearing, sudden movements and pressure.
Progressive bone demineralisation leads to thinning and weakening
of the bones, with lytic lesions involving the skull ('salt and pepper'
radiographic aspect) or subperiostal resorptions.

Pathogenic factors for bone lesions associated with 2°HPT are deficiency of vitamin D and/or its receptors, skeletal resistance to the
calcaemic effects of PTH (Fig 1.4), aluminium toxicity, osteoporosis
linked to ageing and the recently described dialysis-associated
amyloidosis of the beta2-microglobulin type.[76] In contrast, low serum
PTH levels accompany the dynamic bone disease, whose pathogenesis as part of renal osteodystrophy is poorly understood. Parathyroid
hormone (PTH) binds to its receptors on the osteoblasts. PTH together
with tumour necrosis factor α (TNF-α) and interleukin-1 (IL-1) activate the remodeling cycle through actions on the layer of osteoblasts
covering bone surfaces. PTH stimulates osteoblastic proliferation at a
discrete undetermined point in osteoblast ontogeny, in part by stimulating the production of insulin-like growth factor (IGF-1). Activated
osteoblasts release soluble factors (as IL-6, IL-11, granulocyte-
macrophage colony-stimulating factor), that induce the proliferation
and differentiation of osteoclast precursors and activate the function
of osteoclasts.

Aluminium associated osteomalacia is a serious complication of
advanced renal disease and should be differentiated from the effects
of 2°HPT. In an experimental model of azotaemic rats, aluminium
appeared to alter the relationship between serum PTH and calcium.
Sources of aluminium include the water used for haemodialysis and
the gastrointestinal absorption of aluminium from some phosphate-
binders. Serum aluminium levels and bone biopsy may be necessary
to confirm this diagnosis.

Figure 1.4
Role of parathyroid hormone in modulating the bone metabolism.

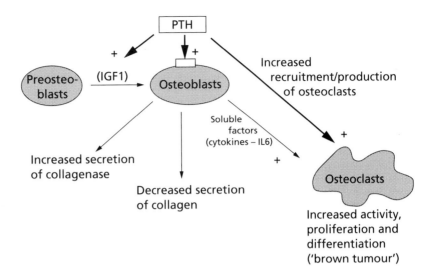

Soft tissue calcification

This is a frequent manifestation of $2°$HPT, affecting 27% of patients with renal failure at the outset of dialysis and 58% of those who have been dialysis-dependent for more than 5 years.[77] Calcification may involve soft tissues, blood vessels, kidneys (nephrocalcinosis), lungs, heart and skin. Calcification in soft tissues may compress adjacent structures, causing pain, organ dysfunction and cosmetic deformities.

Although debatable, a likely mechanism for metastatic calcification is the increased serum calcium × phosphate product and values greater than 70 (4.5–5, respectively) are considered an indication for parathyroidectomy.

Calciphylaxis

Calciphylaxis is a rare condition associated with haemodialysis or transplantation, high PTH values and an increased serum calcium × phosphate product. Patients present with severe calf pain and tenderness due to extensive non-ulcerating large, hard and tender subcutaneous plaques in the calves. These painful, violaceous, mottled cutaneous lesions progress to skin and subcutaneous necrosis, deep non-healing ulcers and gangrene. The lesions are reticular in pattern and may be very large (up to 20 cm). Involvement of the distal fingers and toes is characteristic; lesions less commonly involve the forearms, arms, trunk, buttocks, thighs and legs. This severe complication can threaten digits, limbs and a patient's life. Calcium deposition can be confirmed radiologically and by bone scanning. Before urgent parathyroidectomy is performed, medical treatment with phosphate binders might be useful. The condition is no longer rare and is not confined to patients on haemodialysis; it has been described in predialysis renal failure.[78]

Pruritus

Pruritus can be severe, intractable and disabling. It is attributed to increased calcium levels in the skin and usually improves after parathyroidectomy.

Other symptoms

Muscle weakness, proximal myopathy, easy fatigability are often disclosed by careful history. Peptic ulcer disease (20%) and neuropathy (10%) can be associated.

'Cardiotoxicity' of PTH

In a five-year longitudinal echocardiographic study including 52 patients dependent on haemodialysis, one of the best clinical predictors for the presence of left-ventricular hypertrophy was raised PTH. This direct effect is mediated by specific receptors for PTH in the cardiomyocytes and by a permissive role on activation of interstitial cells in the heart. Increased cytosolic calcium concentration in the cardiomyocytes contributes to reduced myocardial performance and a raised calcium-phosphate product leads to myocardial and valve calcification.[79]

Investigative techniques

- Hyperphosphataemia with normo/hypercalcaemia is demonstrated in all patients.
- Increased levels of intact PTH are decisive for diagnosis and this excludes diagnostic confusion created by measuring C-terminal fragments of PTH (as in previous assays), which accumulates due to decreased renal clearance. Because uraemia induces a bone resistance to the effects of PTH, the target range of optimal plasma intact PTH concentration for these patients is not necessarily the absolute range recommended for healthy non-uraemic patients. Some centres therefore consider optimal concentrations for patients on haemodialysis to be 2–3 times the upper limit of normal and 2–5 times the upper normal limits when they are on continuous ambulatory peritoneal dialysis (CAPD).
- Increased alkaline phosphatase levels confirm bone disease.
- Serum levels of vitamin D can be measured to confirm adequate substitution.
- Serum aluminium levels are monitored to exclude aluminium toxicity as a cause of bone disease.
- The typical histopathological findings are asymmetric enlargement, nodularity and increased numbers of oxyphil cells. Diffuse and nodular hyperplasia can coexist within the same gland. The macroscopic difference in involvement of each gland (i.e. size and degree of nodularity) is striking.

Because of the chronicity of the process, a prolonged period of biochemical surveillance allows the disease to be seen in evolution.

Radiological investigations

Subperiosteal bone resorption is seen in up to 86% of these patients, especially in the phalanges, pelvis, distal clavicles, ribs, femur, mandible or skull. Classically, the earliest radiographic lesion seen is an irregularity of the radial aspect of the second digit middle phalanx. Elevated alkaline phosphatase levels correlate well with the severity of bone disease. In a patient maintained on dialysis with appropriate medical treatment, progressive radiographic findings of bone disease should serve as an indication for operation.

Management options

Medical treatment
Goals: to maintain calcium and phosphate levels close to normal levels, to suppress PTH secretion and to ameliorate the bone disease.

Methods available: diet, calcium supplementation, phosphate binders, routine vitamin D, bisphosphonates

- Dietary phosphate restriction (< 1000 mg/24 h) is complemented with phosphate-binding agents in a dose adapted to the meals' content of phosphate. Calcium acetate and calcium carbonate are preferred to aluminium hydroxide (to reduce the risk of aluminium toxicity).
- Daily calcium intake of at least 1500 mg is necessary and eventually can be assured using oral supplementation. If the patient is still hypocalcaemic, calcium may be added to the dialysis bath to achieve normocalcaemia.
- Long-term treatment with calcium-alpha-ketoglutarate (4.5 g/day) is reported to normalise 2°HPT by simultaneously phosphate-binding and correcting serum Ca/P ratio without vitamin D treatment.[80]
- Routine vitamin D supplementation is now started before a patient commences dialysis and its plasma levels should be monitored to ensure adequate dosage.[81] High peak plasma levels are more efficient to suppress PTH secretion and once weekly intravenous bolus administration seems to be a safe and cost effective protocol.[82,83] Good results have been reported also with oral therapy. The risks of vitamin D treatment include the development of hypercalcaemia and persistent hyperphosphataemia.
- Aluminium toxicity has been treated successfully with desferoxamine.
- Pruritus is ameliorated by charcoal haemoperfusion in conjunction with standard haemodialysis.

Table 1.5 *Improvement of symptoms after parathyroidectomy*

Symptoms	Improvement after parathyroidectomy (%)	Comments
Bone pain	85	Alkaline phosphatase levels generally correlate with the extent of bone resorption
Joint pain	80	
Pruritus	85	
Malaise	73	
[Ca] × [P] > 70 (in mg dl^{-1})		
C-terminal PTH fragments > 3000 μEq l^{-1}		Associated with resolution of symptoms after parathyroidectomy[70]

- The use of diphosphonates in the treatment of 2°HPT is still experimental. Details about their properties are presented in Table 1.3.
- PTH removal during continuous ambulatory peritoneal dialysis (CAPD) is greater than with haemodialysis, but CAPD has the disadvantage that protein losses are greater and vitamin D and its binding protein are lost in the peritoneal dialysate.

Surgical treatment for 2°HPT
Conservative medical therapy fails in 5–10% of patients on long-term dialysis and surgical treatment becomes necessary.

Indications for operation are based in part on the knowledge of which symptoms and signs are likely to improve after parathyroidectomy (Table 1.5) and from an assessment of the rate of progression of biochemical abnormalities. When offering a surgical option patients should be informed of its potential risks (recurrent hyperparathyroidism, injury to the recurrent laryngeal nerves).

Perioperative care
Patients should undergo dialysis within 1 day of operation and then 48 hours postoperatively or as needed. The risk of bleeding should be kept in mind since heparin is used during haemodialysis and platelets are dysfunctional in severely uraemic patients. Preoperative vitamin D treatment should continue since it decreases the chance of postoperative hypocalcaemia.

Marked hypocalcaemia may occur after parathyroidectomy, due to the hungry bone syndrome, hypomagnesaemia and hypofunction of parathyroid remnants or grafts. Oral supplementation (up to 6 g of elemental calcium can be given daily) suffices for mild symptoms, whereas more severe hypocalcaemia is treated with intravenous calcium and magnesium.

'Technical options'

Standard transverse neck incision. All four glands are located and resected tissue confirmed by frozen section. Transcervical thymectomy (by dissection along the thyrothymic ligament) should be routine, aiming to remove supranumerary glands or embryonic rests.

If all four glands are not found in the 'classical' locations, the retro-oesophageal space, superior thyroid pedicles and areas along the carotid sheath should be explored. If after a rigorous search all four glands are not identified, the operation should be concluded. Median sternotomy is not performed as part of the initial operation. The pathology report, postoperative PTH and calcium levels and the clinical response should influence further decisions about localisation studies (see previous section) in anticipation of re-exploration.

Surgical strategies

Subtotal parathyroidectomy

This involves resection of 3½ glands, leaving approx. 50 mg of viable tissue *in situ*. If permanent dialysis is anticipated the remnant should be small (due to long-term hypertrophy of the remnant) whereas it should be larger if renal transplant is likely (to avoid subsequent hypoparathyroidism). The disadvantage of this approach is that a second cervical exploration would be needed if persistent or recurrent hyperparathyroidism occurs.

Total parathyroidectomy plus autotransplantation

This technique was introduced around 1975 by Wells. The gland which macroscopically looks most normal and on frozen sections shows predominantly diffuse hyperplasia (and not nodular hyperplasia) is selected for autografting. The gland is sliced into $3 \times 1 \times 1$ mm pieces which are placed in a bath of ice-cold saline. The forearm flexor mass is exposed through a longitudinal incision below the antecubital fossa and about 15 such parathyroid fragments are placed – each in its own muscle pocket. Each pocket is closed by reapproximating the fascia with a non-absorbable suture (to prevent graft extrusion, mark the site of implantation and aid re-exploration if necessary). Some fragments can be cryopreserved.

Primary graft failure is extremely rare. Graft function can be evaluated by measuring PTH levels in the ipsilateral antecubital vein and comparing this with the contralateral non-grafted forearm. A gradient between grafted versus non-grafted arm proves graft viability and function; lack of gradient suggests either failure of the graft (when PTH levels are low) or persistent HPT due to missed gland in the neck. Grafting of cryopreserved cells is successful in only 60% of patients.

Total parathyroidectomy alone

This option may now be preferred and in small series recently reported it appears to be a safe and effective option with all patients having symptomatic and biochemical improvement. If followed-up for several years, most patients are found to have detectable levels of PTH,[84] suggesting that total parathyroidectomy was not 'complete' and residual parathyroid cells or parathyroid cell rests become activated under the continued biochemical stimulus of chronic renal failure.

Results

Both subtotal parathyroidectomy and total parathyroidectomy plus autograft have been preferred before in the hope of avoiding the need for long-term calcium supplementation and equivalent results have been cited with both procedures. In 1991, a randomised trial[85] concluded that total parathyroidectomy is superior to subtotal parathyroidectomy in terms of recurrence rate (no recurrence vs. 4/20) and symptom amelioration scores (pruritus, 100% vs 45%, weakness, 83% vs 20%).

A wide range of recurrence rates has been reported for both procedures (10–70%). In an analysis of 73 patients with chronic renal failure, recurrent HPT was diagnosed in four of 39 patients who underwent total parathyroidectomy with autograft and two out of 34 patients who underwent subtotal parathyroidectomy, indicating that there is little to choose between the two techniques.[86]

Persistent HPT is diagnosed if hypercalcaemia recurs within 6 months after initial surgery. The most common reasons for recurrent hypercalcaemia include: unrecognised asymmetric hyperplasia of all four glands; too large a remnant left behind; unrecognised hyper-functioning supernumerary glands; hyperfunction of the auto-transplanted parathyroid tissue. Reoperation of such patients can be extremely successful, a recurrence rate of only 10.5% being reported for a large series of 152 such patients.[87]

A rare cause is **parathyromatosis**, where multiple rests of hyper-functioning parathyroid tissue are scattered throughout the fibrofatty tissue of the lower neck and superior mediastinum. Various authors speculate that abnormally placed parathyroid tissue is either inadvertent autoimplantation of tissue from the handling of abnormal glands during previous operations or hyperfunction of tissue left behind during ontogenesis.[88]

Permanent hypocalcaemia can ensue after reoperations for persistent or recurrent hyperparathyroidism. If cryopreserved material is available it may subsequently be used to restore normocalcaemia, sometimes long after surgery.

Tertiary HPT is the condition in which 'reactive' parathyroid hyperplasia results in autonomous hypersecretion such that HPT continues despite correction of the underlying renal disease. Based on calcium levels it is estimated to occur in 25–50% of patients, but PTH levels and bone biopsies suggest a prevalence of up to 70%. These early postrenal transplant findings improve with time, such that 60% of these patients become normocalcaemic within 12 months and only few require operation.

Transplant patients usually present with less severe disease, have better normalisation of biochemical parameters after parathyroidectomy, and rarely develop recurrent hyperparathyroidism compared with those on haemodialysis.

References

1. Mundy GR, Cove DH. Primary hyperparathyroidism: changes in the pattern of clinical presentation. Lancet 1980; i: 1317–20.
2. Arnold A, Staunton CE, Kim HG *et al.* Monoclonality and abnormal PTH genes in parathyroid adenomas. N Engl J Med 1988; 318: 658–62.
3. Friedman E, Bale AE, Marx SJ *et al.* Genetic abnormalities in parathyroid adenomas. J Clin Endocrinol Metab 1990; 71: 293–7.
4. Thakker RV, Bouloux P, Wooding C *et al.* Association of parathyroid tumours in MEN type 1 with loss of alleles on chromosome 11. N Engl J Med 1989; 321: 218–24.
5. Friedman E, Sakaguci K *et al.* Clonality of parathyroid tumours in familial MEN type 1. N Engl J Med 1989; 321: 213–18.
6. Arnold A, Brown MF, Urena P *et al.* Monoclonality of parathyroid tumours in chronic renal failure and in primary parathyroid hyperplasia. J Clin Invest 1995; 95: 2047–53.
7. Rosenberg CL, Kim HG, Shows TB *et al.* Rearrangement and overexpression of D11S287E, a candidate oncogene on chromosome 11q13 in benign parathyroid tumors. Oncogene 1991; 6: 449–53.
8. Motokura T, Bloom T, Kim HG *et al.* A novel cyclin encoded by a bc11-linked candidate oncogene. Nature 1991; 350: 512–15.
9. Bates S, Peters G. Cyclin D1 as a cellular proto-oncogene. Semin Cancer Biol 1995; 6: 73–82.
10. Cryns VL, Thor A, Xu HJ *et al.* Loss of the retinoblastoma tumor-suppressor gene in parathyroid carcinoma. N Engl J Med 1994; 330: 757–61.
11. Weinberg RA. The retinoblastoma protein and cell cycle control. Cell 1995; 81: 323–30.
12. Cryns VL, Yi SM, Tahara H *et al.* Frequent loss of chromosome arm 1p DNA in parathyroid

adenomas. Genes Chrom Cancer 1995; 13: 9–17.
13. Tahara H, Smith AP, Gaz RD *et al.* Genomic localization of novel candidate tumor suppressor gene loci in human parathyroid adenomas. Cancer Res 1996; 56: 599–605
14. Hakim JP, Levine MA. Absence of p53 point mutations in parathyroid adenoma and carcinoma. J Clin Endocrinol Metab 1994; 78: 103–6.
15. Cryns VL, Rubio MP, Thor AD *et al.* p53 abnormalities in human parathyroid carcinoma. J Clin Endocrinol Metab 1994; 78: 1320–4.
16. Brown EM, Gamba G, Riccardi D *et al.* Cloning and characterisation of an extracellular Ca^{2+}-sensing receptor from bovine parathyroid. Nature 1993; 366: 575–80
17. Pollak MR, Brown EM, Chou YHW. Mutations in the human calcium-sensing receptor gene cause familial hypocalciuric hypercalcaemia and neonatal severe hyperparathyroidism. Cell 1993; 75: 1297–303.
18. Hosokawa Y, Pollak MR, Brown EM *et al.* The extracellular calcium-sensing receptor gene in human parathyroid tumours. J Clin Endocrinol Metab 1995; 80: 3107–10.
19. Thomson DB, Samowitz WS, Odelberg S *et al.* Genetic abnormalities in sporadic parathyroid adenomas: loss of heterozygosity for chromosome 3q markers flanking the calcium receptor locus. J Clin Endocrinol Metab 1995 80: 3377–80.
20. Kifor O, Moore FD, Wang JP *et al.* Reduced immunostaining for the extracellular Ca^{2+}-sensing receptor in primary and uremic secondary hyperparathyroidism. J Clin Endocrinol Metab 1996; 81: 1598–606.
21. Saito A, Pietromonaco S, Kwor-Chieh Loo A, Farquhar MG. Complete cloning and sequencing of rat gp330/'megalin', a distinc-

tive member of the low density lipoprotein receptor gene family. Proc Natl Acad Sci USA 1994; 91: 9725–29.

22. Juhlin C, Klareskog L, Nygren P et al. Hyperparathyroidism is associated with reduced expression of a parathyroid calcium receptor mechanism defined by monoclonal antiparathyroid antibodies. Endocrinology 1988; 122: 2999–3001.

23. Schneider AB, Gierlowski TC, Shore-Freedman E et al. Dose–response relationships for radiation-induced hyperparathyroidism. J Clin Endocrinol Metab 1995; 80: 254–7.

24. Harms HM, Schlinke E, Neubauer O. Pulse amplitude and frequency modulation of parathyroid hormone in primary hyperpara-thyroidism. J Clin Endocrinol Metab 1994; 78: 53–7.

25. Brown EM, Segre GV, Goldring SR. Serpentine receptors for parathyroid hormone, calcitonin and calcium ions. Bailliére's Clin Endocrinol Metab 1996; 123–61.

26. Carling T, Kindmark A, Hellman P et al. Vitamin D receptor genotypes in primary hyperparathyroidism. Nature Med 1995; 1: 1309–11.

27. Elvius M, Lagrelius A, Nygren A et al. Seventeen year follow-up study of bone mass in patients with mild asymptomatic hyperparathyroidism some of whom were operated on. Eur J Surg Acta Chir 1995; 161: 863–9.

28. Benishin CG, Lewanczuk RZ, Shan J, Pang PKT. Purification and structural characterization of parathyroid hypertensive factor. J Cardiovasc Pharmacol 1994; 23(S2): S9–S13.

29. Lewanczuk RZ, Benishin CG, Shan J, Pang PKT. Clinical aspects of parathyroid hypertensive factor. J Cardiovasc Pharmacol 1994 23(S2): S23–S26.

30. Hedback G, Oden A, Tissel LA. Parathyroid adenoma weight and the risk of death after treatment for primary hyperparathyroidism. Surgery 1995; 117: 134–9.

31. National Center for Health Statistics: vital statistics of the United States, 1986, Vol 2, Part A, Mortality. Washington, DC, US Government Printing Office, DHHS Publ No (PHS) 1986; 88–1122.

32. Monchik JM. Presidential address: normocalcemic hyperparathyroidism. Surgery 1995; 118: 917–23.

33. Fitzpatrick LA, Bilezikian JP. Acute primary hyperparathyroidism. Am J Med 1987; 82: 275–82.

34. Suva LJ, Winslow GA, Wettenhall RE et al. A parathyroid hormone related peptide implicated in malignant hypercalcaemia: cloning and expression. Science 1987; 237: 893–6.

35. White TF, Farndon JR, Conceicao SC et al. Serum calcium status in health and disease: a comparison of measured and derived parameters. Clin Chim Acta 1986; 157: 199–214.

36. Taylor J, Fraser W, Banaszkiewicz P et al. Lateralization of parathyroid adenomas by intraoperative parathyroid hormone estimation. Br J Surg 1995; 82: 1428–9.

37. Farndon JR, Geraghty JM, Dilley WG et al. Serum gastrin, calcitonin, and prolactin as markers of multiple endocrine neoplasia syndromes in patients with primary hyperparathyroidism. World J Surg 1987; 11: 253–7.

38. Carlson GL, Farndon JR, Shenton BK et al. Thallous chloride uptake and DNA profile in parathyroid adenomas. Br J Surg 1990; 77: 1302–4.

39. Mitchell BK, Kinder BK, Cornelius E, Stewart AF. Primary hyperparathyroidism: preoperative localisation using technetium-sestamibi scanning. J Clin Endocrinol Metab 1995; 80: 7–10.

40. Mitchell BK, Merrell RC, Kinder BK. Localisation studies in patients with hyperparathyroidism. Surg Clin North Am 1995; 75: 483–94.

41. Wright AR, Goddard PR, Nicholson S et al. Fat-suppression magnetic resonance imaging in the preoperative localisation of parathyroid adenomas. Clin Radiol 1992; 46: 324–8.

42. Hellman P, Ahlstrom H, Bergstrom M et al. Positron emission tomography with ^{11}C-methionine in hyperparathyroidism. Surgery 1994; 116: 974–81.

43. Wei JP, Burke GJ. Analysis of savings in operative time for primary hyperparathyroidism using localization with technetium 99m sestamibi scan. Am J Surg 1995; 170: 488–91.

44. Irvin GL, Prudhomme DL, Deriso GT et al. A new approach to parathyroidectomy. Ann Surg 1994; 219: 574–81.

45. Zmora O, Schachter PP, Heyman Z et al. Correct preoperative localization: does it permit a change in operative strategy for

primary hyperparathyroidism? Surgery 1995, 118: 932–5.

46. Sacks BA, Pallotta JA, Cole A, Hurwitz J. Diagnosis of parathyroid adenomas: efficacy of measuring parathormone levels in needle aspirates of cervical masses. Am J Roentgenol 1994; 163: 1223–6.

47. Tezelman S, Shen W, Siperstein AE *et al.* Persistent or recurrent hyperparathyroidism in patients with double adenomas Surgery 1995; 118: 1115–24.

48. August DA, Flynn SD, Jones MA *et al.* Parathyroid carcinoma: the relationship of nuclear DNA content to clinical outcome. Surgery 1993; 113: 290–6.

49. Bondeson L, Sandelin K, Grimelius L. Histopathological variables and DNA cytometry in parathyroid carcinoma. Am J Surg Pathol 1993; 17: 820–9.

50. Yoshimoto K, Yamasaki R, Sakai H. Ectopic production of parathyroid hormone by small cell lung cancer in a patient with hypercalcaemia. J Clin Endocrinol Metab 1989; 68: 976–81.

51. Nussbaum SR, Gaz RD, Arnold A. Hypercalcaemia and ectopic secretion of parathyroid hormone by an ovarian carcinoma with rearrangement of the gene for parathyroid hormone. N Engl J Med 1990; 323: 1324–8.

52. Pearce SHS, Brown EM. Calcium-sensing receptor mutations: insights into a structurally and functionally novel receptor. J Clin Endocrinol Metab 1996; 81: 1309–11.

53. McKane WR, Khosla S, Egan KS *et al.* Role of calcium intake in modulating age-related increases in parathyroid function and bone resorption. J Clin Endocrinol Metab 1996; 81: 1699–703.

54. Lucarotti ME, Hamilton JA, Farndon JR. Somatostatin and primary hyperparathyroidism. Br J Surg 1994; 81: 1141–3.

55. Hasse C, Zielke A, Bruns C *et al.* Influence of somatostatin to biochemical parameters in patients with primary hyperparathyroidism. Exp Clin Endocrinol Diab 1995; 103: 391–7.

56. Bilezikian JP. Management of hypercalcaemia. J Clin Endocrinol Metab 1993; 77: 1445–9.

57. Hamdy NAT, McCloskey EV, Kanis JA. Role of bisphosphonates in the medical management of hyperparathyroidism. Acta Chir Aust 1994; 26(S112): 6–7.

58. Lind L, Ljunghall S. Pre-operative evaluation of risk factors for complications in patients with primary hyperparathyroidism. Eur J Clin Invest 1995; 25: 955–8.

59. Albright F, Reifenstein EC. The parathyroid glands and metabolic bone disease. Baltimore: Williams & Wilkins, 1948.

60. Gunn A. Parathyroid exploration. London: Wolfe, 1988.

61. Wells SA, Leight GS, Ross AJ. Primary hyperparathyroidism. Chicago: Year Book Medical Publishers, 1980.

62. Tommasi M, Brocchi A, Benucci A *et al.* Intraoperative fall in plasma levels of intact parathyroid hormone in patients undergoing parathyroid adenomectomy. Int J Biol Markers 1995; 10: 206–10.

63. Wong NACS, Wong WK, Farndon JR. Early postoperative calcium concentrations as a predictor of need for calcium supplementation after parathyroidectomy. Br J Surg 1996; 83: 532–4.

64. Thompson NW, Sandelin K. Primary hyperparathyroidism caused by multiple gland disease (hyperplasia) long-term results in familial and sporadic cases. Acta Chir Aust 1994; 26(S112): 44–7.

65. Grant CS, Weaver A. Treatment of primary parathyroid hyperplasia: representative experience at Mayo Clinic. Acta Chir Aust 1994; 26(S112): 41–4.

66. Vetto JT, Brennan MF, Woodruf J, Burt M. Parathyroid carcinoma: diagnosis and clinical history. Surgery 1993; 114: 882–92.

67. Bergenfelz A, Valdermarsson S, Ahren B. Functional recovery of the parathyroid glands after surgery for primary hyperparathyroidism Surgery 1994; 116: 827–36.

68. Muller H. True recurrence of hyperparathyroidism: proposed criteria for recurrence. Br J Surg 1975; 62: 556–559.

69. Llach F, Felsenfeld A, Coleman M *et al.* Renal osteodistrophy in 131 unselected hemodialysis patients. Kidney Int 1984; 25: 187.

70. Demeure M, McGee D, Wilkes W *et al.* Results of surgical treatment for hyperparathyroidism associated with renal disease. Am J Surg 1990; 160: 337–40.

71. Loda M, Lipman J, Cukor B *et al.* Nodular foci in parathyroid adenomas and hyperplasia: an immunohistochemical analysis of proliferative activity. Hum Pathol 1994; 25: 1050–6.

72. Tominaga Y, Sato K, Tanaka Y *et al.* Histopathology and pathophysiology of secondary hyperparathyroidism due to chronic renal failure. Clin Nephrol 1995; 44(S1): S42–S47.

73. Goodman WG, Belin T, Gales B *et al.* Calcium-regulated parathyroid hormone release in patients with mild or advanced secondary hyperparathyroidism. Kidney Int 1995; 48: 1553–8.

74. Schaefer L, Malchow M, Schaefer RM *et al.* Effects of parathyroid hormone on renal tubular proteinases. Miner Electrolyte Metab 1996; 22: 182–6.

75. Rao DS, Shih MS, Mohini R. Effect of serum parathyroid hormone and bone marrow fibrosis on the response to erythropoietin in uremia. N Engl J Med 1993; 328: 171–5.

76. Hruska KA, Teitlebaum SL. Rena osteodistrophy. N Engl J Med 1995; 333: 166–74.

77. Nichols P, Owen JP, Ellis HA *et al.* Parathyroidectomy in chronic renal failure: a nine years follow up study. Q J Med, New Series 1990; 77: 1175–3.

78. Fine A, Fleming S, Leslie W. Calciphylaxis presenting with calf pain and plaques in four continuous ambulatory peritoneal dialysis patients and in one predialysis patient. Am J Kidney Dis 1995; 25: 498–502.

79. Timio M. Cardiotoxicity of parathyroid hormone in chronic renal failure. Ital J Miner Electrolyte Metab 1995; 9(2): 119–24.

80. Zimmermann E, Wassmer S, Steudle V. Long-term treatment with calcium-alpha-ketoglutarate corrects secondary hyper-parathyroidism. Miner Electrolyte Metab 1996; 22: 196–9.

81. Llach F, Hervas J, Cerezo S. The importance of dosing intravenous calcitriol in dialysis patients with severe hyperparathyroidism. Am J Kidney Dis 1995; 26: 845–51.

82. Stim JA, Lowe J, Arruda JAL, Dunea G. Once weekly intravenous calcitriol suppresses hyperparathyroidism in hemodialysis patients. ASAIO J 1995; 41:M693–M698.

83. AlaHouhala M, Holmberg C, Ronnholm K *et al.* Alphacalcidol oral pulses normalize uremic hyperparathyroidism prior to dialysis. Pediatr Nephrol 1995; 9: 737–41.

84. Nicholson ML, Feehally J. Br J Surg 1995; 82: 1427.

85. Rothmund M, Wagner P, Schark C. Subtotal parathyroidectomy vs. total parathyroidectomy and autotransplantation in secondary hyperparathyroidism – a randomised trial. World J Surg 1991; 15: 745–50.

86. Nichols P, Owen JP, Ellis HA, Farndon JR, Kelly PJ, Ward MK. Parathyroidectomy in chronic renal failure: a nine-year follow-up study. Q J Med 1990; 77: 1175–93.

87. Henry J-FR, Denizot A *et al.* Results of reoperations for persistent or recurrent secondary hyperparathyroidism. World J Surg 1990; 14: 303–7.

88. Kollmorgen CF, Aust MR *et al.* Parathyromatosis – a rare yet important cause of persistent or recurrent hyperparathyroidism. Surgery 1994; 116: 111–15.

2 The thyroid gland

Malcolm H. Wheeler

Embryology

The median thyroid diverticulum in the floor of the pharynx gives rise to the thyroid gland and grows downwards between the ventral ends of the first and second pharyngeal arches, the stalk of the diverticulum elongating to become the thyroglossal duct. This duct, later obliterated, extends from the foramen caecum at the base of the tongue to the isthmus, its distal part remaining as the pyramidal lobe of the thyroid. The ultimobranchial bodies, arising from the fourth pharyngeal pouch on each side, become applied to the lateral portion of the thyroid gland and contribute the parafollicular C-cells. These cells of neural crest origin, become secondarily involved with the thyroid but may later assume clinical significance as the cells giving rise to medullary thyroid carcinoma.

Investigation of the thyroid

Thyroid hormones

Measurement of thyroid hormones in the serum allows precise assessment of thyroid status to confirm the clinical diagnosis or clarify a difficult diagnostic problem. The thyroid hormones thyroxine (T4) and triiodothyronine (T3) are stored in colloid bound to thyroglobulin. The immediate control of synthesis and release of these hormones is achieved by thyroid stimulating hormone (TSH) released from the anterior pituitary. TSH secretion is regulated by the level of thyroid hormones in blood by a negative feedback mechanism. Thyrotrophin releasing hormone (TRH) from the hypothalamus also influences TSH secretion. In the circulation the thyroid hormones are bound to thyroxine-binding globulin (TBG), thyroxine binding pre-albumin (TBPA) and albumin. The principal metabolic effects of the thyroid hormones are due to unbound free T4 and T3 (0.03–0.04% and 0.2–0.5% of the total circulating hormones, respectively). Because almost all T4 and T3 is protein bound measurement of total hormones is influenced by conditions which change the serum levels of thyroxine binding proteins. For example, elevated levels are seen in pregnancy and in women taking oral contraceptives and low levels in the nephrotic syndrome. Drugs such as salicylates and some antibiotics compete for protein binding. Radioimmunoassays for free T4 and T3 are now readily available and give a precise assessment of thyroid function. T3 is the more active physiological hormone with 80% being produced in the periphery by mono deiodination of T4. Measurement of T3 is particularly important in T3 toxicosis when there is a clinical picture of thyrotoxicosis with normal serum T4 levels.

Thyroid stimulating hormone (TSH) can also be measured precisely by a sensitive immunochemiluminometric assay (normal range 0– 5 mU l⁻¹). Raised TSH levels are seen in primary hypothyroidism (e.g. autoimmune thyroiditis) and after treatment of thyrotoxicosis by surgery or radioiodine. Reduced TSH levels occur in hyperthyroidism.

Thyroid antibodies

Thyroglobulin
Antibodies to this major constituent of colloid and precursor of thyroid hormones are found in most people with Graves' disease and virtually all those with Hashimoto's thyroiditis.[1] Thyroglobulin measurement is used either in place of or as an adjunct to radioiodine scanning to detect residual or recurrent tumour in patients who have undergone total thyroidectomy for differentiated thyroid malignancy[2] and who are receiving replacement thyroxine.

Thyroid peroxidase (TPO)
Antibodies to thyroid peroxidase, previously know as thyroid micro-somal antigen, are found in most patients with Graves' disease or Hashimoto's thyroiditis.[3] Raised titres are also detected in post partum thyroiditis and non-organ specific autoimmune diseases such as rheumatoid arthritis.

TSH receptor antibodies (TRAbs)
Most TSH receptor autoantibodies have a stimulatory action but in some instances antibodies bind to the receptor and block activity. Measurement of TRAbs is especially valuable in the diagnosis of Graves' disease, being detected in approximately 90% of patients.[4] Neonatal hyperthyroidism may result from transplacental passage of TRAbs.

Calcitonin

Increased serum levels of calcitonin, produced by the parafollicular C-cells, are found in medullary thyroid carcinoma (MTC).[5] Measurement of basal or stimulated calcitonin levels provides a method to assess the completeness of surgical resection of medullary thyroid carcinoma and is valuable in the follow-up and detection of metastases after thy-roidectomy. Screening for the detection of familial medullary thyroid carcinoma, usually as part of the MEN 2A or 2B syndrome, has until recently been dependent on measurement of stimulated calcitonin levels. Identification of germ line mutations in the RET proto-oncogene on chromosome 10[6] is now replacing biochemical screening.

Carcinoembryonic antigen (CEA)

Carcinoembryonic antigen measurement is a useful adjunct to calcitonin assay in the follow-up of patients with medullary thyroid carcinoma.

Thyroid isotope scanning

Traditionally the thyroid gland has been scanned either with ^{123}I or technetium pertechnetate ^{99m}Tc, classifying nodules into those that are non-functioning 'cold', normally functioning 'warm' and hyperfunctioning 'hot'. Although the finding of a 'hot' nodule is usually consistent with benign pathology more than 80% of nodules are cold and only 20% of these will be malignant. Iodine scanning is therefore not helpful in the diagnosis of malignancy and has only a limited role in investigation of the euthyroid patient with a solitary nodule. Discrepant imaging is well documented with hot ^{99m}Tc images being cold on ^{123}I scanning.[7] It has therefore been suggested that all ^{99m}Tc hot scans should be re-evaluated with ^{123}I. Isotope scanning has most utility in the investigation of a solitary autonomous toxic nodule or toxic multinodular goitre. Iodine scanning identifies patients with metastatic thyroid tumours and aids localisation of ectopic thyroid tissue. Other isotopes are occasionally used especially in the evaluation of medullary thyroid carcinoma. These include pentavalent dimercaptosuccinic acid (DMSA),[8] thallium[9] and meta-iodobenzyl guanidine (MIBG).[10]

Radioiodine uptake

Measurement of the 4 and 48 h uptake of an administered dose of radioactive ^{123}I is useful in the assessment of thyrotoxicosis. Increased uptake is seen in most forms of the disorder with the notable exceptions of thyrotoxicosis due to subacute thyroiditis and following excessive T4 intake.

Ultrasonography

This technique is operator dependent but is capable of identifying impalpable nodules as small as 0.3 mm in diameter, will discriminate cystic from solid lesions but cannot distinguish benign from malignant disease. Cystic nodules constitute 15–25%[11] of all thyroid nodules and when 4 cm or more in diameter may have a malignancy rate of approximately 20%.[12]

CT scanning and MRI

These techniques have an increasingly important role in the assessment of thyroid disease particularly in the evaluation of retrosternal goitres and glands producing significant pressure effects and distortion of adjacent structures.

Needle biopsy

This technique is a most valuable complement to clinical examination particularly in the assessment of thyroid nodular disease. There are two quite distinct types of needle biopsy.

Cutting needle biopsy

This method produces a core of tissue suitable for histological examination. It has high diagnostic accuracy but is a painful procedure with poor compliance and may cause haematoma, tracheal puncture and recurrent laryngeal nerve damage. Lesions less than 3 cm in size may not be amenable to this technique. The risk of seeding malignancy along the needle tract has been greatly exaggerated.[13]

Fine needle aspiration cytology (FNAC, ABC)

This technique employs a fine gauge (21 or 23) needle to obtain a thyroid sample suitable for cytological assessment. First used in Scandinavia in the early 1950s[14] it is now universally accepted as being a highly accurate, cost-effective method with low morbidity and good patient compliance. The method can accurately diagnose:

- Colloid nodules
- Thyroiditis
- Papillary carcinoma
- Medullary carcinoma
- Anaplastic carcinoma
- Lymphoma

Its major limitation is its inability to distinguish benign from malignant follicular neoplasms,[15] this distinction being dependent on the histological criteria of capsular and vascular invasion.

Four possible results are available from FNAC:

- Malignant
- Benign
- Suspicious
- Inadequate

The first two categories are well defined and indeed Lowhagen *et al.*[15] reported no false positive results with respect to malignancy and a false negative rate of 2.2% which later fell to 0. Grant *et al.*[16] found a false negative rate of only 0.7% in 439 patients studied and concluded that FNAC was a safe, reliable and accurate means of discriminating between benign and malignant lesions of the thyroid. Suspicious lesions are mostly the follicular tumours and because of the inability of the technique to provide histological data all such lesions should be resected. An inadequate sample rate of 15% is not uncommon and such a result should not be regarded as being benign but is an indication for repeat aspiration.

Goitre The term goitre, derived from the Latin guttur, meaning throat, is used as a non-specific term to indicate enlargement of the thyroid gland. A classification of goitre is shown in Table 2.1.

Simple goitre Simple goitre is the result of TSH stimulation, usually secondary to inadequate levels of circulating thyroid hormones. In these circumstances TSH stimulation causes diffuse hyperplasia of the thyroid and an elevation in hormone output. Iodine deficiency is a key factor in simple endemic goitre, associated with a low iodine content of water and food.[17] There are 5–10 mg of iodine in the thyroid pool with a turnover rate of 1% daily. The minimum daily dietary requirements of iodine are therefore small, being approximately 50–100 mg. Endemic goitrous areas are in mountainous regions such as the Alps, Andes and Himalayas. In Britain recognised regions include the Chiltern's, Cotswolds, Derbyshire and South Wales.

Table 2.1 *Classification of goitre*

Simple goitre (endemic or sporadic)	Diffuse hyperplastic goitre Nodular goitre
Toxic goitre	Diffuse (Graves' disease) Toxic multinodular goitre Toxic solitary nodule
Neoplastic goitre	Benign Malignant
Thyroiditis	Subacute (granulomatous) – de Quervain's Autoimmune (Hashimoto's) Riedel's Acute suppurative
Miscellaneous	Chronic bacterial infection (e.g. TB or syphilis) Actinomycosis Amyloidosis Dyshormonogenesis

Iodine deficiency in its most extreme form is associated with cretinism, congenital hypothyroidism and various degrees of mental impairment. Usually an endemic goitre commences as a soft diffuse enlargement appearing in childhood and eventually becoming a colloid goitre at a later stage when TSH stimulation has fallen off. Times of physiological stress such as puberty and pregnancy result in increased demands for thyroxine and are accompanied by TSH stimulation of the thyroid and diffuse hyperplasia. The natural history of thyroid stimulation by TSH is such that there are fluctuating levels of stimulation but eventually active and inactive lobules co-exist. At this stage nodules form and throughout the thyroid there are changes of hyperplasia, cystic degeneration, haemorrhage, colloid-filled follicles, fibrosis and later calcification. Simple goitre occurring in a non-endemic area is usually described as sporadic. The nodules of endemic goitre appear earlier than those in sporadic glands. All types of goitre occur more often in women.

Environmental factors such as the dietary goitrogen thiocyanate in cassava or vegetables of the brassica family may cause thyroid enlargement.[18] The interaction of environmental goitrogens and iodine deficiency may explain some of the differences in the prevalence of endemic goitre seen with similar degrees of iodine deficiency. Other environmental agents including calcium and drugs such as the antithyroid agent carbimazole are capable of acting at various sites within the thyroid gland, interfering with the process of hormone synthesis, and leading to hyperplasia of the thyroid with goitre formation.

Paradoxically excess iodine intake can inhibit proteolysis and release of thyroid hormones leading to an iodine goitre and hypothyroidism.[18]

Deficiency of one or more of the enzymes in the thyroid responsible for thyroxine synthesis may be the cause of sporadic goitre. These deficiencies, either complete or partial, are usually genetically determined and are well illustrated by the dyshormonogenetic Pendred's syndrome in which thyroid enlargement progresses to nodular goitre and is associated with deafness. Severe forms of dyshormonogenesis result in hypothyroidism and cretinism in the infant. Treatment consists of thyroxine and eventually thyroidectomy if the goitre enlarges giving rise to pressure symptoms or cosmetic difficulties.

Prevention and treatment of simple goitre

Prevention of the development of simple endemic goitre can be achieved by the addition of iodine to table salt. At the prenodular stage a hyperplastic goitre can be made to regress in size by giving thyroxine 0.1–0.15 mg daily often continuing for several years. Thyroidectomy may be indicated for cosmetic reasons or because of pressure effects if the gland does not regress.

Thyroid nodules

Thyroid nodules are common, being a feature of many different thyroid diseases. In a non-goitrous area the prevalence of palpable thyroid nodules in a population aged 30–59 years was 4.2%.[19] At adult autopsy the prevalence of thyroid nodules (many less than 1 cm in diameter) is perhaps as high as 50%.[20] Although the vast majority of thyroid nodules are benign and include colloid lesions, follicular adenomas, nodular thyroiditis and degenerative cysts, the essential clinical problem, particularly when the lesion is solitary, remains the distinction between benign and malignant disease.

Clinical assessment

Most thyroid nodules are asymptomatic but the acute development of a painful swelling in the thyroid usually suggests haemorrhage into a pre-existing colloid nodule. This is an important condition to recognise as spontaneous resolution, sometimes aided by aspiration, will occur in a few weeks without any action.

Rapid growth of an existing nodule, with discomfort radiating into the face or jaw, may be due to malignancy. A malignant nodule, however, may grow slowly over many years before a diagnosis is made. Thyroid nodules also occur more often in women but a solitary nodule in a male carries a greater risk of malignancy. In the elderly, a rapidly growing firm painful lesion is likely to be an anaplastic carcinoma. The young are particularly at risk for malignancy, for example, a solitary nodule is likely to be malignant in 50% of children under 14 years of age.[21, 22] A positive family history of thyroid or other endocrine disease may be relevant to the diagnosis of medullary thyroid cancer in MEN 2A, 2B and non-MEN familial syndromes (Chapter 4).

Several key environmental and geographic factors require consideration in that the incidence of follicular cancer is increased in endemic goitrous areas,[23] iodine-rich regions such as Iceland have an increased incidence of papillary cancer[24] and the recent Chernobyl nuclear reactor accident demonstrates the tumour-inducing effects of irradiation. Although the association between thyroid carcinoma and a previous history of head and neck irradiation in children was first recorded in 1950[25] the true magnitude of the problem was only identified by DeGroot and Paloyan in the Chicago area in 1973.[26] Irradiation also increases the incidence of benign thyroid nodules but the reported risk of malignancy in a palpable nodule found in a previously irradiated thyroid ranges from 20 to 50%. High dose external irradiation to the neck for conditions such as Hodgkin's lymphoma may also increase the risk of thyroid malignancy.[27] The latent period for developing post-irradiation tumours ranges from 6 to 35 years. Therapeutic radioiodine used in the treatment of Graves' disease and the administration of diagnostic isotopes are not associated with any increased risk of malignancy.

A preliminary clinical examination of the patient is directed towards assessment of thyroid status, although most patients with a solitary thyroid nodule are euthyroid. A nodule in a hyperthyroid patient is highly unlikely to be malignant. Previously much emphasis was placed on the distinction between a clinically solitary nodule and a multi-nodular gland in the belief that multinodular goitres were unlikely to contain malignancy. When a dominant lesion is present within a multinodular gland, however, the malignancy rate may be similar to that of the true solitary nodule.

A hard fixed nodule is likely to be malignant but it is not uncommon for papillary lesions to be cystic and follicular lesions to be soft as a result of haemorrhage. A very hard lesion may be an entirely benign calcified colloid nodule. Lymphadenopathy in the central paratracheal groups or in the lateral deep cervical region is a common finding in papillary and medullary carcinomas.

Although voice change and hoarseness may be non-specific, a proven recurrent laryngeal nerve palsy on the side of a palpable thyroid nodule is likely to indicate malignant infiltration. Rarely direct pressure from a benign lesion produces vocal cord paralysis. Although the presence of pressure symptoms, tracheal deviation or retrosternal extension will not aid the distinction of malignant from benign lesions these features will be considerations in the selection of patients for surgery.

Following a careful clinical assessment an opinion will be formed as to the likelihood of malignancy. Further supportive and diagnostic tests become appropriate. The thyroid status will be confirmed by measurement of T4 and TSH and a radiograph of the neck and chest delineate retrosternal extension or airway distortion. Most calcified thyroid nodules are benign but some papillary and medullary neoplasms have a characteristic fine stippled or punctate calcification. Measurement of calcitonin is not routinely performed but this determination can facilitate the identification of an unsuspected medullary carcinoma.[28] Hypercalcitonaemia is not absolutely specific for medullary tumours and raised levels may be seen in patients with carcinoma of the breast, pancreas, lung and with carcinoid tumours, phaeochromocytoma and bony metastases.

Positive thyroid antibody titres are non-specific and can be raised in malignancy.

Thyroglobulin measurement although valuable in the follow-up of patients with malignant tumours has no value in their initial diagnosis.

Diagnostic investigation

Isotope scanning
Unless the patient has thyrotoxicosis, scintigraphy of the thyroid either with ^{123}I or technetium pertechnetate ^{99m}Tc has little value in the investigation of the patient with a thyroid nodule.

Ultrasonography

This technique has limited diagnostic value in the assessment of thyroid nodules.

Needle biopsy and aspiration cytology (FNAC)

This highly accurate and cost-effective technique is the method of choice for precisely diagnosing most patients with thyroid nodular disease. A recent refinement of the method using an immunocyto-chemical technique for the detection of thyroid peroxidase (TPO) may be a useful adjunct to FNAC in the preoperative diagnosis of follicular malignancy.[29] Delbridge *et al.*[30] have shown that proton magnetic resonance spectroscopy (PMRS) analysis of FNAC specimens helps to make the distinction between benign and malignant lesions.

Treatment

Thyroid hormone administration

There is little evidence that the administration of thyroxine is capable of reducing the size of benign nodules. It is a concern that TSH suppression by T4 is a component in the management of thyroid malignancy and reducing the size of an incorrectly diagnosed malignant nodule by T4 is clearly a potential pitfall.

Summary of indications for surgery

Selection for surgery is based primarily on clinical features aided by preoperative aspiration biopsy cytology yielding either a diagnostic or suspicious appearance of malignancy. Another large proportion of patients undergo surgery because of pressure and mechanical symptoms including dyspnoea, choking and dysphagia, often associated with progressive increase in size of the nodule. A scheme of management for patients with solitary thyroid nodular disease is shown in Fig. 2.1. Clinical features such as characteristics of nodule, lymphadenopathy, recurrent laryngeal nerve palsy, family history, history of irradiation may all override cytological findings in the decision for surgery.

Surgery for thyroid nodules

The minimum surgical procedure for adequate treatment of the solitary thyroid nodule is a unilateral total lobectomy with removal of the isthmus and pyramidal lobe. This is a safe operation with minimal risk of damaging either the parathyroids or the recurrent laryngeal nerve. A full histological examination of the nodule is permitted with no risk of tumour spillage in the operative field. This surgical procedure usually obviates the need to reoperate and remove a posterior thyroid lobe remnant if the definitive histology should be returned as malignant or if there should be any benign nodule recurrence at a

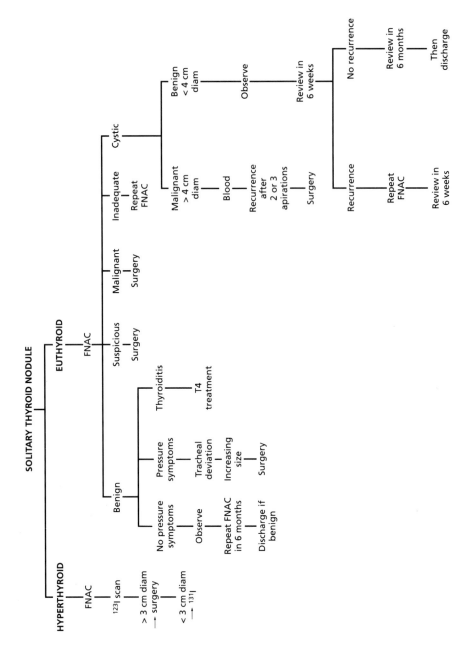

Figure 2.1 *Scheme of management for solitary thyroid nodule.*

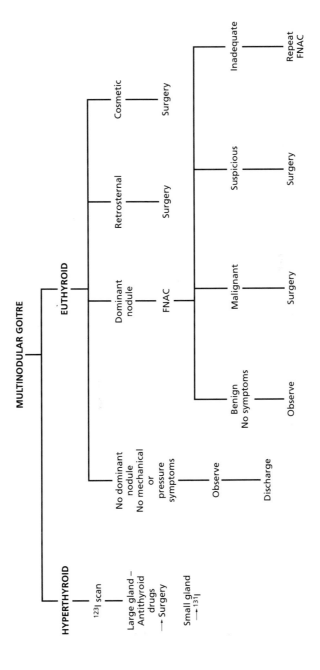

Figure 2.2 *Scheme of management for multinodular thyroid.*

later date. These are most important benefits compared with the time-honoured, but out-moded, operation of unilateral subtotal lobectomy.

Frozen section histology can be used to confirm the preoperative diagnosis and aid decision making particularly with respect to benign pathology where lobectomy alone will be sufficient.

Thyroid cysts

Confirmation of the diagnosis of a thyroid cyst is usually made by fine needle aspiration and this simple technique can be both diagnostic and therapeutic. A full cytological assessment usually requires sampling thyroid tissue adjacent to the cyst for fear of missing a carcinoma in the cyst wall. If a cyst refills it is appropriate to reaspirate but after two or three such manoeuvres surgery is likely to be indicated. A large cyst (greater than 4 cm in diameter), a significantly blood-stained aspirate, cytological findings of neoplasia or a previous history of irradiation are all indications for surgery.

Multinodular disease

The usual indications for surgery are cosmetic or pressure effects, a dominant nodule perhaps increasing in size or showing cytological features which raise the possibility of malignancy, thyrotoxicosis or retrosternal extension (Fig. 2.2). The surgical procedure will be tailored to the situation found at surgery and although frequently a bilateral subtotal thyroidectomy is appropriate, if there is asymmetrical nodularity with one lobe significantly larger than the other then a unilateral total lobectomy with a subtotal procedure on the opposite side may be indicated.

There has been some support for the more radical approach of performing a total thyroidectomy when the multinodularity is both bilateral and extensive often with no normal thyroid tissue to be left as a remnant.[31]

Retrosternal goitre

Almost all retrosternal goitres arise from growth of the lower half of the thyroid lobes extending down into a substernal position. The degree of descent of the gland is variable but when palpable in the neck it is usually classified as substernal whereas a gland entirely within the chest is intrathoracic. In some instances a retrosternal goitre may be quite asymptomatic being found as a coincidental observation on a chest radiograph. Many patients are symptomatic with problems of airway compression, 'asthma', dysphagia, hoarseness of the voice and even thyrotoxicosis. Recurrent laryngeal nerve palsy rarely occurs as a direct pressure effect of a benign lesion but more dramatic pressure effects can lead to superior vena cava compression syndrome. The incidence of malignancy in retrosternal glands is probably no different from that of other nodular goitres but of course a gland behind the sternum is not amenable to palpation or fine needle aspiration cytology for diagnosis.

Confirmation of the diagnosis can be made by a combination of plain radiograph and either CT or MRI. These latter investigations will give precise information concerning airway compromise. Respiratory function tests with flow loop studies are helpful in assessment.

The diagnosis of a retrosternal goitre is usually an indication for surgery both to obtain a precise histological diagnosis and to remove the significant risk of progressive airway obstruction resulting from growth of the gland or from haemorrhage into a benign colloid lesion.

Thyroid cancer

Thyroid cancer is rare (3.7–4.7 per 100 000 of population)[32] accounting for fewer than 1%[33] of all malignancies and 0.5% of all cancer death.[34] The thyroid cancers constitute an extremely heterogeneous group of tumours with a wide spectrum of biological behaviour but, remarkably, in most instances are well treated by appropriate therapy, with a high survival rate. Disappointingly, because of the lack of long-term follow-up studies and large randomised trials comparing various surgical procedures, the optimal management for many of these tumours remains controversial.

Papillary carcinoma

Introduction
This is the commonest thyroid tumour which shows an increased incidence in iodine-rich areas and usually affects children and young adults. Previous neck irradiation particularly in the young may predispose to thyroid cancer and approximately 85% of such irradiation-induced tumours are papillary.[26] A rare familial form of the disease has also been described.[35]

Pathology
This tumour which has a propensity for lymphatic spread both within the thyroid and to the paratracheal and cervical lymph nodes is usually a hard whitish lesion infiltrating the thyroid gland and presents as a thyroid nodule. The lesion is frequently multifocal (30–87.5%),[36] rarely encapsulated and blood-borne spread is usually a late feature.

These tumours can be divided into three main types based on their size and extent.

Minimal
These are lesions 1 cm or less in size, usually not clinically obvious and often called papillary microcarcinoma. They readily metastasise to regional lymph nodes and are a frequent finding at autopsy being detected in 6–13% of thyroid glands of patients dying from causes other than thyroid disease. The older term for small tumours was

occult, describing lesions 1.5 cm or less in size. Many of these were clinically apparent with cervical lymphadenopathy (lateral aberrant thyroid). Although rarely associated with metastatic disease, deaths have been reported, the Mayo Clinic group describing four fatalities in 396 patients with tumours 1.5 cm or less in diameter.[37]

Intrathyroidal
These lesions are larger than minimal tumours, have a less favourable prognosis, are situated totally within the thyroid and do not invade adjacent structures.

Extrathyroidal
This is a locally advanced condition extending through the thyroid capsule often involving adjacent structures such as the trachea, oesophagus and recurrent laryngeal nerve. The prognosis of this disease is the least favourable for papillary carcinoma.

Histology
The typical lesion has a mixture of papillary projections and follicular structures. The cuboidal cells with pale abundant cytoplasm have intranuclear cytoplasmic inclusions, nuclear overlapping and grooves (Orphan Annie cells). Psammoma bodies occur and are associated with a high incidence of lymphatic spread. The presence of involved lymph nodes, however, does not seem to affect the prognosis adversely. Follicular, encapsulated, diffuse sclerosing and tall cell varieties of papillary carcinoma have also been described.

Clinical presentation
The commonest presentation of papillary carcinoma is a thyroid nodule frequently associated with enlarged cervical lymph nodes, especially in children. Cystic change in metastases is not unusual such that the differential diagnosis may include a branchial cyst. Involvement of adjacent structures by a locally invasive tumour may cause hoarseness of the voice due to recurrent laryngeal nerve palsy, airway symptoms because of tracheal involvement and dysphagia as a result of oesophageal invasion. Less than 1% of patients at the time of initial presentation will show features of distant metastases. The highest frequency of metastases at initial presentation is seen in children, but up to 20% of patients overall will ultimately develop distant spread.[38]

Diagnosis
Diagnosis is based on a combination of careful clinical assessment and fine needle aspiration cytology.

Follicular carcinoma

Introduction
This tumour, less common than papillary carcinoma, has a higher incidence in iodine-deficient areas due to chronic TSH stimulation and can also be caused by previous irradiation. The disease has a female to male ratio of 3:1, affects an older age group (mean age 50 years) than papillary carcinoma and rarely occurs in familial form.[39]

Pathology
Follicular carcinoma is invariably encapsulated, solitary, readily exhibiting vascular invasion and spread via the bloodstream. In contrast to papillary tumours lymphatic spread is usually a late phenomenon seen with advanced tumours. Follicular carcinoma is classified into two types according to histopathological features.

1. Minimally invasive: this tumour is seen on histology to demonstrate only slight capsular or vascular invasion in contrast to the second type.
2. Frankly invasive: this more aggressive tumour, the diagnosis of which depends on histological confirmation of capsular and vascular invasion, may demonstrate venous extension particularly into the middle thyroid and internal jugular veins. Although most well-differentiated tumours have a well-formed follicular structure the oxyphilic Hurthle cell lesion is composed mostly of cells with eosinophilic granular cytoplasm, large clear nuclei and trabecular architecture. Some consider this variety to be a particularly aggressive form of follicular carcinoma with a greater propensity for multifocality and lymph node metastases.[40] Furthermore, therapeutic options in Hurthle cell tumours are limited by the inability of the lesion to concentrate radioactive iodine. Nevertheless they do synthesise thyroglobulin.

Clinical features
Follicular thyroid cancer presents as a discrete solitary thyroid nodule increasing in size. Although many tumours are firm a follicular carcinoma is often soft because of haemorrhage within the lesion. Metastatic disease may already be present at the time of diagnosis with bone and lung involvement.

Diagnosis
Unlike papillary thyroid carcinoma follicular carcinoma cannot be diagnosed precisely by FNAC. The cytology report will describe a follicular tumour, usually showing a microfollicular pattern, the majority of such lesions being entirely benign. Only 20% of these will be subsequently identified as follicular carcinoma.

Treatment of differentiated thyroid cancer

There is general agreement that thyroidectomy is the treatment of choice but the precise extent ranging from excisional biopsy to total thyroidectomy remains controversial.[41] The treatment objectives are to irradicate primary tumour, reduce the incidence of distant or local recurrence, facilitate treatment of metastases, cure the maximum number of patients and achieve all of these objectives with minimal morbidity.

Papillary carcinoma can be separated into high and low risk groups in terms of risk for recurrence and long-term survival primarily on the basis of the age of the patient at the time of diagnosis, younger subjects usually having a more favourable outlook. Several more sophisticated prognostic scoring systems have been introduced to identify high risk tumours and aid comparison between different surgical therapies. The AGES score system from the Mayo Clinic considers *Age* of patient, histological *Grade*, *Extent* and *Size* of tumour.[42] The majority of patients being assessed by the scoring system fit into the low risk group with an excellent long-term prognosis. Other scoring systems include AMES (*Age*, *Metastasis*, *Extent* and *Size*) and MACIS (*Metastasis*, *Age*, *Completeness* of resection, *Invasion*, *Size*).

Total thyroidectomy has been advocated because of its ability to treat multifocal tumour, decrease local recurrence, decrease distant recurrence, reduce the risk of anaplasia in remaining remnants, facilitate treatment with ^{131}I and permit postoperative thyroglobulin measurements for monitoring the patient's subsequent progress. In the case of papillary carcinoma there is a high incidence of multifocality which clearly would not be treated by a unilateral or even near total thyroidectomy. It is likely, however, that many small foci of microscopic tumour remaining after less than total thyroidectomy stay dormant and do not necessarily progress and achieve clinical significance. Nevertheless local tumour recurrence is a serious event carrying a high risk of death from the thyroid cancer. Retrospective studies of thyroidectomy for papillary tumours have demonstrated a reduced local recurrence rate when total thyroidectomy was performed compared with a subtotal resection.[43] With respect to mortality risk it has been shown that high risk patients have a lower mortality rate at 25 years when treated by bilateral resection rather than an ipsilateral lobectomy.[42] The life-threatening complication of anaplastic transformation in an inadequately resected papillary carcinoma may be avoided by initial total thyroidectomy.

Most patients with differentiated thyroid cancer will have presented with a unilateral thyroid nodule and should be treated by the minimum surgical procedure of total lobectomy on the side of the lesion, isthmusectomy and removal of the pyramidal lobe. If papillary carcinoma is confirmed usually by combination of preoperative FNAC and intraoperative frozen section a total thyroidectomy is the most appropriate surgical treatment for intrathyroidal and extrathyroidal tumours. Thyroidectomy must always include clearance of pretracheal and paratracheal lymph nodes. The thymus should not be disturbed for fear of devascularising the inferior parathyroids often situated within the superior thymic horns. Lymph nodes in the lateral carotid chain group are biopsied and if positive on frozen section histology should be cleared by a modified neck dissection leaving the internal jugular vein and sternomastoid muscle intact. There is no evidence to support more extensive dissection. More extensive extrathyroidal papillary carcinomas, however, may require radical excision of adjacent structures even including part of the trachea with construction of a temporary tracheostomy.

A unilateral total lobectomy and isthmusectomy is adequate for minimal (less than 1 cm) lesions and the rare encapsulated papillary cancers which generally have an excellent prognosis. The recurrent laryngeal nerve must be identified throughout its course in these procedures so that damage may be avoided. Rarely is it necessary to sacrifice the nerve to achieve tumour clearance. The incidence of postoperative hypoparathyroidism should be no more than 3%, care being taken to identify the parathyroid glands and leave their blood supply intact.

Follicular tumours diagnosed on fine needle aspiration cytology are treated by total lobectomy, isthmusectomy and removal of the pyramidal lobe. Frozen section is usually unhelpful, failing to demonstrate capsular or vascular invasion, because of sampling difficulties. If the definitive histology is returned as a minimal lesion then a unilateral procedure is all that is required. A lesion shown to be frankly invasive will require a total thyroidectomy either performed within a few days of the initial lobectomy or after a period of three to four months. Lymph node dissection is not routinely performed for follicular tumours. A decision to proceed to a total thyroidectomy can often be made at the time of surgery on the basis of the macroscopic appearances of the lesion and especially when the tumour size is in excess of 4 cm.

Hurthle cell lesion considered by some to have a bad prognosis should be treated by total thyroidectomy and central neck node dissection.[40]

Postoperative treatment

Thyroxine
Any patient who has undergone total thyroidectomy will require replacement treatment with thyroxine. In patients with papillary carcinoma prescribing thyroxine will suppress TSH levels which may well influence the biological behaviour of the tumour.

Thyroglobulin

Thyroglobulin measurement is a sensitive indicator of residual or recurrent differentiated thyroid cancer when a total thyroidectomy has been performed and the patient is on full replacement/suppressive thyroxine dosage.[2] This measurement is now performed routinely at each postoperative clinic attendance and has markedly reduced the need for routine serial radioactive iodine scanning.

Radioactive iodine

Radioactive iodine is a most useful means of detecting metastatic disease when total thyroidectomy has been performed for differentiated thyroid cancer but approximately 20% of papillary carcinomas in patients older than 50 years of age are incapable of concentrating ^{131}I.[38] Most follicular carcinomas, with the exception of the Hurthle cell variety, can be imaged by radioiodine. If total thyroidectomy has been performed for differentiated cancer, patients are initially placed on triiodothyronine (T3) 20 µg tds and sent home to await an ^{131}I scan approximately six weeks later. T3 is discontinued two weeks before the scan to allow a rise in TSH level before administering 2–5 mCi of ^{131}I. If there are no metastases and the total thyroidectomy has been successful the uptake at 24 h should be less than 1%. When there is significant uptake in the thyroid bed this can be ablated with radio-iodine and any metastatic disease subsequently treated with a therapeutic dose of 150–200 mCi ^{131}I. Patients are then placed on thyroxine (0.15–0.2 mg daily), scanning is repeated at six monthly intervals and repeated therapeutic doses of ^{131}I given as necessary until all residual uptake is ablated. The maximum cumulative dose of ^{131}I should be no greater than 800–1000 mCi. Patients whose metastases are visible only on radioiodine scanning despite negative chest radiography or tomography have an excellent prognosis.[44] Once stable and disease free, subsequent follow-up is achieved by a combination of clinical examination and serum thyroglobulin measurement.

Anaplastic carcinoma

This highly aggressive tumour usually affects the elderly with a peak incidence between 60 and 70 years of age. Anaplastic carcinoma occurs slightly more often in females than males and the tumour has a higher incidence in areas of endemic goitre. The tumour rapidly infiltrates local structures and metastases via the bloodstream and lymphatics. The frequent finding of foci of papillary or follicular carcinoma in anaplastic tumours suggests that this disease originates in an unrecognised or untreated differentiated tumour.[45] The clinical findings are typically those of an elderly female often with a long history of goitre that suddenly starts to grow rapidly with hoarseness, dysphonia, dysphagia and a compromised airway.

Although the clinical findings are virtually diagnostic, confirmation may be obtained by FNAC, the aspirate showing bizarre giant cells, multinucleated cells and pleomorphic tumour cells. Resection of the thyroid is rarely possible because of the local extent of disease. Incision biopsy for diagnostic purposes should be avoided for fear of initiating an uncontrollable local spread of the disease. If surgery is possible it should relieve an obstructed airway by excision of the isthmus. Radiotherapy and doxorubicin are the main modalities of treatment but invariably the tumour rapidly progresses usually leading to death of the patient within six months.

Malignant lymphoma

Thyroid lymphoma, usually of the non-Hodgkin's B-cell type, can develop as part of a generalised lymphomatous process but can be confined as a primary tumour to the thyroid. The majority of such lymphomas arise in a background of long-standing autoimmune Hashimoto's thyroiditis[46] although only a tiny minority of patients with this relatively common disorder will ultimately go on to develop lymphoma.

These tumours infiltrate throughout lymphatics and blood vessels of the thyroid spreading directly into adjacent tissue and involving cervical nodes.

As in the case of anaplastic carcinoma this is primarily a disease of elderly females, a typical patient presenting with a painless firm thyroid mass, rapidly increasing in size. There may be a history of goitre or autoimmune disease, some patients being either frankly hypothyroid or perhaps already receiving thyroxine medication. This tumour grows to involve adjacent cervical structures and lymphadenopathy is invariably present. The diagnosis can be confirmed by FNAC although full characterisation may require histological assessment of a core biopsy. Radiotherapy and chemotherapy are the main treatment modalities. Chemotherapy is of most value for extrathyroidal and disseminated disease. Surgery may be necessary to free the trachea when there is impending airway obstruction. Although five-year survival of 85% has been reported[47] the overall prognosis of the disease is significantly influenced by the histopathological grade of the lesion and the presence of locally extensive or disseminated disease.

Squamous cell carcinoma

This is a rare tumour, distinct from the squamous metaplasia often seen in papillary carcinomas. It is an aggressive disease with a clinical course similar to that of anaplastic carcinoma; most tumours are unresectable.

Metastatic carcinoma of the thyroid

The thyroid gland can be the site of metastatic spread from primary tumours in the breast, kidney and lung. Careful clinical assessment may suggest the correct diagnosis but confirmation is usually obtained by FNAC. In some instances resection of the thyroid gland is indicated if the primary disease is otherwise well controlled.

Medullary carcinoma (MTC)

Introduction
This is a tumour which arises from the C-cells, derived from neural ectoderm, and accounts for approximately 8% of malignant thyroid tumours. Hazard in 1959[48] described the tumour as a solid non-follicular carcinoma with co-existing amyloid. Williams[49] proposed that the disease arose from the parafollicular C-cells, which were later shown to secrete calcitonin, a peptide capable of lowering the blood calcium and amenable to measurement by radioimmunoassay.[50] MTC is a sporadic tumour in 80% of patients and familial in 20%. The familial syndromes are inherited in an autosomal dominant manner with almost complete penetrance but variable expressivity and consist of the MEN 2A and 2B syndromes and the rarer non-MEN familial form.

Pathology
MTC is a solid tumour located in the upper two thirds of the thyroid and is usually both multicentric and bilateral when occurring in the familial form. The typical histological picture is one of infiltrating neoplastic cells invading the thyroid, forming glandular and solid areas with amyloid stroma. Variants of this histological pattern frequently occur. The tumour grows locally but readily spreads by lymphatics to regional nodes and via the bloodstream to distant sites such as liver, lungs and bones. This tumour synthesises and secretes calcitonin, a most valuable histochemical marker for MTC. Calcitonin gene-related peptide (CGRP) is also produced by C-cells but has little clinical value as a tumour marker. Carcinoembryonic antigen (CEA) is another tumour marker.

Clinical features
As with most thyroid tumours the disease typically presents as a mass in the neck often with enlarged cervical and mediastinal lymph nodes. Involvement of adjacent organs and the recurrent laryngeal nerve may cause respiratory or swallowing difficulties and voice changes. Sporadic disease has a peak incidence at 40–50 years of age whereas inherited familial disease is usually seen at a younger age. Diarrhoea is often a prominent clinical feature but the ability of this tumour to secrete a range of hormones and peptides including calcitonin, prostaglandins, 5-hydroxytryptamine and ACTH can give rise to a range of clinical syndromes which may include Cushing's syndrome.

Although the familial varieties of the disease can present in an identical manner to sporadic disease biochemical and more recently genetic screening can detect the condition at a preclinical stage before there is histological or macroscopic evidence of the disease.

Diagnosis
Clinical assessment and the taking of a careful family history are fundamental to establishing a precise diagnosis and confirmation is obtained by FNAC and measurement of serum calcitonin. Because of the close association of phaeochromocytoma and MTC in the MEN familial forms measurement of urinary VMA and metanephrines should be carried out in all patients with MTC before progressing to any invasive measures such as surgery.

Familial disease (see Chapter 4)

Treatment
Total thyroidectomy is the appropriate procedure to adequately treat multicentric and bilateral disease. The central and paratracheal lymph nodes are cleared from the level of the thyroid cartilage to the upper mediastinum including thymectomy. The lateral nodes in the carotid sheath are sampled and if involved with tumour a modified radical node dissection is performed preserving the internal jugular vein, sternomastoid muscle and spinal accessory nerve. Even when the primary tumour is extensive the recurrent laryngeal nerve can usually be preserved. Because of the multifocal nature of hereditary tumours a bilateral lymph node clearance is advised.

Prognosis
The presence or absence of distant metastases and lymph node positivity are major factors in determining the ultimate prognosis. Excellent 10-year survival figures of approximately 90% have been reported[51] but when lymph node metastases are present this survival rate is reduced to 45%. It is likely that sporadic disease and MEN2B tumours have the worst prognosis with the best outlook being seen in the non-MEN familial and MEN2A patients.

Follow-up
After surgery regular clinical and biochemical follow-up is carried out with measurement of the two tumour markers calcitonin and carcinoembryonic antigen (CEA). When raised levels of these agents persist after thyroidectomy or develop at a later stage this may signify persistent and recurrent disease. Ultrasonography, CT, MRI and scanning with MIBG, octreotide or DMSA can be utilised to detect this disease. For occult disease selective venous catheterisation and sampling for calcitonin measurement have been used.[52] Laparoscopic assessment of the liver can detect small metastases not visible by conventional scanning. A proportion of these patients can be helped by re-operative surgery but the benefits of radical re-operative surgery remain controversial. External irradiation can occasionally produce some benefit but chemotherapy with doxorubicin is both toxic and disappointing.

Hyper-thyroidism

Hyperthyroidism is a condition in which there are increased levels of thyroid hormones in the blood and has a prevalence in the UK of approximately 27 per 1000 women and 2.3 per 1000 men.[53] Although Graves' disease is the most common cause of hyperthyroidism (thyrotoxicosis), other causes require consideration (Table 2.2). Graves' disease (diffuse toxic goitre) is an immunological disorder in which thyroid stimulating antibodies (TsAb) of the IgG type bind to the TSH receptor and stimulate the thyroid cell to produce and secrete an excess of thyroid hormones. HLA studies demonstrate that those positive for HLA B8 and HLA DW3 have an increased susceptibility to the disease. The thyroid gland hypertrophies producing diffuse enlargement although nodular varieties of the condition are recognised. An important subgroup is that of internodular hyperplasia in a background of multinodular goitre. Histologically there is acinar hyperplasia, high columnar epithelium, increased vascularity and frequently lymphoid infiltration.

Table 2.2 *Causes of thyrotoxicosis*

Common	Diffuse toxic goitre (Graves' disease)
	Toxic multinodular goitre (Plummer's disease)
	Toxic solitary nodule
	Toxic multinodular goitre with internodular hyperplasia
	Nodular goitre with hyperthyroidism due to exogenous iodine
	Exogenous thyroid hormone excess (factitious)
	Thyroiditis (subacute and autoimmune) – transient
Rare	Diffuse thyroid autonomy
	Metastatic thyroid carcinoma
	Struma ovarii
	Pituitary tumour secreting thyroid stimulating hormone
	Choriocarcinoma and hydatidiform mole
	Neonatal thyrotoxicosis
	Post partum hyperthyroidism
	Following ^{131}I therapy

Clinical features (Table 2.3)

Most of the symptoms and signs of thyrotoxicosis result from excess thyroid hormones stimulating metabolism, heat production and oxygen consumption. Cardiac features are caused by β adrenergic sympathetic activity. Although Graves' disease can occur at any age it is especially common in young woman between 20 and 40. The onset

Table 2.3 Clinical features of thyrotoxicosis

Palpitations, tachycardia, cardiac arrhythmias, cardiac failure
Sweating
Tremor
Hyperkinetic movements
Nervousness
Myopathy
Tiredness and lethargy
Weight loss (occasional weight gain due to increased appetite)
Heat intolerance
Diarrhoea
Vomiting
Irritability
Emotional disturbance
Behavioural abnormalities
Ophthalmic signs
Irregular menstruation and amenorrhoea
Pretibial myxoedema
Thyroid acropathy
Vitiligo
Alopecia

---

may be gradual or abrupt with an extremely variable subsequent course often characterised by exacerbations and remissions. Clinical features due to hypermetabolism tend to predominate although in the elderly the cardiovascular and neurological features are usually prominent. Hyperthyroidism can be severe and fatal. In children the condition often causes growth abnormalities.

The immunological changes in Graves' disease are complex and undoubtedly cause many of the ophthalmic symptoms and signs, but the precise mechanisms are yet to be determined. Ophthalmopathy has two major components:

1. Non-infiltrative ophthalmopathy resulting from increased sympathetic activity leading to upper lid retraction, a stare and infrequent blinking.
2. Infiltrative ophthalmopathy causing oedema of the orbital contents, lids and periorbital tissues, cellular infiltration and deposition of mucopolysaccharide material within the orbit. Although the ophthalmopathy is usually bilateral it may affect only one eye. Diplopia particularly on upward outward gaze results from weakening and paralysis of the external ocular muscles. The cornea is vulnerable to damage and ulceration may occur. Papilloedema, retinal haemorrhage and optic nerve damage (malignant exophthalmos) can progress to blindness.

Investigation

Measurement of free T4, T3 and TSH will confirm the diagnosis (in T3 toxicosis T4 levels will be normal but T3 raised and TSH suppressed). A radioactive iodine or technetium scan is not essential in patients with Graves' disease although it is necessary in the assessment of toxic solitary and multinodular goitre to determine the site of nodular overactivity. Radioactive iodine uptake studies are particularly appropriate when a diagnosis of thyroiditis or factitious hyperthyroidism is being considered.

In Graves' disease three treatment modalities can be used either alone or in combination to restore the euthyroid state:

- Antithyroid drugs
- Radioactive iodine
- Surgery

Each treatment has an important role but medical, personal and social factors should be considered and a particular treatment plan individualised for each patient.

Medical treatment

Antithyroid drugs (propylthiouracil, carbimazole and methimazole)

These drugs interfere with the incorporation of iodine into tyrosine residues and prevent the intrathyroglobulin coupling of iodotyrosines into iodothyronines. Carbimazole may also have some immunosuppressive action on TsAb production as well as its immediate biochemical effects. Medical treatment with thionamides has two principal roles:

1. Treatment of newly diagnosed patients with Graves' disease in the hope of inducing a permanent remission;
2. To render the toxic patient euthyroid in preparation for surgery.

Although most patients can be rendered euthyroid with antithyroid drugs there is unfortunately a less than optimum remission rate after an 'adequate' course of medication. A relapse rate of approximately 43% is seen in the first year after cessation of drugs and approximately 20% of the remaining patients relapse in each of the subsequent five years.[54] Antithyroid drugs are therefore only a satisfactory long-term solution to the problems of hyperthyroidism for less than 50% of patients overall. Carbimazole is prescribed in a dose of 10–15 mg eight hourly reducing to 5 mg eight hourly once the euthyroid state has been achieved. Iatrogenic hypothyroidism may be prevented by the administration of a small dose of thyroxine in a so-called blocking/replacement regimen. Patients must be monitored carefully with regular clinical assessment and measurement of thyroid function tests. All patients are warned concerning side effects, particularly those relating to effects on the bone marrow resulting in leucopenia, agranulocytosis and aplastic anaemia. Instructions are given to discontinue carbimazole and seek medical advice immediately should buccal ulceration or a sore throat develop. Other side effects include rashes, pruritis, arthritis and nausea.

Propylthiouracil is more widely used in the USA and can be used effectively if mild side effects have occurred with carbimazole. The other major indication for administration of antithyroid drugs is to render the patient euthyroid once a decision has been made to proceed with surgery.

β-adrenergic blockers
Many of the manifestations of hyperthyroidism, particularly those relating to the cardiovascular system, can be ameliorated by the administration of beta blockers such as propranolol. This agent also reduces peripheral conversion of T4 into T3. Beta blockers are usually used in combination with one of the thionamides particularly in patients who are severely toxic and in those patients being prepared for surgery. The usual dose of propranolol is 20–40 mg eight hourly. New long-acting beta blockers can be administered once daily. Beta blockers are absolutely contraindicated in patients with asthma. When used as a preoperative preparation propranolol must not be omitted on the morning of surgery and must be continued for 5 days postoperatively because of the 8 day half-life of circulating thyroxine.

Radioactive iodine
[131]I used to control thyrotoxicosis achieves its effect by destruction of overactive thyroid tissue. There would appear to be no adverse effects of ^{131}I treatment with respect to leukaemia, thyroid carcinoma, fetal damage or genetic mutation and in the USA the therapy is given to children. [131]I (555 MBq) is administered as an ablative dose and the patient is given carbimazole 10 mg tds started 3 days after the administration and continued for approximately 1 month in order to counter the effects of thyroid hormone release which might precipitate a thyroid crisis. Although some patients require additional doses of ^{131}I, as a result of an inadequate response to the first, the majority of patients will be cured of toxicity. An ablative dose (555 MBq) will render more than 60% of patients hypothyroid in one year.[55] Regular long-term surveillance is required and thyroxine replacement given as necessary.

Surgery

Thyroidectomy in patients with Graves' disease is safe and rapidly renders the patient euthyroid. The principal indications for surgery are:

- Relapse after an adequate course of antithyroid drugs;
- Severe thyrotoxicosis with a large goitre;
- Difficulty in controlling toxicity with antithyroid drugs;
- High T4 levels (T4 > 70 pmol l^{-1}).

Surgery would be offered to the majority of patients under 40 years of age fulfilling the above criteria.

Operative strategy

Details of thyroidectomy are covered in the section dealing specifically with surgical technique but essentially the procedure is one of bilateral subtotal thyroidectomy leaving a 3–4 g posterior remnant of thyroid tissue on each side of the trachea. When there is a very small goitre (less than 20 g) much smaller remnants should be left.

Special circumstances in Graves' disease

Children

Treatment should be started with antithyroid drugs and continued for up to 2 years. When treatment is discontinued relapse may occur in up to 50% of patients. These children are usually candidates for surgery and the resection must be more radical than in adults because remnant growth and recurrent hyperthyroidism are more likely.

Pregnancy

Radioactive iodine is absolutely contraindicated. Antithyroid drugs are used, propylthiouracil being the drug of choice as it crosses the placenta less readily than carbimazole. Once control of thyrotoxicosis has been achieved the dose of antithyroid drugs should be reduced as far as possible and the thyroid status of the mother carefully measured. A blocking/replacement regimen must not be used as thyroxine does not cross the placenta in sufficient amounts to avoid fetal hypothyroidism. In a patient still requiring high doses of antithyroid drugs or difficult to control, surgery may be safely performed in the second trimester.

Recurrent hyperthyroidism after surgery

Further surgery is not indicated as it is likely to be unsuccessful and carries a significant risk of damage to recurrent laryngeal nerves and parathyroid glands. Over the age of 40 ^{131}I is the treatment of choice whereas under 40 years of age antithyroid drugs are prescribed in the hope of achieving lasting remission.

Neonatal hyperthyroidism

TsAbs crossing the placenta may stimulate the fetal thyroid to produce a transient hyperthyroidism. Active supportive treatment with antithyroid drugs is necessary and the whole process is usually self-limiting within a period of one to two months.

Ophthalmic Graves' disease

The effect of surgery on this condition is somewhat unpredictable although in the past total thyroidectomy has been advocated in an attempt to arrest the progress of the eye disease. Patients must be warned that effective treatment of the thyrotoxicosis is not a guarantee that ophthalmopathy will regress. Mild symptoms can be treated by the administration of methyl cellulose eye drops but more severe disease may require steroids, lateral tarsorrhaphy or even orbital decompression.

Toxic multinodular goitre

Antithyroid drugs are of no value as a long-term treatment because thyrotoxicity is due to autonomy and will recur once any medication is discontinued. [131]I can be used for small goitres but usually a subtotal thyroidectomy is most appropriate after achievement of the euthyroid state.

Toxic solitary nodule

This condition caused by a single autonomous thyroid nodule can be treated by either a unilateral thyroid lobectomy or [131]I.

Follow-up

Because of the risk of developing postoperative hypothyroidism patients who have undergone any form of treatment for hyperthyroidism must be followed on a long-term basis with regular clinical and biochemical assessment.

Thyroiditis

The thyroid gland may be subject to inflammatory change in a variety of conditions, the process being either focal or diffuse and often associated with thyroid dysfunction.

Subacute thyroiditis

This condition, often called granulomatous or de Quervain's thyroiditis is probably of viral origin. It is characterised by painful swelling of one or both thyroid lobes with associated malaise and fever. Frequently there is a preceding history of sore throat or viral infection a week or two before the onset of thyroid symptoms. Approximately one third of patients are asymptomatic apart from enlargement of the thyroid gland but 10–15% have a more acute illness with symptoms and signs of hyperthyroidism resulting from loss of thyroid hormones from the damaged, inflamed thyroid. Thyroid hormone levels are raised but in contrast to Graves' disease there is low uptake of radioactive iodine on scintigraphy. The ESR is invariably raised. The disease process of subacute thyroiditis is usually self-limiting with resolution of local symptoms and thyroid dysfunction. A few patients, however, pass through a mild hypothyroid phase.

Local symptoms can be controlled with aspirin but if severe and prolonged a course of steroids can be helpful. The transient hyperthyroidism does not require treatment with antithyroid drugs.

Autoimmune thyroiditis

Focal thyroiditis is often seen in association with other thyroid disease particularly Graves' hyperthyroidism and is a not infrequent finding in autopsy studies. A condition of lymphomatous thyroiditis was described by Hashimoto and occurs as a diffuse process throughout the thyroid gland which usually enlarges to several times normal size. Although classically the gland enlargement is diffuse there may be nodularity and lobulation making the distinction from simple multinodular goitre or even malignant disease difficult. Histologically there is infiltration of the thyroid by lymphocytes and plasma cells, frequently secondary lymphoid nodules and adjacent stromal fibrosis. The condition is due to an immunological disorder characterised by thyroid antibodies (antithyroglobulin and antimicrosomal (TPO)) in the serum. A positive family history of other autoimmune disease such as pernicious anaemia, gastritis, vitiligo, diabetes mellitus, Addison's disease, autoimmune liver disease and thyrotoxicosis is frequently obtained.[56] As a result of destructive changes within the infiltrated thyroid, hypothyroidism usually ensues and when present requires treatment with thyroxine. This medication suppresses TSH and leads to shrinkage of the thyroid gland with relief of any local symptoms. Surgery is not usually required since pressure symptoms and involvement of adjacent structures occurs rarely. Occasionally a satisfactory reduction in the size of the goitre can be achieved by the administration of steroids. The risk of developing lymphoma of the thyroid, although small, is increased several times in the presence of Hashimoto's thyroiditis.[46] When the thyroid, involved with autoimmune disease, is seen to rapidly enlarge or develop a firm asymmetrical nodular area exclusion of lymphoma by FNAC or core biopsy is required.

Riedel's thyroiditis

This condition, sometimes called invasive fibrous thyroiditis, is characterised by a dense fibrous inflammatory infiltrate throughout the thyroid, sometimes extending through the capsule to involve adjacent structures. The condition is rare but is important because the clinical picture mimics thyroid malignancy. Sclerosing cholangitis, retroperitoneal, mediastinal and retro-orbital fibrosis may co-exist. Needle biopsy is likely to be uninformative and often an open incision biopsy is required to establish a precise diagnosis. Surgical resection of the isthmus may be required to free a compromised airway. Steroid medication has been tried without much success and recently there have been reports of benefit from tamoxifen.[57]

Acute suppurative thyroiditis

The thyroid can be infected by a variety of bacterial or fungal agents producing clinical features of an acute painfully inflamed gland. Confirmation of diagnosis and bacteriology is obtained by needle aspiration and appropriate antibiotics administered. The condition is rare in Western practice.

Postpartum thyroiditis[58]

This condition is now recognised much more frequently and is characterised by an early thyrotoxic phase usually with mild symptoms and transient dysfunction.[59] There is a later hypothyroid phase sometimes requiring treatment with thyroxine, long-term hypothyroidism occurring in up to 25% of patients.

Developmental abnormalities of the thyroid

Thyroglossal cyst

This condition results from persistence of part of the thyroglossal duct and is usually found as a midline cyst (occasionally more laterally) just below the hyoid bone or above the thyroid cartilage. Less commonly the cyst is found at a higher level above the hyoid bone. The essential diagnostic feature is that of upward movement on swallowing and because of the attachment of the thyroglossal tract to the foramen caecum the cyst rises on protrusion of the tongue. These cysts are prone to infection and should be excised. The most appropriate and successful operation is the Sistrunk's procedure with excision of the central portion of the hyoid bone. Malignancy usually of a papillary type, can occur within the thyroglossal cyst as a primary phenomenon.[60]

Thyroglossal fistula

This results from infection or inadequate removal of a thyroglossal cyst, the opening being found at a lower level in the neck than the original cyst. Complete excision of the fistula is achieved by careful tracing of the tract superiorly forwards to the foramen caecum with excision of the central portion of the hyoid bone.

Lingual thyroid

When the thyroid gland fails to descend it may be found in the back of the tongue close to the foramen caecum. If large it can result in respiratory or swallowing difficulties and haemorrhage. Diagnosis is confirmed by radioactive iodine scanning and treatment with thyroxine or radioactive iodine should result in shrinkage of the gland without the need to resort to surgery.

Ectopic thyroid

Arrested descent of the thyroid will result in the gland being found at any point along the line of the thyroglossal tract and in these circumstances may be the only thyroid tissue present. If excision is carried out full replacement thyroxine dosage is required.

Hypo-thyroidism

Hypothyroidism is a hypometabolic state resulting from insufficient thyroid hormone or a resistance of the tissues to thyroxine. Causes can be classified as congenital to which the term cretinism is usually applied and acquired (adult type). Retardation of growth and mental development are the serious features of hypothyroidism in the infant. The child fails to thrive, is constipated and displays the classical physical signs of a puffy face, large tongue and protuberant abdomen. In the adult type the extreme presentation is that of myxoedema characterised by weight gain, facial puffiness and pallor, dry skin, hair loss, hoarseness of the voice, declining intellect and in extreme cases psychiatric disturbance and even coma.

The causes of hypothyroidism are given in Table 2.4.

The diagnosis of primary hypothyroidism is confirmed by measurement of low free T4 and T3 levels and high TSH levels. Treatment is by thyroxine starting cautiously in myxoedematous and elderly patients who may already be suffering from heart disease, with a low dose (0.025 mg) increasing gradually over a period of two to three months to a full replacement level.

Table 2.4 *Causes of hypothyroidism*

Primary hypothyroidism
Thyroid agenesis
Disorders of thyroid hormone synthesis
Iodine deficiency
Dyshormonogenesis
Antithyroid drugs
Thyroid gland damage
Hashimoto's thyroiditis
Surgical resection of the thyroid
Radioactive iodine ablation
Postsubacute thyroiditis
Secondary hypothyroidism (pituitary)
Pituitary tumour
Autoimmune hypophysitis
Tertiary hypothyroidism (hypothalamic)
Hypothalamic tumour
Generalised or peripheral thyroid hormone resistance

Thyroidectomy The term 'thyroidectomy' embraces a variety of surgical procedures on the thyroid, the precise operation being tailored according to the existing pathology (Table 2.5).

Technique of unilateral total thyroid lobectomy

After obtaining informed consent from the patient the preoperative preparation should include examination of the vocal cords by indirect laryngoscopy to exclude an unsuspected pre-existing unilateral nerve palsy; this being particularly important if the patient has undergone previous thyroid surgery.

General anaesthesia with endotracheal intubation and muscle relaxation is used and the patient is placed supine on an operating table tilted 15 degrees upwards at the head end in order to reduce venous engorgement. Neck extension and access to the thyroid are facilitated by the placing of a sand bag pillow in the interscapular region. The head must be well supported and care taken, particularly in the elderly, not to overextend the neck.

A curved skin incision is placed 3–4 cm above the sternal notch extending laterally to the sternomastoid muscles. The incision is deepened through the platysma and upper and lower skin flaps are raised by a combination of sharp and blunt dissection in the plane anterior to the anterior jugular veins. The upper flap is freed to the level of the thyroid notch and the lower to the suprasternal notch. These skin flaps are held apart with two wishbone self-retaining retractors and a midline incision made through the fascia over the thyroid. It is the length of this vertical incision which determines access to the thyroid. The strap muscles will be separated, dissected from the thyroid and

Table 2.5 *Thyroid surgery*

Procedures	Indications
Unilateral total lobectomy including pyramidal lobe and isthmus	Solitary nodules Unilateral multinodular disease
Bilateral subtotal thyroidectomy (unilateral lobectomy and contralateral resection)	Diffuse toxic goitre of Graves' disease Bilateral non-toxic and toxic multinodular goitre Hashimoto's thyroiditis
Total thyroidectomy	Most cases of papillary, follicular and medullary carcinoma
Excision of isthmus	May be only procedure possible in anaplastic carcinoma or lymphoma to free airway. Riedel's thyroiditis

retracted laterally. These muscles are not divided routinely but can be if greater exposure is required to gain safer access to a large or vascular goitre.

The thyroid lobe is dislocated and delivered forward by the insertion of the index finger between the thyroid lobe and strap muscles. The middle thyroid veins, if apparent at this stage, should be ligated and divided. Any adhesions lateral to the thyroid lobe are divided by a combination of sharp and blunt dissection and the thyroid lobe retracted further medially usually with a gauze swab between the operator's thumb and the gland. Tissue forceps must not be placed on the thyroid when performing surgery for a solitary nodule, in case the lesion should prove to be malignant and cell spillage occur.

Full mobilisation of the thyroid lobe is then achieved by ligation and division of the superior thyroid vessels at the upper pole. To gain access to these vessels it is often helpful to pass a finger upwards in the plane behind the vessels, breaking down adhesions, and then with gentle downward traction on the thyroid the vessels come clearly into view. The space medial to the superior thyroid artery is carefully opened with a pledget or artery forceps to expose the external branch of the superior laryngeal nerve (ESLN) which is usually easily identified on the inferior pharyngeal constrictor before entering the cricothyroid muscle. A non-toothed forcep is then passed under the vascular pedicle to lift the vessels forward. The branches of the superior thyroid artery and vein must be individually tied close to the thyroid gland in order to avoid damage to the ESLN. In approximately 20% of patients this nerve may pass between the

Figure 2.3
(a) The external superior laryngeal nerve (ESLN) passing medial to the superior thyroid artery before entering the cricothyroid muscle. (b) The ESLN is in a vulnerable position when passing between branches of superior thyroid artery.

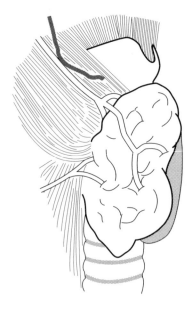

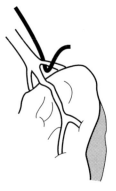

(a)

(b)

Figure 2.4
Recurrent laryngeal nerve held in a vulnerable anterior position by fork of inferior thyroid artery branches.

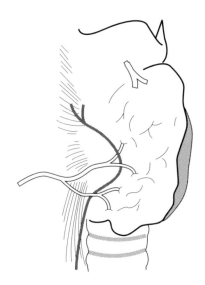

branches of the vessels and is in danger if mass ligation is carried out (Fig 2.3). In a further 20% of patients the nerve runs its distal course through the inferior pharyngeal constrictor muscle, is not visible at surgery and indeed is at no risk of damage.

The recurrent laryngeal nerve (RLN) should now be identified before further dissection of the thyroid lobe takes place. The nerve may run close to the tracheo-oesophageal groove but there is enormous variability of its position, course and relationship to key anatomical structures in the neck. If damage is to be avoided an accurate knowledge of the normal anatomy and these variations is of paramount importance. Palpation of the RLN as a cord-like structure against the trachea is frequently a useful initial guide to the nerve's location. The nerve can then be exposed by gentle dissection of the overlying fascial layers with a small artery clip. It often has a small blood vessel running on its surface. Vulnerability is somewhat greater on the right than the left because of the obliquity of the nerve's course. The nerve usually lies deep to the inferior thyroid artery but can be vulnerable by anterior fixation by the glandular branches of this artery (Fig. 2.4). Precise definition of the nerve/artery relationship is most important. A potential pitfall for the unwary exists when the recurrent laryngeal nerve passes superficial to the inferior thyroid artery, appears to pulsate, and may therefore be mistaken for a vessel and ligated.

It can be displaced from its usual position by nodules, particularly in the posterior part of the thyroid lobe and occasionally is displaced anteriorly close to the lower pole of the thyroid into a dangerous position where it may be ligated and divided with the inferior thyroid veins. Clearly these veins must not be clipped until the nerve has been identified in its lower third. In the operation of unilateral lobectomy the small arterial branches to the thyroid must all be individually

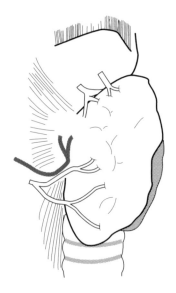

Figure 2.5 *Non-recurrent laryngeal nerve passing in close proximity to the inferior thyroid artery before ascending to the larynx.*

clipped and tied close to the gland staying on the thyroid capsule. The main inferior thyroid artery trunk is not ligated.

The nerve is at most risk close to its point of entry into the larynx as it passes through Berry's ligament, often adopting a curving looping course before entering the larynx. To identify the nerve in this region the suspensory fascia must be carefully divided, staying close to the thyroid and picking up superficial layers one at a time with fine haemostats, being absolutely certain, at each stage, that only fascia and small arterial branches are included. The nerve is soon seen at a deeper level glistening with its fine accompanying arterial blood vessel aiding identification. The inferior cornu of the thyroid cartilage is a most dependable land mark for the point of entry of the RLN into the larynx.

In approximately 1% of patients the nerve is non-recurrent on the right side of the neck arising from the vagus and passing medially close to the inferior thyroid artery before turning to ascend and enter the larynx (Fig. 2.5). Ligation of the main trunk of the inferior thyroid artery in these circumstances could obviously result in permanent damage to the nerve. It is well recognised that the RLN can divide into several branches before entering the larynx and therefore clear identification of all divisions is necessary for their preservation.

The parathyroid glands must now be identified and when they are in their usual positions, the inferior gland can be located close to the lower pole of the thyroid anterior to the recurrent laryngeal nerve. The superior gland is usually seen just above the inferior thyroid artery, in more than 90% of patients being within a 1 cm radius of the junction of the inferior thyroid artery and the recurrent laryngeal nerve. The dissection of the thyroid should continue close to the capsule of the gland with ligation and division of the individual branches of the inferior thyroid artery, preserving those branches which supply the parathyroid glands. It is possible to tease the parathyroid glands away from the thyroid with their blood supply intact, leaving them free but viable. Enlargement of the thyroid can carry the parathyroid glands far forward onto the anterolateral surface of the gland and they may then be devascularised or inadvertently excised. In these circumstances they should be diced into 1 mm cubes and autotransplanted into several pockets in the sternomastoid muscle.

It is important to keep diathermy usage to a minimum as heat conduction may damage the recurrent laryngeal nerve, the blood supply to the parathyroids or the delicate joints within the larynx.

The thyroid lobe is now almost completely free and is dissected further medially by dividing the vascular fascia binding it to the trachea and larynx. The division of Berry's ligament is completed, taking care to re-identify the recurrent laryngeal nerve. Small vessels close to the nerve at this point require careful clipping and ligation otherwise troublesome bleeding may obscure the nerve's entry point to the larynx. Safe thyroidectomy is dependent on careful haemostasis as it is only by this discipline that the recurrent nerve and parathyroid glands can be identified and left undamaged.

The thyroid lobe mobilisation is now complete and the resection must include the isthmus and pyramidal lobe. The cut surface of the contralateral thyroid lobe is usually oversewn to obtain haemostasis.

The sand bag pillow is removed from under the patient's interscapular area and the neck space re-examined for bleeding. The wound is closed in layers with absorbable material to the muscle layers and the skin is closed with a subcuticular prolene suture or skin clips which can be removed at three days.

Total thyroidectomy

In total thyroidectomy, usually performed for cancer but occasionally for gross multinodular disease, the opposite thyroid lobe will also be mobilised in a similar manner to that described for unilateral lobectomy with identification of recurrent laryngeal nerve, external branch of superior laryngeal nerve and both parathyroid glands. If the procedure is for cancer an appropriate lymph node clearance will also be necessary.

Subtotal thyroidectomy

When subtotal thyroidectomy is performed, perhaps for Graves' disease, the principles of identification of the vital structures are exactly the same as those employed in a unilateral total lobectomy. In Graves' disease a small remnant, usually 3–4 g, of tissue is left *in situ* on each side of the trachea and haemostasis secured by oversewing the lateral edge of each remnant. As in unilateral lobectomy the main trunk of the inferior thyroid artery is not ligated but individual small bleeding vessels on the surface of the remnant may require ligation. Unilateral total lobectomy and a contralateral resection leaving a larger single remnant may be an acceptable alternative strategy.

Retrosternal goitre

In retrosternal goitre, the blood supply to the thyroid derived from the superior and inferior thyroid arteries, is usually accessible in the neck. Ligation and division of the superior pole vessels is an essential, preliminary step before mobilisation of the gland is attempted. The retrosternal portion can then be delivered from behind the sternum by gentle traction aided by the introduction of a finger alongside the gland. Placement of traction sutures in the thyroid or the gentle introduction of a desert spoon alongside the gland may also facilitate delivery. Median sternotomy is rarely necessary to remove a retrosternal thyroid.

Recurrent goitre

Surgery for recurrent thyroid disease is particularly hazardous with respect to recurrent laryngeal nerve and parathyroid gland damage as identification of these structures is likely to be impeded by the presence of scar tissue. A lateral approach to the thyroid lobe to be resected can be gained by dissecting in the plane between the strap muscles and the anterior border of the sternomastoid where there may be fewer adhesions.

Complications of thyroidectomy

The most important complications of thyroidectomy are shown in Table 2.6. Those complications relating to damaged individual struc-

Table 2.6 *Complications of thyroid surgery*

Recurrent laryngeal nerve injury
External superior laryngeal nerve injury
Hypoparathyroidism
Laryngeal oedema – airway obstruction
Bleeding – haematoma
Hypothyroidism
Hyperthyroidism
Wound infection
Keloid
Suture granuloma

tures can be kept to a minimum by operating in a bloodless field and performing a meticulous anatomical dissection.

Recurrent laryngeal nerve

Damage to the recurrent laryngeal nerve should be extremely rare following routine thyroidectomy[61] although the risk of damage is increased when performing re-operative thyroid surgery.[62] Identification of the recurrent laryngeal nerve at surgery is the fundamental step to avoiding damage. When this policy is employed any nerve damage is likely to be a transient neuropraxia and recovery will occur after a few weeks or months. If the nerve has not been identified then paralysis will be permanent in up to one third of nerves injured. Extremely low nerve injury rates have been reported even when performing extensive surgery for thyroid cancer.[63]

External branch of superior laryngeal nerve

Assessment of damage to the external superior laryngeal nerve (ESLN) is difficult as the changes may be subtle and easily overlooked. Disability results in changes of voice pitch, range, fatiguability and particularly affects the quality of the singing voice. The nerve is most likely to be damaged at the time of ligation and division of the superior thyroid vessels.[64] To avoid this complication the arterial branches should be individually ligated close to the thyroid and the nerve identified whenever possible.

Hypoparathyroidism

This complication can be avoided by careful identification of the parathyroid glands and preservation of their delicate arterial blood supply. In bilateral subtotal resection for Graves' disease the incidence of hypoparathyroidism should be no more than 0.5%. The complication is more frequent after total thyroidectomy for cancer but even in these circumstances the incidence has been reported within the range of only 1–3%.[63]

Hypothyroidism

This sequal of thyroidectomy is inevitable after major resections and occurs in Graves' disease at an incidence of about 50%. This is not a true complication but an acceptable feature of the treatment of hyperthyroidism and is easily managed by the administration of thyroxine.

Recurrent hyperthyroidism

If this occurs after surgery for Graves' disease it represents a failure of the operation. The incidence is approximately 5% and will vary depending on the size of the thyroid remnants left *in situ*, be influenced by the complex immunological processes taking place in primary hyperthyroidism and may also be related to iodine intake.

Thyroid crisis

This potentially life-threatening condition is rarely seen but classically occurs in the postoperative period in a patient who has undergone surgery without adequate preoperative preparation. Hormones released by gland manipulation result in an acute postoperative thyrotoxicosis. The condition may also result from stress of infection or other unrelated surgery in the untreated, undiagnosed thyrotoxic patient. The clinical picture is one of;

- Extreme distress
- Dyspnoea
- Tachycardia
- Hyperpyrexia
- Restlessness
- Confusion
- Delirium
- Vomiting
- Diarrhoea

Propylthiouracil (200–250 mg) is given every 4 h, by nasogastric tube if necessary and Lugol's iodine 0.3 ml p.o. eight hourly or sodium iodide 1.5 g i.v. over 24 h should be given commencing an hour later. Adrenergic effects are treated by careful administration of propranolol 1–2 mg i.v. under ECG-monitored control. General supportive measures consist of rehydration with intravenous fluids, cooling with ice packs, the administration of oxygen, digoxin if there is evidence of cardiac failure, appropriate sedation and corticosteroids.

Haemorrhage

Bleeding into the wound is a serious complication of thyroidectomy. When the bleeding and haematoma occur deep to the strap muscles the situation can rapidly develop into a life-threatening emergency because of associated airway obstruction resulting from laryngeal and subglottic oedema.

Airway obstruction

Although mortality from thyroidectomy is extremely rare today airway obstruction remains the most potentially dangerous of the complications. It was once thought that airway obstruction caused by postoperative bleeding was due to compression of the trachea by the expanding haematoma. This is unlikely to be the case except in the rare condition of tracheomalacia. Subglottic and laryngeal mucosal oedema consequent upon venous and lymphatic obstruction occludes the airway from within. It must be appreciated that airway obstruction can occur by this mechanism as a result of operative manipulation of the trachea without any postoperative bleeding or haematoma deep to the strap muscles. It is crucial that early signs of airway obstruction (patient distress and stridor) should be recognised and immediate action taken. If symptoms are mild and there is no haematoma, conservative measures of humidified oxygen and intravenous steroids may suffice. An anaesthetist must be consulted immediately because intubation may subsequently prove necessary to restore an occluding airway. If a skilled anaesthetist is not immediately available the situation can be retrieved by insertion of a Medicut 12 (blue) needle percutaneously directly into the trachea. Any obvious haematoma should be evacuated and this should ideally be performed under general anaesthesia with endotracheal intubation in the operating room. Rarely is it necessary to remove sutures on the ward.

Wound complications
The use of absorbable suture material has virtually abolished the complication of suture granuloma following thyroidectomy. Keloid scars may still occur in susceptible individuals.

References

1. Beever K, Bradbury J, Phillips D et al. Highly sensitive assays of autoantibodies to thyroglobulin and to thyroid peroxidase. Clin Chem 1989; 35: 1949–54.
2. van Herle AJ, Uller RP. Elevated serum thyroglobulin: a marker of metastases in differentiated thyroid carcinoma. J Clin Invest 1975; 56: 270–7.
3. Doullay F, Ruf J, Codaccioni JL, Carayon P. Prevalence of autoantibodies to thyroperoxidase in patients with various thyroid and autoimmune diseases. Autoimmunity 1991; 9: 237–44.
4. Rees-Smith B, McLachlan SM, Furmaniak J. Autoantibodies to the thyrotropin receptor. Endocr Rev 1988; 9: 106–21.
5. Melvin KEW, Tashjian AH. The syndrome of excessive thyrocalcitonin produced by medullary carcinoma of the thyroid. Proc Nat Acad Sci USA 1968; 59: 1216–22.
6. Mulligan LM, Kwok JBJ, Healey CS et al. Germ-line mutations of the RET proto oncogene in multiple endocrine neoplasia type IIA. Nature 1993; 363: 458–60.
7. Turner JW, Spencer RB. Thyroid carcinoma presenting as a pertechnetate hot nodule without ^{131}I uptake. Case report. J Nucl Med 1976; 17: 22–3.
8. Ochi H, Yamamoto K, Endo K et al. A new imaging agent for medullary carcinoma of the thyroid. J Nucl Med 1984; 25: 323–5.
9. Hoefnagal CA, Delprat CC, Marcuse HR, Vijlder JMM. Role of thallium-201 total-body scintigraphy in follow up of thyroid carcinoma. J Nucl Med 1986; 27: 1854–7.
10. Clarke SEM, Lazarus CR, Wraight P et al. Pentavalant (99mTc) DMSA, ^{131}I MIBG, and (99mTc) MDP. An evaluation of three imaging techniques in patients with medullary carcinoma of the thyroid. J Nucl Med 1988; 29: 33–8.
11. Rosen IB, Walfish PG, Miskin M. The ultrasound of thyroid masses. Surg Clin North Am 1979; 59: 19–33.
12. Rosen IB, Wallace D, Strawbridge HG, Walfish PG. Re-evaluation of needle aspiration cytology in detection of thyroid cancer. Surgery 1981; 90: 747–56.
13. Miller JH. Needle biopsy of the thyroid: methods and recommendations. Thyroid Today 1982; 5: 1–5.
14. Soderstrom N. Aspiration biopsy punctures of goitres for aspiration and biopsy. Acta Med Scand 1952; 144: 237–44.
15. Lowhagen T, Granberg PO, Lundell G et al. Aspiration biopsy cytology (ABC) in nodules of the thyroid gland suspected to be malignant. Surg Clin North Am 1979; 59: 3–18.
16. Grant CS, Hay ID, Gough IR et al. Long term follow up of patients with benign thyroid FNA cytologic diagnosis. Surgery 1989; 106: 980–91.
17. Gaitin E, Nelson NC, Poole GV. Endemic goitre and endemic thyroid disorders. World

J Surg 1991; 15: 205–15.

18. Gaitin E. Aetiology of benign thyroid disease – environmental aspects. In Wheeler MH, Lazarus JH (eds) Diseases of the thyroid. Pathophysiology and management. London: Chapman & Hall Medical, 1994, pp. 73–84.

19. Vander JB, Gaston EA, Dawber TR. The significance of non toxic thyroid nodules: Final report of a 15 year study of the incidence of thyroid malignancy. Ann Intern Med 1968; 69: 537–40.

20. Hellwig CA. Thyroid gland in Kansas. Am J Clin Pathol 1935; 5: 103–11.

21. Hayles AB, Johnson LM, Beahrs OH, Woolner LL. Carcinoma of the thyroid in children. Am J Surg 1963; 106: 735–43.

22. Harness JK, Thompson NW, Nishiyama RH. Childhood thyroid carcinoma. Arch Surg 1971; 102: 278–84.

23. Cuello C, Correa P, Eisenberg H. Geographic pathology of thyroid carcinoma. Cancer 1969; 23: 230–9.

24. Williams ED, Doniach I, Bjarnason O, Michie W. Thyroid cancer in an iodine rich area: a histopathological study. Cancer 1977; 39: 215–22.

25. Duffy BJ, Fitzgerald PJ. Cancer of the thyroid in children: a report of 28 cases. J Clin Endocrinol Metab 1950; 10: 1296–308.

26. De Groot LJ, Paloyan E. Thyroid carcinoma and radiation: a Chicago endemic. JAMA 1973; 225: 487–91.

27. Naunheim KS, Kaplan EL, Straus FH et al. High dose external radiation to the neck and subsequent thyroid carcinoma. In: Kaplan EL (ed.) Surgery of the thyroid and parathyroid glands. Edinburgh: Churchill Livingstone, 1983, pp. 51–62.

28. Henry JF. 1995 Personal communication.

29. Henry JF, Denizot A, Procelli A et al. Thyroperoxidase immunodetection for the diagnosis of malignancy on fine-needle aspiration of thyroid nodules. World J Surg 1994; 18: 529–34.

30. Delbridge L, Lean CL, Russell P et al. Proton magnetic resonance and human thyroid neoplasia II: Potential avoidance of surgery for benign follicular neoplasms. World J Surg 1994; 18: 512–17.

31. Reeve TS, Delbridge L, Cohen A. Total thyroidectomy: the preferred option for multinodular goitre. Ann Surg 1987; 206: 782–6.

32. Thompson NW, Nishiyama RH, Harness JK. Thyroid carcinoma. Current controversies. Curr Probl Surg 1978; 15: 1–67.

33. Thompson NW. The thyroid nodule: surgical management. In: Johnston IDA, Thompson NW (eds) Endocrine surgery. London: Butterworths, 1983, pp. 14–24.

34. Reeve TS. Operations for non medullary cancer of the thyroid gland. In: Kaplan EL (ed.) Surgery of the thyroid and parathyroid glands. Edinburgh: Churchill Livingstone, 1983, pp. 63–74.

35. Lote K, Anderson K, Nordal E, Brennhoved IO. Familial occurrence of papillary thyroid carcinoma. Cancer 1980; 46: 1291–7.

36. Pasieka JL, Thompson NW, McLeod MK et al. The incidence of bilateral well differentiated thyroid cancer found at completion thyroidectomy. World J Surg 1992; 16: 711–16.

37. McConahey WM, Hay ID, Woolner LB et al. Papillary thyroid cancer treated at the Mayo Clinic, 1946 through 1970: initial manifestations, pathologic findings, therapy and outcome. Mayo Clin Proc 1986; 61: 978–96.

38. Thompson NW. Differentiated thyroid carcinoma. In Wheeler MH, Lazarus JH (eds) Diseases of the the thyroid. Pathophysiology and management. London: Chapman & Hall, Medical, 1994, pp. 367–77.

39. Ozaki O, Ito K, Kobayashi K et al. Familial occurrence of differentiated non-medullary thyroid carcinoma. World J Surg 1988; 12: 565–71.

40. Thompson NW. Total thyroidectomy in the treatment of thyroid carcinoma. In: Endocrine surgical update. New York: Grune & Stratton, 1983, pp. 71–84.

41. Stephenson BM, Wheeler MH, Clark OH. The role of total thyroidectomy in the management of differentiated thyroid cancer. In Daly JM (ed.) Current opinion in general surgery. Philadelphia: Current Science, 1994, pp. 53–9.

42. Hay ID, Grant CS, Taylor WF, McConahey WM. Ipsilateral lobectomy versus bilateral lobe resection in papillary thyroid carcinoma: a retrospective analysis of surgical outcome using a novel prognostic scoring system. Surgery 1987; 102: 1088–95.

43. Mazzaferri EL, Young RL. Papillary thyroid carcinoma: a 10-year follow-up report of the impact of therapy in 576 patients. Am J Med 1981; 70: 511–18.

44. Vassilopoulou-Sellin R, Kline MJ, Smith TH *et al.* Pulmonary metastases in children and young adults with differentiated thyroid cancer. Cancer 1993; 71: 1348–52.

45. Backdahl M, Hamberger B, Lowhagen T, Lundell G. Anaplastic giant cell thyroid carcinoma. In: Wheeler MH, Lazarus JH (eds) Diseases of the thyroid. Pathophysiology and management. London: Chapman & Hall, 1994, pp. 379–85.

46. Sirota DK, Segal RL. Primary lymphomas of the thyroid gland. JAMA 1979; 242: 1743–6.

47. Devine RM, Edis AJ, Banks PM. Primary lymphoma of the thyroid: a review of the Mayo Clinic experience through 1978. World J Surg 1981; 5: 33.

48. Hazard JB, Hawk WA, Crile G. Medullary (solid) carcinoma of the thyroid. A clinicopathologic entity. J Clin Endocrinol Metab 1959; 19: 152–61.

49. Williams ED. Histogenesis of medullary carcinoma of the thyroid. J Clin Pathol 1966; 19: 114–18.

50. Tashjian AH, Howland BG, Melvin KEW *et al.* Immunoassay of human calcitonin: clinical measurement, relation to serum calcium and studies in patients with medullary carcinoma. N Eng J Med 1970; 283: 890–5.

51. Pyke CM, Hay ID, Goellner JR *et al.* Prognostic significance of calcitonin immunoreactivity, amyloid staining and flow cytometric DNA measurements in medullary thyroid carcinoma. Surgery 1991; 110: 967–71.

52. Sizemore GW. Medullary carcinoma of the thyroid. Semin Oncol 1987; 14: 306–14.

53. Tunbridge WMG, Evered DC, Hall R *et al.* The spectrum of thyroid disease in a community: the Whickham survey. Clin Endocrinol 1977; 7: 481–93.

54. Sheldon J, Reid DJ. Thyrotoxicosis: changing trends in treatment. Ann R Coll Surg Engl 1986; 68: 283–5.

55. Kendall-Taylor P, Keir MJ, Ross WM. Ablative radioiodine therapy for hyperthyroidism: long term follow up study. Br Med J 1984; 289: 361–3.

56. Furmaniak J, Rees-Smith B. Diagnostic tests of thyroid function and structure – thyroid antibodies. In: Wheeler MH, Lazarus JH (eds) Diseases of the thyroid. Pathophysiology and management. London: Chapman & Hall Medical, 1994, pp. 117–30.

57. Few J, Thompson NW, Angelos P, Simeonle D, Giordando T, Reeve T. Riedels Thyroiditis: Treatment with Taxoxyfen. Surg 1996; 120: 993–99.

58. Lazarus JH, Othman S. Thyroid disease in relation to pregnancy. Clin Endocrinol 1991; 34: 91–8.

59. Amino N, Miyai K, Onishi T *et al.* Transient hypothyroidism after delivery in autoimmune thyroiditis. J Clin Endocrinol Metab 1976; 2: 296–301.

60. Stephenson BM, Wheeler MH. Carcinoma of the thyroglossal duct. Aust NZ J Surg 1994; 64: 212.

61. Wade JSH. Vulnerability of the recurrent laryngeal nerves at thyroidectomy. Br J Surg 1955; 43: 164–80.

62. Beahrs OH, Vandertoll DJ. Complications of secondary thyroidectomy. Surg Gynecol Obstet 1963; 117: 535–9.

63. Clark OH. Total thyroidectomy: the treatment of choice for patients with differentiated thyroid cancer. Ann Surg 1982; 196: 361–70.

64. Lennquist S, Cahlin C, Smeds S. The superior laryngeal nerve in thyroid surgery. Surgery 1987; 102: 999–1008.

3 The adrenal glands

Anthony E. Young
W. James B. Smellie

Adrenal diseases comprise the third commonest group of illness seen by the endocrine surgeon after thyroid and parathyroid disease and as such represent less than 5% of the endocrine surgeon's operative workload. The bulk of the diagnostic preliminaries will have been undertaken by an endocrinologist or general clinician prior to referral, but the complexity of these diseases, the potential for misdiagnosis and the systemic changes that can make surgery dangerous must all be understood by the surgeon and the communication between surgeon and physician must be of high quality.

Surgical adrenal disease essentially falls into two categories.

1. Endocrinologically significant disease of the cortex and medulla, e.g. Conn's Syndrome, phaeochromocytoma;
2. Non-functioning tumours; malignant or benign including those incidentally discovered on scanning ('incidentalomas').

These categories will be considered separately, though they are not mutually exclusive. The operative procedure of adrenalectomy will be dealt with at the end of the chapter.

Adrenal physiology

The understanding of adrenal endocrine disease is only achievable when the basic physiology of the adrenal cortex and the adrenal medulla is understood (Figs 3.1–3.3). The knowledge allows a rational testing for endocrine disease and a comprehension of the mechanism of the physical effects that are seen.

The adrenal gland consists of two embryologically separate parts. The outer cortex, giving the characteristically yellow colour seen at operation, is derived from coelomic epithelium and is concerned with steroid synthesis and secretion. The inner medulla is derived from neuroectoderm and is responsible for the adrenal component of the sympathoadrenomedullary system.

Figure 3.1
Physiological pathways for the production and control of cortisol secretion.

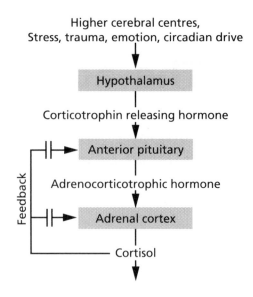

Figure 3.2
Physiological pathways for the production and control of aldosterone secretion.

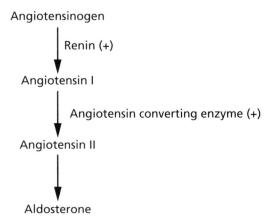

The adrenal cortex

The cortex is separated into three histological layers: the outer zona glomerulosa which produces mineralocorticoids, e.g. aldosterone; the poorly developed zona fasciculata which produces glucocorticoids, e.g. cortisol and the inner zona reticularis which produces sex steroids. The cortex also contains neuroendocrine fibres responsible for some neural control of endocrine function.

Aldosterone, the predominant mineralocorticoid, is secreted under the control of renin, via angiotensin II. It has the effect of retaining Na^+ and water and causing the loss of K^+ and H^+ from the renal tubules. In the normal adrenal, secretion of the glucocorticoids is under the direct control of ACTH (adrenocorticotrophic hormone). ACTH is secreted from the anterior pituitary gland at a rate determined by the stimulant effect of CRF (corticotrophin releasing factor) and by the

Figure 3.3
Biochemical pathways of the metabolism of adrenaline and noradrenaline.

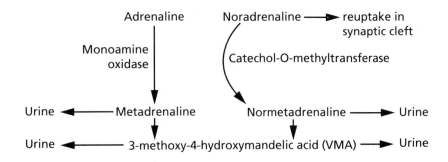

inhibitory effect of circulating natural or synthetic glucocorticoids. The rate of release of CRF from the median prominence of the hypothalamus is dependent on neural stimuli from the brain and is inhibited by glucocorticoids. Glucocorticoids have a wide range of effects on many systems of the body and absence of circulating glucocorticoid is incompatible with life. Adrenal androgen production is under the control of ACTH and possibly a pituitary adrenal androgen-stimulating hormone. The predominant androgen, dehydro-epiandrosterone, is weakly androgenic. Another weakly androgenic product, androstenedione, is aromatised outside the adrenal to oestrogen and is a significant source of oestrogen in postmenopausal women.

Adrenaline, dopamine and noradrenaline are synthesised in the adrenal medulla from common precursors. The majority of catechol-amines are synthesised from dietary tyrosine although a pathway of conversion of phenylalanine into tyrosine in the liver also exists. The tyrosine is concentrated in the neuroendocrine cells and is converted into dopamine via DOPA (dihydroxyphenalanine) in the cytoplasm. The dopamine is then transported into granulated vesicles and is converted into noradrenaline. Some neurones and adrenal medullary cells contain a further enzyme, PNMT (phenylethanol-amine-N-methyltransferase) to catalyse the conversion of noradrenaline into adrenaline. The adrenaline is then stored in storage vesicles. Adrenaline and noradrenaline are released in response to direct neural stimuli to the adrenal medulla.

Functioning adrenal abnormalities

These are in the form of benign or malignant tumours or hyperplasia. The categories are as follows.

1. Cortex
   (a) Cortical tumours; cortisone secreting tumours leading to Cushing's syndrome; aldosterone secreting tumours leading to Conn's syndrome; sex hormone secreting tumours leading to virilisation or feminisation.

(b) Diffuse hyperplasia either as a primary disease or a consequence of stimulation by trophic hormones leading to hypercortisolism (Cushing's syndrome), hyperaldosteronism (Conn's syndrome), virilisation (adrenogenital syndrome)

2. Medulla
   Tumours secreting adrenaline/noradrenaline
   (Phaeochromocytoma)

Cushing's syndrome and disease

Excess circulating cortisol leads to physiological and bodily changes described as Cushing's syndrome. The commonest cause of this is the iatrogenic administration of steroids for the treatment of other disease. This chapter will however only consider hypercortisolism caused by the following:

1. Primary adrenal disease
   (a) Adenoma
   (b) Carcinoma
   (c) Macronodular cortical hyperplasia
   (d) PPND – primary pigmented nodular adrenal cortical disease

2. Secondary adrenal disease
   (a) True Cushing's disease, i.e. the disease described by Harvey Cushing in 1932 is adrenocortical hyperplasia due to excess ACTH secretion from a pituitary microadenoma.[1]
   (b) Adrenocortical hyperplasia secondary to excess ACTH secretion from a non-pituitary source, 'Ectopic ACTH syndrome'.

The incidence of the different types varies from centre from centre depending on referral patterns, but essentially 50% of Cushing's disease is attributable to a primary adrenal source, 25% to primary pituitary disease and 25% to an ectopic source of ACTH.

Clinical presentation

The clinical presentation after iatrogenic administration of steroids is not, in most instances, gross; the patient gains weight, the cheeks become rounded and pink, the patient's appetite increases as does their sense of well-being. Slight hirsutism may be noted. Only after long-term high-dose steroid administration do the serious sequelae of muscle weakness, osteoporosis, hypertension and diabetes become problematic. By contrast primary hypercortisolism tends to declare itself late with the symptoms and signs fully developed. The inexorable slow progression of the signs can often only be appreciated when the family photograph album is produced and the current habitus compared to that seen in the past. An exception to this slow progression are the syndromes produced by an ectopic ACTH source and in cortisol secreting carcinoma when the signs appear rapidly and are severe early. The signs and symptoms of other forms of primary

Table 3.1 *Presenting symptoms and signs in 70 patients with Cushing's syndrome*

Symptoms	%	Signs	%
Weight gain	71	Obesity	95
Menstrual irregularities	84	Truncal	45
Hirsutism in women	80	Generalised	52
Lethargy/depression	48	Plethora	94
Headache	48	Facial rounding	88
Thirst/frequency	44	Hypertension	84
Backache	41	Bruising	62
Muscular weakness	27	Striae	56
Shortness of breath	26	Buffalo hump	55
Recurrent infections	26	Myopathy	55
Abdominal pain	21	Ankle oedema	47
Fractures	18	Acne	21
Loss of scalp hair	12	Osteoporosis	52

From: Ross EJ, Lynch CD.[3]

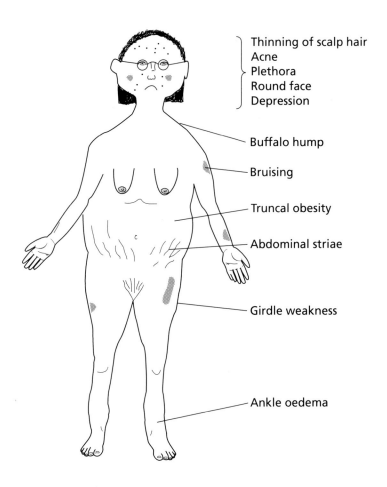

Figure 3.4 *The typical stigmata of Cushing's syndrome.*

Thinning of scalp hair
Acne
Plethora
Round face
Depression

Buffalo hump

Bruising

Truncal obesity

Abdominal striae

Girdle weakness

Ankle oedema

hypercortisolism, together with frequencies, are shown in Table 3.1. The detailed changes are complex[2,3] but the overall pattern familiar (Fig. 3.4).

Obesity
This may be gross and the patient may increase by 50% of body weight. It is predominantly truncal especially in the form of a protuberant abdomen and a 'buffalo hump' on the shoulders. The overall appearances have sometimes be likened to a 'lemon on sticks'. The wasting of the thigh and upper arm muscles and oedema of the ankles contributing to this appearance.

Loss of connective tissue
Thinning of the skin leads to a purple, plethoric face and purple, abdominal striae. The changes in the walls of venules and capillaries allow prompt bleeding in response to trauma and the lack of subcutaneous connective tissue allows spread of this haemorrhage into large, blotchy haematomas. Blood clotting is normal.

Hirsutism and virilism
In females this is not due to increased cortisol but to an increase in testosterone. This testosterone originates from excessive synthesis in the adrenal cortex and increased transformation of androstenedione or dehydroepiandrostenedione to testosterone in the periphery. The effect is an increase in the growth of hair, particularly noticeable as facial hair in females. As the disease progresses the skin becomes oily and acne is prominent. The hair becomes dishevelled and greasy and scalp hair is lost. The typical facies of the patient is one of obesity, plethora, acne, hirsutism and a receding hair-line. About 80% of premenopausal women develop menstrual disorders and many will develop amenorrhoea.

Whereas plasma testosterone is increased in women it is decreased in men as cortisol decreases not only gonadotrophin moderation but also testicular response to gonadotrophins. Men, therefore, show loss of libido, testicular atrophy and gynaecomastia.

Muscle weakness
Increased protein catabolism occurs predominately in proximal muscle groups with weakness and loss of muscle bulk. The result is a change in the contour of the body and the patient has difficulty rising from sitting and difficulty moving around.

Osteoporosis
Cortisol inhibits the development of osteoid and lowers the serum calcium, thus producing secondary hyperparathyroidism with increased reabsorption of calcium from bone. This together with proximal muscle loss frequently leads to backache and can even be severe enough to cause crush fractures of vertebrae or spontaneous fractures of other bones.

Hypertension

About 80% of patients with Cushing's syndrome have a degree of hypertension. This is not usually severe but it may have been present for long enough to lead to a cerebrovascular accident or coronary heart disease.

Glucose intolerance

This occurs in most patients and may progress to frank diabetes. Increased cortisol reduces the peripheral utilisation of glucose and stimulates gluconeogenesis in the liver. Initially there is a good insulin response, but this eventually fails and the patient becomes frankly diabetic.

Psychological changes

These are common and frequently overlooked. They may be interpreted as a natural response to the change in the appearance of the body, to weakness and to malaise. The psychological changes are a genuine, endogenous psychosis in many patients commonly in the form of depression but often with paranoid ideas and even hallucinations. The patient may become retarded and even mimic schizophrenia. Some patients will attempt or commit suicide. The usual observation that therapeutic steroids may produce euphoria is not reflected in the patient with overt Cushing's syndrome.

Differential diagnosis

Most fat, plethoric, hairy women with erratic menstrual habits will not have Cushing's syndrome. Biochemical investigation will distinguish between those who are simply hypertensive diabetics and those with polycystic ovaries. Greater difficulty may initially be experienced in separating out the depressive who may have a raised cortisol and loss of circadian rhythm or the alcoholic who may also have a raised serum cortisol not suppressible by dexamethasone.

Clinical presentation of ectopic ATCH syndrome

The majority of these patients have a small cell carcinoma of the lung. The next commonest cause is a carcinoid usually of the thymus or the lung. Rare causes include medullary carcinoma of the thyroid and the syndrome has been reported in association with primary carcinomas in most organs of the body. The secretion of corticotrophins is usually very high and the symptoms develop rapidly partly as a consequence of the malignancy and partly of the Cushing's. These include weight loss, oedema due to sodium retention, gross muscle weakness from steroid myopathy combined with paraneoplastic myopathy, pigmentation due to an MSH-like substance and psychological changes. Investigation usually discloses very high circulating cortisol levels, glycosuria and marked hypokalaemia.

Occasionally a Cushing's adenoma of the adrenal will undergo spontaneous haemorrhage and this may be the presenting event (Fig. 3.5).

Figure 3.5
Spontaneous haemorrhage from a large, benign cortisol-producing tumour of the right adrenal. The CT shows not only the tumour but also the haemorrhage filling much of the peritoneal cavity.

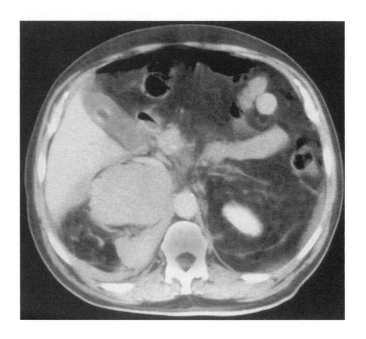

Investigation of Cushing's syndrome

As the clinical presentation does not necessarily yield the underlying cause of the Cushing's syndrome, more extensive investigation is usually required. It is important that the surgeon should be involved as early as possible in the diagnostic process. Patients with Cushing's syndrome are often poor candidates for anaesthesia and surgery and the longer the investigation is allowed to run without a clear treatment plan, the more ill the patient may become. There are three phases to the investigation of a patient with Cushing's syndrome:[4]

1. Is it definitely Cushing's syndrome on biochemical testing?
2. Is the primary lesion in the adrenal, pituitary or ectopic?
3. What are the anatomical details of the primary lesion?

Endocrine investigations

Diagnosis of Cushing's syndrome

The diagnosis of Cushing's syndrome is normally suspected in a patient as a result of the characteristic body habitus and biochemical abnormalities that are associated with the syndrome. The diagnosis of Cushing's syndrome depends predominantly on demonstrating a persistent, inappropriate elevation in serum glucocorticoids. The reason for this elevation may be as a result of ACTH-independent hypersecretion of glucocorticoids by the adrenal gland or glands, inappropriately elevated ACTH secretion by the pituitary, ACTH secretion from ectopic sources outside the pituitary, inappropriate secretion of CRF, or administration of glucocorticoids.

Establishment of the biochemical diagnosis of Cushing's syndrome

Some alternative medicines contain steroids and it is necessary to take a detailed drug history to exclude exogenous steroid administration. The diagnosis of endogenous Cushing's syndrome depends upon demonstrating the loss of normal circadian rhythm as well as a persistent elevation of cortisol. It is necessary to take at least three serum samples to demonstrate the loss of rhythm. The mean 24 h cortisol levels can be estimated by collecting and measuring the 24 h urinary free cortisol (UFC) which gives an integrated measure of the cortisol production. As a screening test this is 95% accurate.[5,6] Having established the presence of elevated serum glucocorticoids it is then necessary to establish whether the normal regulation of the hypothalamopituitary–adrenal axis has been disturbed. In a normal individual, administration of dexamethasone at low doses (0.5 mg) results in total suppression of the serum cortisol. This suppression is lost in patients with Cushing's syndrome but is normal in patients with obesity in whom elevated UFC is demonstrated. Patients with depression may also lose cortisol suppression in response to dexamethasone but the insulin tolerance test will distinguish between these conditions. Patients with Cushing's syndrome are resistant to insulin and therefore do not become hypoglycaemic in response to 0.3 u kg^{-1} i.v. This will usually distinguish the two conditions. Patients with alcoholic pseudo-Cushing's usually have an obvious history and may show deranged liver function tests.

Establishment of the cause of Cushing's syndrome

If the ACTH is low a diagnosis of adrenal disease can be made and the patient imaged to establish the anatomical location of a functioning adrenal neoplasm. If the ACTH is high, a diagnosis of ACTH-dependent adrenal hyperplasia is made and the source of the ACTH must be established. The two tests that are most reliable in determining the source of the ACTH are the CRH test and the high-dose dexamethasone test. Since few ectopic sources of ACTH, e.g. a small-cell carcinoma of the lung, are CRH dependent, the serum ACTH will not rise in patients with an ectopic source after the administration of CRH, whereas most pituitary adenomas remain CRH dependent. Patients with Cushing's disease (pituitary-dependent) will have a rapid rise in serum ACTH in response to CRH. The high-dose dexamethasone test relies on the fact that most patients with pituitary-dependent Cushing's syndrome partially suppress the serum cortisol levels in response to high doses of exogenous steroids whereas ectopic sources of ACTH and adrenal tumours do not.

A rare cause of Cushing's syndrome is ectopic CRH production.[7] Nephroblastomas, bronchogenic carcinomas, medullary carcinomas of the thyroid, pancreatic tumours, phaeochromocytomas and pituitary carcinomas can release a peptide with CRH-like activity. These patients 'appear' biochemically as though there is a source of ectopic ACTH.

Other rare causes of Cushing's disease are macronodular hyperplasia of the adrenals as a result of prolonged stimulation of the glands by ACTH resulting in the autonomous secretion of cortisol by the adrenal.[8] In primary pigmented nodular hyperplasia (PPND) there are pigmented micronodules as a result of stimulation by an abnormal immunoglobulin.[8] Carney's syndrome is a cluster of abnormalities including mesenchymal tumours, skin pigmentation, peripheral nerve tumours and endocrine abnormalities including autonomous hypersecreting multinodular adrenal glands.[9]

Imaging in ACTH-dependent Cushing's syndrome

Pituitary radiograph, chest radiograph, CT or MRI of the pituitary or whole-body and whole body or inferior petrosal venous ACTH assays have been used to find the source of ACTH.

Anatomical details

Pituitary

Pituitary microadenomas causing Cushing's disease are usually very small. The overall change in pituitary size cannot, therefore, be seen on conventional skull radiograph even with tomography. CT scanning will identify about 50% of tumours but the intravenous contrast does not 'light up' microadenomas. Interpretation is confused by the fact that many normal people have non-functioning pituitary microadenomas. Currently the most useful test is magnetic resonance imaging (MRI) with or without gadolinium enhancement. Where there is doubt as to whether high levels of ACTH are being secreted by the pituitary or an ectopic source, bilateral inferior petrosal sinus venous sampling may be undertaken.[10] This is, however, technically difficult and very operator dependent. Two catheters must be manipulated by the Seldinger technique from the right femoral vein to the petrosal sinuses and ACTH samples obtained simultaneously from both catheters and from a peripheral vein. These tests are repeated after administration of corticotrophin releasing hormone.

Adrenals

The advent of CT rendered obsolete the assessment of the adrenals by plain radiographs with tomography. Ultrasonography is a useful, quick screening test to determine whether there is an adrenal lesion. If this is known early in the investigative process, tests can be targeted to determine if this is the cause of the Cushing's syndrome.

CT is undertaken with contrast and maximum information is given if 2 mm slices are taken through the adrenal area (Fig. 3.6). A large tumour, one with indeterminate edges or areas of necrosis within it, suggests malignancy (Fig. 3.7).

MRI is increasingly used to assess the adrenals (Fig. 3.8), but is of little additional value over CT when the tumour is small and well

Figure 3.6
CT scan showing an adenoma in the right adrenal gland in association with Cushing's syndrome.

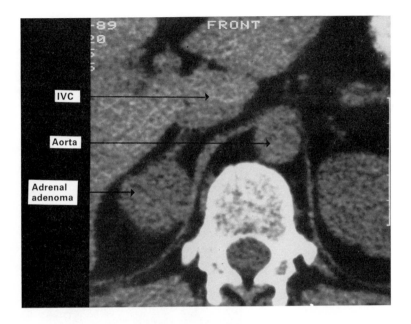

Figure 3.7 *CT scan of the abdomen of a patient with gross Cushing's syndrome of rapid onset showing a large tumour of the left adrenal gland with irregular margins and necrosis. This was a malignant tumour.*

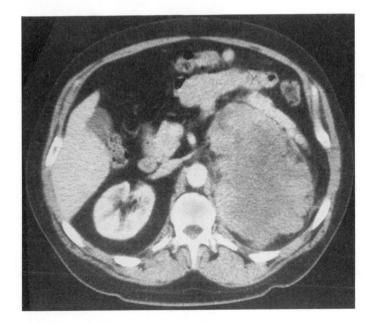

circumscribed. It is, however, valuable for very small tumours not clearly defined on CT or in larger tumours where there is a suspicion of malignancy. It is particularly valuable at showing invasion of the vena cava. It has been claimed that there is a higher signal intensity in T2 weighted images with malignant tumours than benign.

Figure 3.8
MRI scan of a left adrenal tumour showing brightly in relation to surrounding structures.

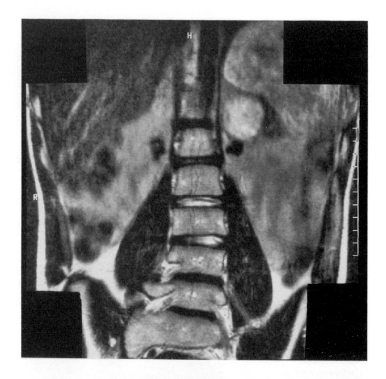

Figure 3.9
Cholesterol scan of the adrenal glands. The bottom left hand image is of the kidneys. The top left image is of the adrenals. The top right scan is of the two other images superimposed to identify the position of the 'hot' spot on the adrenal scan (same patient as Figure 3.6).

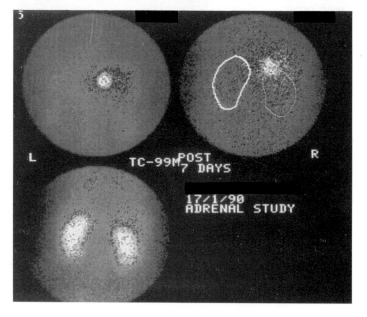

The adrenal cortex can be imaged with scintigraphic cholesterol scans or NP59, but the consequences are a high radiation dose to the adrenals and the test is best avoided if possible. It is a useful functional test because any nodule will 'light up' on the scintiscan and the other adrenal will be suppressed (Fig. 3.9).

Table 3.2 *Results of diagnostic evaluation*

	Serum ACTH	oCRH test	High-dose dexamethasone test	CT/MRI Sella	CT/MRI adrenals	Petrosal sinus sampling	Iodocholesterol scan
Pituitary Cushing's	Normal to mildly elevated	+	>50% suppression	+/–	Mild bilateral enlargement or normal	+	+
Ectopic ACTH	Normal to markedly elevated	–	No suppression	–	Enlarged bilaterally or normal	–	+
Adrenal neoplasms	Undetectable	–	No suppression	–	Unilateral adrenal mass	NA	Adenomas + carcinomas –
Micronodular disease	Undetectable	–	No suppression	–	Minimal diffuse enlargement ('knobby') or normal	–	+/–[a]

[a] At 48 h; may become positive if studied for longer intervals.
+, positive test; –, negative test; +/–, test may be positive or negative. NA, not applicable.
From Perry et al. Primary ádrenal causes of Cushing's ŝyndrone. Ann Surg 1989; 210: 59–68.

Searching for an ectopic ACTH source

The majority of such tumours will be identifiable on CT of the chest. The smaller ectopic ACTH-producing tumours, particularly carcinoids, may be difficult or impossible to visualise. If a suspicious area is seen on CT or MRI then angiography, venous sampling or octreotide isotope scanning may help confirm the diagnosis.[11]

These tests and results are summarised in Table 3.2.

Plan of management

The management of Cushing's disease with a pituitary microadenoma will normally be direct microadenectomy through the trans-sphenoidal route. Larger tumours may require a direct approach through the anterior fossa. Even with good imaging and an experienced operator, the success of microadenectomy may not be greater than 60%. It is possible to destroy the pituitary microadenoma by initial or sub-sequent total pituitary ablation with external or implanted radio-therapy. The benefits of these radical procedures tends to be far outweighed by the disadvantages of total pituitary loss. Failed pituitary surgery is therefore normally best managed by resorting early to bilateral adrenalectomy. The pituitary tumour is left in place and may eventually grow large enough to produce headaches or compro-mise the optic pathways, in which case further surgery may be required. Normally, the unresected adenoma has few side effects apart from causing the development of hyperpigmentation (Nelson's syndrome).

When bilateral adrenalectomy is undertaken for Cushing's disease the route taken will depend on the preference of the surgeon and the habitus of the patient. Bilateral laparoscopic adrenalectomy by the transperitoneal route is feasible though time consuming. The trocars and instruments may not be long enough to reach the adrenals in a very fat patient. A transperitoneal direct approach through a trans-verse upper abdominal incision allows easier access, but the wound is long. Some surgeons prefer a bilateral posterior route or even to undertake removal of one adrenal at a time through separate loin approaches (see section on adrenalectomy).

It is important to remember that these patients are often very sick and even pretreatment with metyrapone or other metabolic blocking agents may not significantly alter their readiness for surgery. At oper-ation, particular care must be directed towards the safe handling of the patient because of their weight, their tissue fragility and spinal osteoporosis. Wounds must be securely sutured in the expectation that healing will be delayed. Prophylactic antibiotics are advised as these patients have an impaired resistance to infection.

Postoperatively, care should be taken to avoid wound infection, to support good respiratory function, to monitor sugar and electrolytes carefully and, most importantly, to replace the cortisol which is now absent from the circulation.

To replace the adrenal function after bilateral adrenalectomy all patients should be given 100 mg of hydrocortisone at the time of induction and the subsequent steroid replacement follows this protocol:

1. 100 mg hydrocortisone sodium succinate in the recovery room and six hourly i.v. until the patient is able to take oral medication.
2. Oral hydrocortisone, 20 mg, with fludrocortisone, 0.1 mg, in the morning and then hydrocortisone, 10 mg, at night. There is no need for mineralocorticoid supplementation until oral feeding has been recommenced.

Patients who are on steroid replacement must be warned of the importance of continuing with therapy, and ideally should wear a bracelet and carry a card with the details of therapy. They should be aware of the need to increase the dose of steroids should intercurrent illness develop and to warn doctors at any hospital to which they are admitted that they are taking steroid medication.

Bilateral adrenalectomy for other causes of Cushing's syndrome

Bilateral adrenalectomy is also required for Cushing's syndrome caused by an ectopic ACTH source (if that source cannot be identified and removed), for PPND and for macronodular adrenal cortical hyperplasia.

Management of Cushing's syndrome due to a solitary adrenal adenoma or carcinoma

Well defined, clearly benign tumours of 10 cm diameter or less may be removed laparoscopically by the transperitioneal or retroperitoneal route. Larger tumours or those in which there is a suspicion of malignancy, should be resected by unilateral adrenalectomy through a loin incision, or if they are very large, through a posterior thoracoabdominal incision. Malignant tumours on the right, if they have invaded the vena cava, may require opening of the vena cava to remove any tumour that has directly invaded it. In some patients partial removal of the vena cava and its replacement by a PTFE tube graft may be needed (Fig. 3.10). The very rare occasion where there is tumour invasion of the hepatic or suprahepatic veins, may require liver transplantation if surgery is contemplated. Large adrenocortical carcinomas on the left may require removal by en bloc excision of the adrenal with surrounding organs, sometimes including the spleen, tail of pancreas and the kidney.

A unilateral cortisol secreting tumour will suppress the opposite adrenal and all such patients will require steroid replacement as described above. The patient may subsequently be weaned from the steroid replacement when the pituitary–adrenal axis function is returned to normal (tested using synacthen). This recovery may take one year or more.

Figure 3.10
(a) CT showing large malignant right adrenal tumour with no symptoms of caval involvement but (b) a cavagram shows extension of the tumour into the lumen of the vena cava.

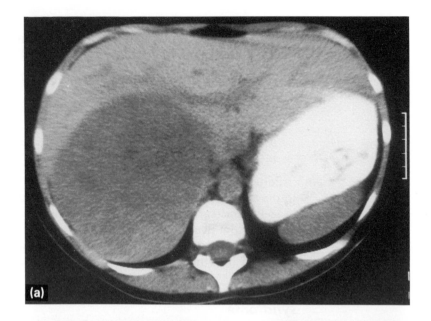

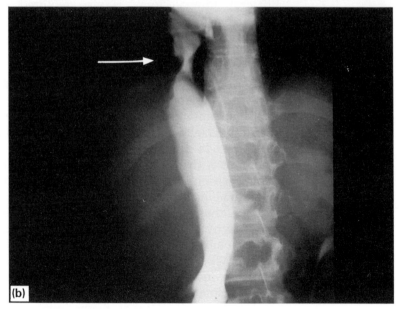

Management of Cushing's syndrome in pregnancy

Patients with Cushing's syndrome rarely become pregnant. When they do the pregnancy is normally complicated and it may be necessary to undertake pituitary surgery or adrenalectomy in the second trimester. For patients with a plasma cortisol over 30 μg dl^{-1} there is no evidence that vaginal delivery is contraindicated if the third trimester is achieved.[12,13]

General management of adrenocortical carcinoma

Adrenocortical carcinoma is rare accounting for 0.02% of cancers. It can occur at any age with a peak incidence in the fourth and fifth decades. About 60% of such tumours have no significant endocrine secretion, and vary in tissue type from those closely approximating normal adrenal cortex to the completely undifferentiated. It is sometimes difficult to distinguish between benign and malignant tumours unless there are clear signs of capsular or vascular invasion. Ploidy studies assessed by flow cytometry may be helpful in predicting malignancy. Functional and non-functional tumours spread by local invasion and by lymphatic and vascular systems.

Non-functioning tumours present by systemic symptoms of weight loss, weakness and occasional fever.

Functional tumours present depending of their type of secretion:

1. Glucocorticoid-secreting tumours present as Cushing's syndrome;
2. Androgen-secreting tumours present as virilisation, hirsutism and amenorrhoea in women, and precocious puberty in boys.
3. Oestrogen-secreting tumours are very rare and in men are an exceptionally rare cause of gynaecomastia. Such gynaecomastia will be associated with testicular atrophy and impotence. Girls will show precocious puberty and women show menstrual irregularities.
4. Aldosterone-secreting malignant adrenal tumours are exceptionally rare and the syndrome produced is identical to that produced by benign tumours.

When possible a surgical resection of adrenocortical malignant tumours must be undertaken and if there are clear histological margins there is little evidence that radiotherapy to the tumour bed is likely to extend the patient's survival or decrease the risk of recurrence.[14] If recurrence occurs debulking surgery may be valuable particularly in hormone-secreting tumours.

Chemotherapy has a limited place in the management of adrenocortical tumours and is reserved for recurrence, inoperable or metastatic disease. The agent of choice is Mitotane (o,p'ddd). This agent has a specific action in interfering with cortisol synthesis but additionally causes regression of the tumour. It appears to be effective in non-functioning adrenocortical tumours. The starting dose is 1–2 g per day increasing gradually to 8–10 g per day. During treatment the patient will require maintenance doses of cortisone and may become hypothyroid, requiring treatment. The side effects may be considerable (nausea, vomiting and fatigue) but if they are not marked, it is worth persisting with treatment as good remissions are sometimes obtained.[15]

There is only limited experience of the treatment of adrenocortical tumours with other chemotherapeutic agents but 110 patients from the MD Anderson Cancer Centre had 5- and 10-year survivals of 23% and 10%, respectively. There is no difference in response between functional and non-functional tumours.[16]

In the palliative care patients with gross Cushing's syndrome blockade with metyrapone or aminoglutethimide is occasionally useful.

Remission of Cushing's syndrome after successful treatment

Almost all the symptoms of Cushing's syndrome will regress after correction of the hypercortisolism. The earliest to respond are the psychological changes which revert to normal within a few days. Within a week of adrenalectomy the blood pressure begins to return to normal but it may be several months before it reaches its final level. About 80% of patients obtain total remission of hypertension. The cardiac and ECG changes improve at the same rate. The skin changes improve slowly over the first few months. The first sign of improvement is often a scaly desquamation at the margin of the scalp. The excess weight is lost but some dieting may be necessary. The muscles only regain full strength after several months. Facial hair becomes less pronounced but the hirsutism never completely disappears. Of the metabolic changes the diabetes usually, but not invariably, is cured and the serum electrolytes return to normal within the first few weeks after surgery. Recalcification of the bones takes many months.

When seen a year after definitive treatment of Cushing's syndrome changes in the patient are usually dramatic with a near total return to previous physical appearance and function.

Adrenogenital syndrome

Adrenogenital syndrome describes a heterogeneous group of disorders that result in abnormalities of the external genitalia. Most patients have congenital adrenal hyperplasia (CAH) in which there is a congenital deficit in one of the enzymes of steroid production. Any enzyme deficit in the pathway to production of aldosterone or cortisol will result in a syndrome characterised by deficit of the end steroid and overproduction of intermediary steroid metabolites. This is due to increased ACTH production as a result of the deficit in the end steroid. Since the path to production of adrenal androgens shares many steroid intermediates with the corticoid production pathway any enzyme block to cortisol production will increase androgen production and virilisation will occur. The clinical presentation of CAH is variable and depends on the site and severity of the block in steroid synthesis. The most common form is as a result of a deficit in the 21-hydroxylase enzyme which causes impairment of the production of cortisol and aldosterone. In its mild form the increased secretion of ACTH results in near normal cortisol levels with normal or raised aldosterone levels. The syndrome includes elevated androgens with ambiguous genitalia and clitoral enlargement in the female and sexual precocity in the male. In its severe form the deficit of cortisol and aldosterone production results in salt-losing, hypoglycaemic crises that require urgent intervention. The mild forms may only present in adult life and are an important differential diagnosis in female patients with virilising features and in men with features of excess androgen production.

The treatment of CAH is by replacement of the deficient steroids, which results in a reduction in ACTH levels and a reduction of the androgens that cause the virilisation. The adrenal hyperplasia does not require surgical intervention but the genital manifestations of excess androgen production, particularly in women, may require specialised surgery.[17]

Aldosteronism (Conn's syndrome)

Aldosteronism (excessive secretion of aldosterone) may occur *primarily* due to tumours, nodularity or hyperplasia of the adrenal glands or *secondarily* as a response to excess stimulation by angiotensin. This latter condition occurs as a response to diminished plasma volume in conditions such as cirrhosis, nephrotic syndrome, diuretic therapy and cardiac failure. It also occurs when increased renin is produced in conditions such as renal artery stenosis, accelerated hypertension and when there is a renin-secreting renal tumour.

In primary aldosteronism one or both adrenals secrete aldosterone in excess, independently of any change in the renin–angiotensin mechanism. Subtypes are:

1. Hypersecretion from a small, benign 'aldosterone producing adenoma' (APA) in the cortex of one adrenal;
2. Bilateral micro- or macronodular hyperplasia of the zona glomerulosa, sometimes described as 'idiopathic hyperaldosteronism' (IHA);
3. Aldosterone-secreting carcinoma is very rare. Most malignant cortical tumours secrete a range of cortical hormones and related substances. It is rare for such tumours to predominantly produce aldosterone;
4. The dominantly inherited 'familial glucocorticoid suppressible hyperaldosteronism'.

Pathology and pathophysiology

Conn's tumours (APA) are more common in women and are more common on the left.[18] Aldosterone is produced by the zona glomerulosa of the adrenal cortex. It promotes the absorption of sodium by the distal renal tubules via the Na/K^+, H^+ ion channel and by this mechanism promotes the retention of water. The secretion of aldosterone is controlled primarily by angiotensin II. Angiotensin II is generated as a result of the activity of renin and angiotensin-converting enzyme (ACE) on angiotensinogen. Renin is a hormone secreted from the juxtaglomerular apparatus of the kidney in response to low blood pressure or volume. The secretion of aldosterone is also increased by ACTH and by an increase in serum K^+ concentrations. Dopamine,

Table 3.3 *Causes of primary hyperaldosteronism*

Type	Frequency (%)	Site	Responsiveness Ang II	Responsiveness ACTH	Surgically correctable
Aldosterone-producing adenoma	64	Uni	−	+	+
Idiopathic hyperaldosteronism	32	Bil	+	−	−
Glucocorticoid-suppressable hyperaldosteronism	1	Bil	−	+	−
Primary adrenal hyperplasia	<1	Uni	−	+	+
Aldosterone-producing, Angiotensin II-responsive adenoma	<1	Uni	+	−	+
Aldosterone-producing carcinoma	<1	Uni	−	−	+

Adapted from reference 19 with permission.

Uni, unilateral pathology; Bil, bilateral pathology.

a putative pituitary aldosterone-stimulating factor, serotonin and atrial natriuretic peptide also influence aldosterone secretion. Aldosterone is metabolised by the liver and plasma concentrations may be pathologically raised as a result of liver impairment.

Primary hyperaldosteronism is a term that describes the inappropriate secretion of aldosterone that is independent of the influence of renin. The causes are listed in Table 3.3.

Low-renin hyperaldosteronism presents with hypertension and hypokalaemic alkalosis due to the direct effect of the excess aldosterone on the distal renal tubules promoting a loss of K^+ and H^+ and a retention of Na^+ and water. The retention of Na^+ and water is partly counteracted by increased secretion of atrial natriuretic peptide (ANP) and the sodium concentrations may be normal and water retention is not generally a feature. A low oral Na^+ intake will mask the hypokalaemia in many patients.

Incidence

Aldosteronism is twice as common in women as men and rarely occurs in children. It predominantly presents between the ages of 30 and 60 years and is discovered in 1% of patients investigated for hypertension. Approximately half the patients will have an adenoma and the other half IHA.

Clinical features

There are no specific clinical features, but clinical suspicion should be aroused when there is a conjunction of hypertension with hypokalaemia. The hypertension is usually moderate or severe and may not have responded satisfactorily to normal medical treatment.

The hypokalaemia will usually have been discovered on routine multichannel analysis or only have declared itself as a consequence of diuretic therapy. However, it may sometimes be marked with severe symptoms of muscle weakness or cramps, malaise, polyuria and polydypsia.

Patients with APA as distinct from IHA usually have more severe hypertension and more profound hypokalaemia and higher aldosterone levels in the plasma.

Investigations

There are three crucial steps in the diagnostic process:

1. Is there primary aldosteronism?
2. Is there one diseased adrenal such that surgery might be appropriate?
3. Is any visualised mass defect the cause of the aldosteronism?

Primary aldosteronism

Investigation to determine this follows complex algorithms outside the scope of this chapter,[20] but remember that one-third of patients with primary aldosteronism may have a normal potassium and hypokalaemia will only be revealed by the prescription of diuretics. Diuretics may, of course, cause hypokalaemia and it is therefore important when investigating these patients to discontinue the diuretic and replace the deficiency in potassium before testing. It is also essential to discontinue aldosterone and calcium channel blocking antihypertensives as these will interfere with results. The diagnosis of primary hyperaldosteronism is therefore based on the concurrence of hypokalaemia, inappropriate increased urinary potassium excretion and a high plasma aldosterone which is not suppressible with an increased intake of sodium chloride. Glucocorticoid levels should be noted as being normal.

Unilateral adrenal pathology

Essentially this is the process of distinguishing APA from IHA. As the glands in IHA may be nodular this is not always an easy sequence of investigations. If there is single, significant-sized adrenal lesion CT scanning is the easiest and cheapest way of assessing this. If a high resolution scan with 3 mm contiguous slices is used approximately 80% of patients with a solitary adenoma will be successfully imaged by CT scan. Contrast enhancement does not improve the value of the films. MRI scanning is equally sensitive but not of any extra value when a single lesion is found. Small equivocal or multiple lesions found on CT or MRI require further evaluation to distinguish between IHA and APA.

Distinction between IHA and APA[21]

One of the best diagnostic tests is to measure blood aldosterone levels after recumbency and after subsequently standing, i.e. on waking in the morning and after the patient has been up and about for three hours. In normal subjects the plasma aldosterone increases by a factor of 2–4 when the patient is upright. In patients with IHA this increase is less pronounced but is more than 33% of the recumbent level. Patients with APA show no change in the postural aldosterone concentrations.

Is the anatomical abnormality a functioning adenoma?

Incompatibility between preliminary biochemical tests and localisation studies requires additional studies such as iodocholesterol isotope scanning with NP59 or adrenal vein sampling for aldosterone. NP59 scanning provides a functional assessment. Scanning must be carried out for five days after the isotope has been given and the results are more likely to be diagnostic if dexamethasone suppression has been given for 7 days previously and if antihypertensive treatment is discontinued. If only one adrenal gland shows on the NP59 scan then there is a good chance that there is a single, significant functioning adenoma. The accuracy of this test is around 80%. The accuracy of adrenal vein sampling is higher, perhaps up to 95% but it is technically difficult especially on the right and is time consuming. It does not need to be combined with retrograde venography.

Treatment

Unequivocal APA is treated by unilateral adrenalectomy if the patient is fit. The tumour is usually small, easily visible and well encapsulated and can be removed laparoscopically or by a posterior approach. The surgery should be preceded by 1–6 weeks of preparation with spironolactone to allow the serum potassium to return to normal. Surgery returns the blood pressure to normal in about 70% of patients. It is important to remember that some adenomas also secrete glucocorticoid and the opposite adrenal may, therefore, be suppressed and replacement treatment with cortisone may be necessary.

The treatment of choice for the relatively benign condition of IHA is treatment with spironolactone at a dose of 100 mg rising to 400 mg per day until the potassium has normalised and the hypertension is under control. The dose may then be gradually reduced. Spironolactone may not control the hypertension when used alone and the addition of calcium channel antagonists, ACE inhibitors or diuretics may be required. Spironolactone affects testosterone synthesis leading to gynaecomastia, reduced libido, impotence and menstrual disorders. It may not be tolerated by the patient and second line therapy with amiloride or triamterene may be preferable.

Familial bilateral glucocorticoid suppressive hyperaldosteronism is rare. It is ideally treated with spironolactone as this is less physiologically disruptive than the glucocorticoid treatment.

The treatment of aldosterone-producing cortical carcinoma is the same as that for predominantly cortisol-secreting carcinomas.

In the rare situation of hyperaldosteronism in pregnancy surgery is preferred to medical therapy unless there is clearly bilateral disease.[22]

Phaeochromo-cytoma

Phaeochromocytoma, neuroblastoma (see later), paragangliomas and ganglioneuromas are derived from the neural crest. Phaeochromo-cytoma may occur wherever neuro-ectodermal tissue is found; hence the occasionally used name chromaffinoma. About 90% are solitary and occur in the adrenal but 5–10% are bilateral and 10% are extra-adrenal. Extra-adrenal phaeochromocytomas are often described as paraganglionomas and can be found in any of the sites identified in Fig. 3.11.

Incidence

The true incidence of phaeochromocytoma is not known, but a phaeochromocytoma was found at 0.3% of autopsies performed at the Mayo Clinic and the incidence has been calculated at 1–2 per 100 000 adults per year.[23] About 0.1% of patients investigated for hypertension will have a phaeochromocytoma. Most phaeochromocytomas are less than 10 cm in diameter when discovered, the average being 5 cm, and they are usually discovered early because of physiological

Figure 3.11
(a) Anatomical distribution of extra-adrenal chromaffin tissue in the newborn. (b) Location of extra-adrenal phaeochromo-cytomas reported in the literature up to 1965.

Modified from Coupland, R. The Natural History of the Chromaffin Cell, Longman Green, 1965.

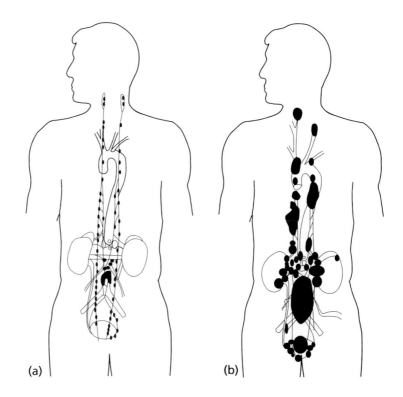

(a)   (b)

catecholamine effects. About 10% of phaeochromocytomas are malignant and these tend to be larger at presentation.

The majority of phaeochromocytomas secrete predominantly adrenaline but some secrete noradrenaline or dopamine, in which case hypotension may be a presenting sign. A range of other physiologically active agents are released from phaeochromocytomas and include serotonin, ACTH, PTH and VIP,[24] but the majority of symptoms are attributable to adrenaline and noradrenaline.

Symptomatology

The symptoms are those of excess circulating adrenaline or noradrenaline but symptoms may be sporadic and paroxysmal against a background of continuing high levels of circulating catecholamines and chronic physiological changes such as hypovolaemia.[25] The continuing high background catecholamine levels do not produce symptoms as a consequence of tachyphylaxis, the desensitisation of alpha- and beta-adrenergic receptors. The presentation of patients with phaeochromocytomas can be dramatic, consisting of severe but transient hypertension, palpitations, tachycardia and sweating with pallor and anxiety. Not all of these may be present and chest pain and weakness may be associated symptoms in about 50% of patients. The attacks may last for minutes or hours and occur at any frequency of from 1–2 times a year to regularly during an hour. They often occur spontaneously but may be precipitated by vigorous exercise, twisting and bending, alcohol, tobacco and certain specific drugs such as anaesthetic agents, phenothiazines, beta blockers and tricyclic antidepressants.

Occasionally the acute effects of hypertension are so severe that the patient may demonstrate fulminating pulmonary oedema or severe arrythmias that may be fatal. In addition to the impressive paroxysmal effects of phaeochromocytoma there are additional chronic effects, most notably a cardiomyopathy. Some patients will only be diagnosed at autopsy but retrospective review of these patients shows that almost all will have had symptoms in life.[26]

Clinical associations

Multiple endocrine neoplasia, type 2 (MEN2)

In MEN2A there is familial occurrence of phaeochromocytoma (which may be bilateral), medullary carcinoma of the thyroid and hyperparathyroidism. Not all patients will develop all three abnormalities but all should be sought in anyone with phaeochromocytoma. In some families only phaeochromocytomas occur and in others there are consistently only medullary carcinomas of the thyroid. In MEN2B, hyperparathyroidism is uncommon but in addition to phaeochromocytoma and medullary carcinoma of the thyroid mucosal neuromas, a marfanoid habitus and sometimes ganglion neuromas in the gastrointestinal tract are added to the phenotype.[27] All forms of MEN2 are autosomally inherited as a dominant gene.

Neurofibromatosis
This is a rare association but phaeochromocytoma will occur in 10% of patients with neurofibromatosis.

Von Hippel Lindau syndrome
About 14% of patients with this syndrome (cerebellar haemangioma) have a phaeochromocytoma.[28] Extra-adrenal paragangliomas or phaeochromocytomas may be associated with adrenal phaeochromocytomas in a few patients. These are not always familial and therefore, even in the supposed sporadic patient, should be sought if the biochemistry does not return to normal after excision of the primary adrenal phaeochromocytoma.

Investigations

If phaeochromocytoma is suspected, a basic screen must always be undertaken to establish the clinical diagnosis by assessing (a) urinary vannilyl mandelic acid (VMA) in a 24-h sample of urine; this test, however, has only a 60% sensitivity in diagnosing phaeochromocytoma; and (b) urinary total catecholamines, a more specific test with 90% sensitivity and specificity in the diagnosis of phaeochromocytoma. If the 24-hour urinary adrenaline level exceeds 35 µg or noradrenaline level exceeds 170 µg then phaeochromocytoma must be suspected. Combining the two amines to give values in excess of 100 µg/24-h will allow a confident diagnosis of phaeochromocytoma. It is possible to measure serum adrenaline and noradrenaline levels, but this is technically more difficult and the results are less specific for the diagnosis of phaeochromocytoma. Any of these determinations can be altered by concurrent administration of drugs such as calcium channel blockers, monoamine oxidase inhibitors, phenothiazines, tricyclic antidepressants, alpha and beta blockers and nalidixic acid.[29]

Localisation

Once an abnormal urinary VMA or catecholamine level has been confirmed, adrenal CT scanning should be undertaken and this will show 90% of tumours. Only rarely will MRI add additional, useful information. If an adrenal tumour is discovered further localisation studies are not needed, particularly if it has a characteristic irregular dark centre. If the patient is pregnant MRI is the preferred imaging modality. If there is a suspicion that there might be multiple or ectopic phaeochromocytomas or if the patient is a known member of an MEN2 family or under the age of 30, then isotopic scanning is indicated. The agent of choice is MIBG (meta-iodobenzylguanidine) which is highly specific for catecholamine-producing tumours whatever the location. Very few false positives are encountered but there is a false negative rate of 5–10% especially with small tumours (see Fig. 3.12).[30]

Occasionally tumours will infarct perhaps in association with a paroxysm and in these circumstances the MIBG may be negative.

Figure 3.12
An ectopic phaeochromo-cytoma.
The MIBG scans suggested that the lesion was in the left adrenal gland but the CT scanning shows the tumour to be located in ganglionic tissue in the lower chest (arrowed)

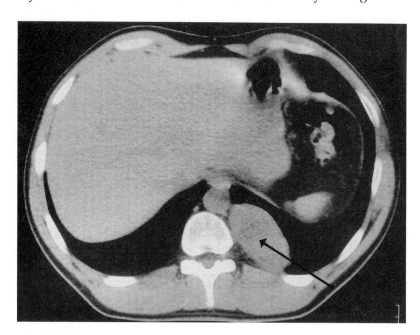

Management

When a phaeochromocytoma has been identified the correct treatment is surgical excision. There is no effective medical treatment but adrenalectomy should not be undertaken without preparation of the patient.

Preoperative management of patients with phaeochromocytoma

The anaesthesia of patients with functioning phaeochromocytomas is highly specialised and even with adequate blockade of catecholamine release may present significant challenges intraoperatively. Close preoperative liason with the anaesthetist responsible for the peroperative management of the patient is mandatory so that the patient is admitted for surgery in the optimal physiological condition.

The introduction of α-adrenergic blockade with appropriate expansion in the intravascular volume resulted in a reduction in the perioperative mortality from 13–45% to 0–3%. The catecholamine excess has a wide range of physiological effects. The most obvious are hypertension, caused by the vasoconstrictive action on blood vessels, sweating and tachycardia. In addition they cause hyperglycaemia and occasionally cardiomyopathy. Patients should be started on an α-adrenergic blocking agent when the diagnosis of phaeochromocytoma is made. Some patients are sensitive to the resulting blockade so the starting dose should be low and increase until blockade is adequate. Phenoxybenzamine is the agent most frequently used starting at a dose of 20–60 mg/day in divided doses. Prazocin or the combined α- and β-blocker labetalol have been used for this purpose. There are no clear rules to assess when the α-blockade is adequate but this is likely to be sufficient when sweating and tachycardia cease and when there is a demonstrable increase in the intravascular volume measured by a drop in the haematocrit associated with an increase in bodyweight. This may require 60–250 mg/day of phenoxybenzamine. If tachycardia or cardiac arrhythmias develop a β-blocker may be added *once α-blockade is adequate*. Pure β-blockade may result in severe hypertensive crisis.

There are no rules as to the duration of treatment with α-blockers prior to surgery but two weeks is probably adequate if there is no evidence of catecholamine-induced cardiomyopathy. If there are ECG abnormalities, e.g. ST-segment elevation, arrhythmias, or evidence of global myocardial dysfunction on an echocardiogram, the treatment may have to continue for as long as 6 months. β-blockade is normally added electively preoperatively if not indicated earlier for control of symptoms. Preoperative preparation with metyrosine (alpha-methyl-*p*-tyrosine), which interferes with catecholamine synthesis, is worthwhile but it has little advantage over traditional regimens using alpha- and beta-blockade.

Close liason between surgeon and anaesthetist is important, since manipulation of the gland may result in catecholamine release and marked hypertension (despite blockade) and devascularisation of the tumour can result in a drop in circulating vasoactive catecholamines with consequent hypotension (Fig. 3.13). Intravenous fluids, hypotensive agents such as nitroprusside and inotropes such as phenylephrine or dopamine are used to control pressure peroperatively. Continuous monitoring of CVP and arterial pressure is required from induction of anaesthesia to the recovery phase. Early in the procedure fluid is given intravenously in a quantity in excess of what the CVP dictates. This deliberate expansion of the circulating blood volume prior to ligation of the adrenal vein and the consequent loss of pressor effect is a valuable prophylaxis against a sudden fall in CVP. This often reduces the need for large doses of pressor agents in the later part of the surgery.[31] If managed well from a pharmacological and circulatory point of view, the patient is usually stable within an hour or so of the end of the operation and does not need prolonged pressor or ventilatory support or monitoring. Overzealous alpha-blockage prior to the operation, however, may lead to postoperative hypotension.

Figure 3.13 *The fluctuations in central venous pressure and blood pressure that may be experienced during operation on a phaeochromo-cytoma. Good preoperation preparation may blunt the severity of peaks and troughs but unpredictably so.*

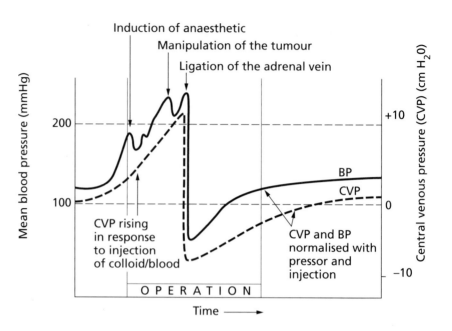

Phaeochromocytoma in pregnancy

Phaeochromocytoma and pregnancy is a dangerous combination for mother and baby. When the diagnosis is not made prepartum maternal mortality exceeds 50%. For those where the diagnosis is made during pregnancy, prognosis is better and standard treatment can be undertaken with alpha blockade followed in the third trimester by synchronous adrenalectomy and caesarean section. Vaginal delivery is contraindicated.[32,33]

Malignant phaeochromocytoma

Malignant phaeochromocytomas are rare and account for less than 10% of phaeochromocytomas. They are no more common in extra-adrenal phaeochromocytoma or in familial forms. As with many other endocrine tumours the histology of the primary lesion may not distinguish benign from malignant, even when ploidy studies are added. The presence of metastases is the only true indicator of malignancy. Many phaeochromocytomas are poorly encapsulated and may seem at operation to be invading local structures but are, nevertheless, benign. Metastases will normally take up MIGB which can be used in localisation and in therapeutic doses which may be palliative. The value of radiotherapy is unproven but a 50% response rate to a chemotherapeutic regimen of cyclophosphamide, vincristine and dacarbazine has been reported.[34]

Adrenal neuro-blastomas: tumours of the developing neuro-endocrine system

Such tumours may develop in neonates and infants wherever such tissue exists and 40% will occur in the adrenal gland and a further 40% in the nearby paraspinal sympathetic tissue. They are the commonest solid tumour of infancy. Neuroblastomas normally present as adrenal masses and are often very large. In children over the age of three there are usually metastases in liver, bone, lung or subcutaneous nodules at the time of presentation. The diagnosis is made by CT scan and primary tumour and metastases may be identified by isotope MIBG or octreotide scans. Urinary catecholamine levels are raised in most patients.

Treatment

The treatment depends on the type and stage but for most patients consists of surgical resection of the adrenal tumour or debulking, followed by chemotherapy. This combination will produce a complete remission in most patients, but many will recur later. In some infants where the primary tumour is completely resected and metastases are limited to the liver, skin or bone marrow (stage IVS), spontaneous remission may occur after resection of the primary tumour, and chemotherapy may not then be needed. In this special subset of children there is an 85% long-term survival rate. For most others survival is worse. Quantification of the N–myc oncogene provides prognostic information and when there is a single copy of the oncogene, a 98% long-term survival rate may be expected. Patients with tumours with more than 10 copies of the gene have an exceptionally poor prognosis regardless of treatment.

Neuroblastoma is a complex condition requiring treatment in a specialist centre.[35,36]

Incidentaloma

About 7% of autospies uncover an unsuspected adrenal tumour and an adrenal mass is an incidental finding in 1% of abdominal CT scans. The term 'incidentaloma' is now in common usage for such coincidentally discovered tumours. When found they should be assessed objectively because they are a potential source of unnecessary and possibly harmful surgery.

About 5% of such tumours are found to be primary adrenal cancers, a further 5% are metastases from an occult primary tumour. About 50% are, however, metastases from known primary tumours. A further 30% are mainly cortical adenomas and may have potential or actual endocrine significance. The remainder consists of haematomas, cysts and myelolipomas (Fig. 3.14). This last group, however, can normally be diagnosed on CT scan and may not require further evaluation. Cysts are normally simple and not associated with malignancy. Haematomas are occasionally a result of trauma but can occur spontaneously in an underlying primary or metastatic tumour. Myelolipomas are benign, non-functioning tumours which only require excision if significant growth occurs.

Figure 3.14
CT scan showing a large tumour in the left adrenal position with the typical features of a myelolipoma. A tumour consisting of areas of dark, fatty tissue divided by thick bands. The tumour was excised and histology confirmed the CT diagnosis.

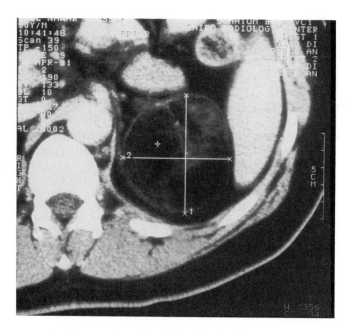

Those patients who have no obvious CT diagnosis and no known malignancy elsewhere require investigation to exclude endocrine disease. It is sufficient to undertake a urinary VMA or catecholamine assay to exclude phaeochromocytoma, a serum potassium to exclude Conn's syndrome and a serum cortisol to exclude Cushing's syndrome. If any one of these screening tests is abnormal then further testing is indicated. If each is normal then the decision whether to remove the adrenal lesion or merely to watch it with serial CT scans is based on the size of the tumour and its CT appearance. CT evidence of irregular contour, invasion of adjacent structures and metastases to retroperitoneal nodes are indications for surgery. In the absence of such signs, size is the best determinant of malignancy; MRI scanning and isotope scanning do not significantly improve the diagnostic power of the CT scan. Tumours less than 6 cm in diameter can normally be watched with serial CT scans. Larger lesions must be excised. If the patient is unfit or unwilling to undergo adrenalectomy then the diagnosis may be improved with CT-guided biopsy (Fig. 3.14). Although the negative predictive value of an adrenal tumour of less than 6 cm being malignant is 99%, the Mayo Clinic recommend that lesions of 4 cm or greater should be excised and smaller tumours re-scanned after three months.[37]

The ease of adrenalectomy is not, an indication for inappropriate surgery and should not encourage departure from the management plan outlined above.[38]

The operation of adrenalectomy

Regardless of the size of the tumour the normal procedure is to undertake total extirpation of the adrenal gland on the affected side. During bilateral adrenalectomy the implantation of part of the residual normal adrenal gland into a muscle (as in parathyroid autotransplantation) has only rarely been shown to be successful at retaining adrenal cortical function and should not normally be attempted.

The routes by which the adrenal may be removed are:

1. Open
   (a) the posterior approach
   (b) the posterolateral approach
   (c) the transperitoneal anterior approach

2. Laparoscopic
   (a) transperitoneal
   (b) retroperitoneal

Open methods (Figs 3.15 and 3.16)

The posterior approach described in 1936 by Hugh Young[39] is the most direct route to the adrenals. It involves a nearly vertical posterior incision in the lumbar muscles with division of the neck of the 12th rib. Both adrenals can be approached synchronously through two parallel incisions with the patient prone. This can be technically difficult especially in obese patients and those with Cushing's syndrome.

The posterolateral loin approach is perhaps the most popular open approach and is familiar as a standard approach to the kidney.

Figure 3.15
CT-guided biopsy of an incidentally discovered non-functioning adrenal tumour.

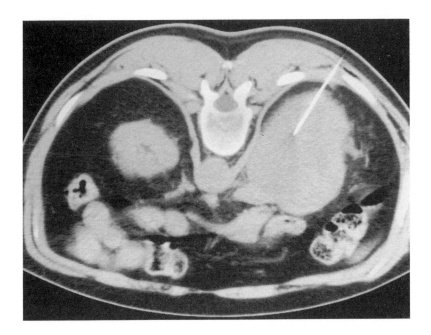

Figure 3.16
Posterior surgical approaches to the adrenal gland. On the left side of the illustration the semivertical curved incision over the necks of the 11th and 12th ribs made in the true posterior (Hugo Young) approach. On the right an incision along the 12th rib. When undertaken with the patient in the side up position, this incision begins more laterally, continues more anteriorly and extends beyond the tip of the 12th rib.

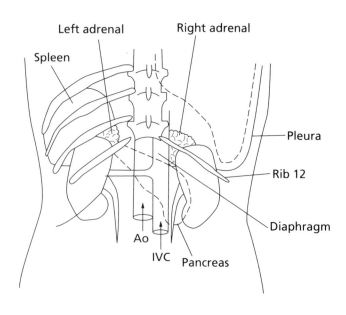

The patient is positioned with the affected side up and the table 'broken'. The incision approaches the adrenal via the bed of the 12th rib or, in thin patients, below it. The approach is extraperitoneal though the peritoneum can be opened if necessary. If the tumour is very large and invasive a higher thoraco-abdominal incision can be used though this is rarely needed.

The open transperitoneal approach is normally only used for bilateral adrenalectomy in Cushing's disease when pituitary surgery has failed. A transverse or 'roof-top' incision allows good access in all but the fattest patients. The open transperitoneal approach was traditionally employed when operating for phaeochromocytoma

Figure 3.17
The three anterior incisions for approach to the adrenal gland. The choice of incision depends on the size and habitus of the patient.

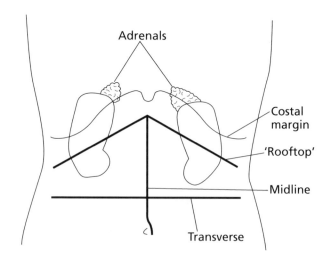

to allow the abdomen to be explored for a second or ectopic phaeochromocytoma. Modern preoperative imaging renders this unnecessary.[40] The technical details of adrenalectomy are outside the scope of this chapter but the following 'tips' are offered in relation to open adrenalectomy.

1. A right adrenalectomy is more difficult than a left.
2. The kidney is invaluable as a retractor and the plane between it and the adrenal should be left undissected until the cranial extremity of the adrenal is freed.
3. The adrenal emerges from the posterior aspect of the IVC and in anterior approaches careful rotation of the cava by an assistant helps to identify the adrenal vein.
4. The clipping or ligature of the short right adrenal vein must be absolutely secure; a slipped ligature or clip may leave an alarmingly large hole in the side of the IVC. A small Satinsky vascular clamp should always be at hand to deal with this eventuality.
5. A dangerous pitfall is the extra or ectopic right adrenal vein arising from the hepatic veins and easily torn during mobilisation.
6. When using the transperitoneal route it is easier to approach from the side after reflecting the splenic flexure of the colon, the spleen and the tail of the pancreas medially than it is to reach the adrenal by way of the lesser sac.
7. Accessory veins may arise from the ascending phrenic vein but are easily controlled.

Laparoscopic route

Laparoscopic adrenalectomy is a new technique.[41] Although the techniques of laparoscopic adrenalectomy are still being developed it can be used for routine, non-malignant tumours less than 10 cm in diameter. The necessary expertise must, however, be available and many centres have found the combination of a surgeon's skills in laparoscopy with a second surgeon skilled in open adrenalectomy to be a safe and effective team. Figures from large series are not yet available by which to judge the expected average operating time (probably about 90 min) and the proportion requiring conversion to open operation (probably about 10%).

The anterior approach can be undertaken with the patient supine or in the side-up position as is used for the standard loin open approach. Four or more 10 mm ports will be needed and crucial implements include an articulated liver retractor, multifire clip applicator and a suction irrigator. There is, as yet, no available instrument suitable for holding the gland effectively without rupturing a delicate adenoma or crushing a functioning phaeochromocytoma. The anterior laparoscopic approach appears to be safe for phaeochromocytoma as

Figure 3.18
Technique of laparoscopic retroperitoneal adrenalectomy showing the use of a balloon to establish an extra peritoneal space adjacent to the adrenal. This technique is currently less commonly used than the straightforward anterior transperitoneal laparoscopic approach. Modified from reference 42.

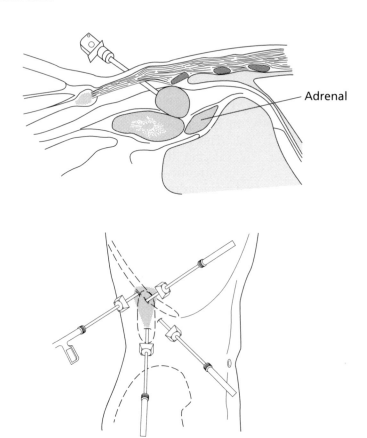

Adrenal

there is minimal manipulation of the gland prior to clipping of the adrenal vein.

Although most surgeons are currently employing the anterior approach, the alternative laparoscopic approach involves the creation of a retroperitoneal space beside the kidney and adrenal gland using an inflatable balloon.[42] No good comparative figures between transperitoneal and retroperitoneal approaches are yet available.

References

1. Cushing HW. The basophil adenomas of the pituitary body and their clinical manifestations. Bull Johns Hopkins Hosp 1932; 50: 137–95.
2. Yanovski JA, Cutler GB. Glucocorticoid action and the clinical features of Cushing's syndrome. Endocrinol Metab Clin North Am 1994; 23: 487–509.
3. Ross EJ, Lynch CD. Cushing's syndrome: killing disease. Lancet 1982; ii: 646–9.
4. Perry RR, Neiman LK, Cutler GB *et al.* Primary adrenal causes of Cushing's syn-

drome. Ann Surg 1989; 210: 59–68.
5. Crapo L. Cushing's syndrome: a review of diagnostic tests. Metab Clin Exp 1979; 28: 955–77.
6. Bouloux P-MG, Rees LH (eds). Diagnostic tests in endocrinology and diabetes. London: Chapman & Hall Medical, 1994.
7. Upton GV, Amatruda TT. Evidence for the presence of tumour peptides with corticotrophin-releasing-factor-like activity in the ectopic ACTH syndrome. N Engl J Med 1971; 285: 419–24.

8. Samuels MH, Loriaux DL. Cushings syndrome and the nodular adrenal gland. Endocrinol Metab Clin North Am 1994; 23: 555–69.

9. Grant CS, Carney JA et al. Primary pigmented nodular adrenocortical disease: diagnosis and management. Surgery 1986; 100: 1178–84.

10. Zovickian J, Oldfield EH, Doppman JL et al. Usefulness of inferior petrosal sinus venous endocrine markers in Cushing's disease. J Neurosurg 1988; 68: 205–10.

11. Becker MB, Aron DC. Ectopic ACTH syndrome and CRH mediated Cushing's syndrome. Endocrinol Metab Clin North Am 1994; 23: 585–606.

12. Sheeler LR. Cushing's syndrome and pregnancy. Endocrinol Metab Clin North Am 1994; 23: 619–27.

13. Watanabe Y, Izumi Y, Yagugi T. Pregnancy in Cushing's syndrome. Folia Endocrinol Japon 1992; 68: 1130–49.

14. Percapio B, Knowlton AH. Radiation therapy of adrenal cortical carcinoma. Acta Radiol Ther Phys 1976; 15: 288–92.

15. Hogan TF, Citrin DL, Johnson BM et al. o'p-DDD (Mitotane) therapy of adrenal cortical carcinoma. Cancer 1978; 42: 2177–81.

16. Venkatesh S, Hickey RC, Sellin RV et al. Adrenal cortical carcinoma. Cancer 1989; 64: 765–9.

17. Young MB, Hughes IA. Response to treatment of congenital adrenal hyperplasia in infancy. Arch Dis Child 1990; 65: 441.

18. Young Jr WFJ, Klee G. Primary aldosteronism. Endocrinol Metab Clin North Am 1988; 17: 367–95.

19. Bouloux LH, Rees LJ (eds). Diagnostic tests in endocrinology and diabetes. London: Chapman & Hall, 1994; pp. 166.

20. Young WF, Hogan MJ, Klee GG et al. Primary aldosteronism: diagnostic treatment. Mayo Clin Proc 1990; 65: 96–110.

21. Gleason PT, Weinberger MH, Pratt JH et al. Evaluation of diagnostic tests in the differential diagnosis of primary aldosteronism. J Urol 1993; 150: 1365–8.

22. Aboud E, De Suriet M, Gordon H. Primary aldosteronism in pregnancy – should it be treated surgically? Irish J Med Sci 1995; 764: 279–80.

23. St John Sutton MC, Sheps SG, Lei JT. Prevalence of clinically unsuspected phaeochromocytoma: review of a 50-year autopsy series. Mayo Clin Proc 1981; 56: 354–60.

24. Bravo EL, Gifford RW, Manger WM. Adrenal medullary tumours; phaeochromocytoma in endocrine tumours. In: Mazzaferri EL, Samaan NA (eds). Endocrine tumours. Boston: Blackwell, 1993; pp. 426–47.

25. Johns VJ, Brunjes S. Phaeochromocytoma. Am J Cardiol 1962; 9: 120–5.

26. Kran NN. Clinically unsuspected phaeochromocytomas: experience at Henry Ford Hospital and a review of the literature. Arch Intern Med 1986; 146: 54–7.

27. O'Riordain DS, O'Brien T, Crotty TB et al. Multiple endocrine neoplasia type 2B: more than an endocrine disorder. Surgery 1995; 118: 926–42.

28. Richard D, Beigelman C, Duclas J-M et al. Phaeochromocytoma as the first manifestations of Von Hippel–Lindau disease. Surgery 1994; 116: 1076–108.

29. Sheps SG, Jiang N, Klee GG, Van Heerdan JA. Recent developments in the diagnosis and treatment of phaeochromocytoma. Mayo Clin Proc 1990; 65: 88–95.

30. Peplinski GR, Norton JA. The predictive value of diagnostic tests for phaeochromocytoma. Surgery 1994; 116: 1101–10.

31. Deoreo GA, Stewart BH, Tarazi RC, Gifford RW. Preoperative blood transfusion in the safe surgical management of phaeochromocytoma. J Urol 194; 111: 715–21.

32. Scheker JC, Chowers I. Phaeochromocytoma and pregnancy. Review of 89 cases. Obstet Gynecol Surv 1971; 26: 729–47.

33. Dreier DT. Thompson NW. Phaeochromocytoma and pregnancy: the epitome of high risk. Surgery 1993; 114: 1148–52.

34. Averbuch SD, Steakley CS, Young RC et al. Malignant phaeochromocytoma. Ann Intern Med 1988; 109: 267–73.

35. O'Dorisio MS, Qualman SJ. Neuroblastoma. In: Mazzaferri EL, Samaan NA (eds). Endocrine tumours. Boston: Blackwell, 1993.

36. Rosen EM, Cassady JR, Frantz CN et al. Neuroblastoma. J Clin Oncol 1984; 2: 719–32.

37. Herrera MF, Grant CS, Van-Heerden JA et al. Incidentally discovered adrenal tumours; an institutional perspective. Surgery 1991; 110: 1014–21.

38. Gajraj H, Young AE. Adrenal incidentalomas. Br J Surg 1993; 80: 422–6.

39. Young HH. A technique for simultaneous exposure and operation on the adrenals. Surg Gynecol Obstet 1936; 63: 179–88.

40. Orchard T, Grant CS, Van-Heerden JA, Weaver A. Phaeochromocytoma, continuing evolution of surgical therapy. Surgery 1993; 114: 1153–9.

41. Gagner M, Haeroix A, Prinz RA *et al.* Early experience with laparoscopic approach to adrenalectomy. Surgery 1993; 114: 1120–3.

42. Parrilla P, Lujan JA, Rodrigues JM *et al.* Initial experience with endoscopic retroperitoneal adrenalectomy. Br J Surg 1996; 83: 987–8.

4 Familial endocrine disease – genetics and early treatment

Radu Mihai
John R. Farndon

Familial endocrine diseases form a group of very rare conditions producing much clinical and scientific interest. Most practitioners should be aware of these problems since some can be life threatening. Recent development of genetic tests allows less invasive screening and this has a major impact on the management of such patients. It is hoped that early detection may translate into more effective therapy.

This chapter will focus on several endocrine diseases with an inherited pattern:

- MEN1 syndrome (multiple endocrine neoplasia syndrome type 1)
- MEN2 syndromes and familial medullary thyroid carcinoma
- Familial papillary carcinoma of the thyroid
- Familial hyperparathyroidism syndromes
- Phaeochromocytoma as part of von Recklinghausen and von Hippel–Lindau syndromes
- Familial primary hyperaldosteronism
- Carney syndrome

MEN1 syndrome

Multiple endocrine neoplasia syndrome (MEN1) is a rare condition, inherited as an autosomal dominant disease with high penetrance and no special geographical, racial or ethnic preferences. Patients present with tumours of the parathyroid glands, pancreatic islets and anterior pituitary. Since 1954 when Wermer reported the first family, considerable insight into the genetics and management of this syndrome has been achieved.

Incidence and geographical distribution

The true incidence of MEN1 is unknown, since there are no long-term, population-based studies. The disease prevalence is estimated to be in the range of 20 to 200 per million but this may be an underestimate of the real penetrance because of the lack of recognition of the syndrome.

The largest-known genealogy of a kindred with MEN1, dating back to 1840, has been constructed in Tasmania. An initial study[1] of over 600 descendants of one English migrant and his spouse suggested that overall, one-quarter of all family members, and one-half of those above the age of 40 manifest one or more endocrine tumours. In the majority, the diagnosis was not suspected until the practitioner was informed of the family history, since symptoms were vague, sometimes bizarre, and overlapped with those of common disorders. More detailed analysis of nearly 2000 descendants of this English immigrant[2] found MEN1 to be highly probable in 130 and moderately probable in 22. Another 242 children and siblings were 50% likely to have inherited this dominant gene. In all age groups, especially the elderly, the majority of affected members had symptoms of only one endocrine disorder or were asymptomatic. In teenagers the most common presentation was pituitary lesions and the second most common insulinomas, and these often developed before hyperparathyroidism. Elevation of gastrin levels, usually associated with hypercalcaemia, was rarely seen in patients younger than 25 years. These data confirm that the familial specificity of the clinical picture varies and the classic presentation (i.e. with symptoms of multiple endocrinopathy) may represent only a small fraction of patients with MEN1 in the community.

In addition to the classical form of MEN1, a related syndrome was first described in the Burin peninsula ($MEN1_{burin}$) and links hyperparathyroidism, prolactinoma and carcinoids and a lower frequency of pancreatic endocrine tumours. All the five families identified in Newfoundland and the Pacific Northwest have the same *PYGM* allele and flanking polymorphic markers of the MEN1 gene.[3]

Morbidity and mortality

Few data are available on the natural history of untreated MEN1 syndrome. In a retrospective study of recorded medical data from 1861 to 1991 the causes of death were determined in a large MEN-1 kindred (159 patients).[4] Of 46 deaths in those classified as 'highly probable' of having MEN1, 20 died of a recognised complication of MEN1 (12 of malignant neoplasm, six of renal calculi and two of peptic ulcer). If accidental deaths are excluded, 50% of the deaths were the result of MEN1, and the mean age of death (50.9 years) was significantly younger than that of other family members. It was concluded that MEN1 leads to premature death, malignant neoplasms being the main cause.

Early diagnosis through prospective screening and the current therapeutic approach should improve the quality of life and decrease the morbidity/mortality associated with MEN1 tumours.

Aetiology

The predisposing genetic defect for MEN1 has been assigned to the long arm of chromosome 11.[5] Loss of heterozygosity at this site has been detected for all typical MEN1 families, proving deletion of the allele at 11q13 derived from the unaffected parent. Inactivation of the wild-type MEN1 allele inherited from the unaffected parent by variable extensive deletions unmasks a constitutional mutation (inherited from the affected parent) in an as yet unidentified gene with tumour suppressor function.[6] Congenital abnormality of one allele of this putative tumour suppressor gene is carried in the germ line of parathyroid, pituitary and pancreatic cells and tumour growth is initiated by a secondary, somatic mutation, affecting the normal allele. Each tumour in MEN1 is thus monoclonal but apparently arises in a background of polyclonal hyperplasia and the patients are prone to have multiple synchronous or asynchronous lesions. Because the secondary mutation occurs randomly, sometimes with an appreciable time lag, the patients may present a variable number of microscopic and macroscopic tumours.

The MEN1 locus is estimated to be one tenth of chromosome 11 and may contain about 30 genes (still to be identified). Efforts to identify the candidate gene(s) for MEN1 continue.

One of the cDNA mapped within the MEN1 locus represents the phospholipase C beta 3 (PLC-β3) gene. PLC-β3 is an enzyme linked to activated subunit of G-proteins and generates inositol trisphosphate (involved in intracellular calcium homeostasis) and diacylglycerol; the last is responsible for the activation of protein kinases C (PKC) involved in cell growth activation and proliferation. The role that PLCβ3 plays in signal transduction makes it a good candidate for being involved in oncogenesis in MEN1 related tumours. Strong evidence is offered by the equal expression of PLCβ3 gene in all tissues affected in MEN1 (parathyroid, pancreatic beta cells, adrenal cortex, anterior pituitary) and the lack of PLCβ3 expression found in some endocrine tumours is consistent with a tumour-suppressor function.

Plasma of MEN1 patients contains a mitogenic factor with structural analogy with bFGF (basic fibroblast growth factor) and a bFGF-related gene is known to be localised at 11q13. Interest was raised by the observation that mitogenic activity is high in known gene carriers; it may precede overt endocrine hyperfunction and the high levels of the mitogen correlate with parathyroid (but not pancreatic or pituitary) function.[7] Even if genetic studies ruled out this bFGF-like gene as the MEN1 gene, it can be speculated that a phase of polyclonal expansion, triggered or sustained by this growth factor may precede the monoclonal expansion of the parathyroid clone precursor. A conclusive model of its role will be offered only when both the MEN1 gene and the growth factor have been cloned and characterised.

Although monoclonality has been described in parathyroid adenomas and hyperplasia in MEN1 patients,[8] it does not correlate with the heterogeneous reduced expression and function of a putative calcium sensing protein regulating parathyroid hormone release.[9]

Presentation

The mode of presentation of MEN1 patients varies according to the index lesion and the nature/quantity of its secreted hormones.

Any of the three clinical components of MEN1 can be the presenting manifestation, but there is a propensity for specific patterns of organ involvement or peptide overproduction with distinct and identifiable family-specific syndromes.[10] Unlike sporadic patients (non-familial), MEN1 tumours are often multicentric, are commonly associated with hyperplasia and have a higher rate of recurrence.

Clinical diagnosis within probands requires identification of at least two lesions classically associated with MEN1 although only one is sufficient in members of established kindreds. Some tumours remain asymptomatic for a long time although associated with hormonal excess.

Because of age-dependent penetrance, most individuals carrying the MEN1 predisposing genetic defect do not develop clinical manifestations until the third decade of life and by the time the clinically overt syndrome appears, most patients are in the fourth decade. The advent of efficient prospective biochemical screening programmes has reduced the age at first diagnosis by two decades, to a mean age of 14–18 years.

Hyperparathyroidism (HPT)

This is the most common lesion in MEN1, with an estimated 90% prevalence in autopsy and screening studies. It is usually the first abnormality detected on screening and parathyroid glands are almost always hyperfunctional by the time islet cell or pituitary involvement becomes clinically evident. Patients are first detected in their teens and by age 40 more than 95% of patients have hypercalcaemia. The onset is gradual and clinically subtle and patients become symptomatic relatively late. The clinical picture is similar to sporadic HPT (see Chapter 1), apart from a greater incidence of peptic ulcer in MEN1 patients (due to occurrence of gastrinomas). Characteristically, multiglandular hyperplasia is found, with possible adenomatous transformation but one or more glands can be macroscopically and microscopically normal (Fig. 4.1).

Pancreatic islet cell tumours

Pancreatic islet cell tumours have a prevalence of 30–75% assessed by clinical screening techniques and 80% in necropsy analyses.[11] They are characteristically multicentric, slow growing and range from nesidioblastosis through adenomas to carcinomas. Multiple peptides might be secreted by a tumour, although usually only one predominates and

Figure 4.1 *One of the four enlarged hyperplastic parathyroid glands from a patient with MEN1 syndrome*

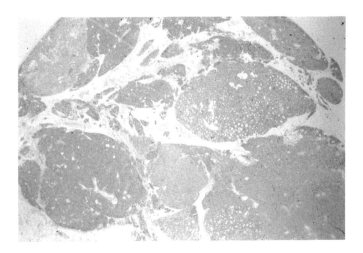

this pattern can vary from one sibling to another.

Most pancreatic tumours are detected by screening imaging of the pancreas or liver but some present after the development of specific symptoms due to hypersecretion of one or more peptide hormones or mechanical effects of a non-functional tumour. A spectrum of islet-cell tumours has been associated with the MEN1 syndrome, from the most frequently encounted insulinoma and gastrinomas, to Vasoactive Intestinal Polypeptide secreting adenoma (VIPoma), glucagonoma, somatostatinoma, Pancreatic Polypeptide (PP)-secreting and ectopic ACTH-secreting tumours.

Gastrinoma

Gastrinomas occur in 30–60% of patients with MEN1. Elevated serum gastrin levels induce gastric acid hypersecretion, which causes recurrent and multiple peptic ulcer, severe reflux oesophagitis and diarrhoea (Zollinger–Ellison syndrome, ZES). Many patients with ZES have small gastrinomas arising within the duodenal wall, which are small in size (1–2 mm), metastasise to the peripancreatic and periduodenal lymph nodes and rarely to the liver (10% of patients).[12]

Insulinoma

Insulinomas occur in up to 35% of patients with MEN1 and in 10–15% it will be the only functional component of pancreatic neuroendocrine disease. They tend to be multiple but multiple tumours in these patients are not always insulinomas unless proven by immunocytochemistry. Only a minority of tumours are metastatic.

Other pancreatic islet cell tumours

Glucagonomas cause hyperglycaemia and a characteristic rash – necrolytic migratory erythema. VIPoma is recognised by the association of watery diarrhoea, achlorhydria and hypokalaemia (Verner Morrison syndrome). hPP (human-pancreatic polypeptide) secretion by pancreatic tumours is frequently detected biochemically but clinically silent.

Pituitary adenomas

These can be detected in 15–40% of patients, although autopsy studies report up to 65% prevalence. Anterior pituitary hyperfunction is most commonly recognised during the fourth decade and manifests as hyperprolactinaemia (prolactinomas) and less commonly as acromegaly (growth hormone (GH) secreting adenoma) or Cushing syndrome *(adenocorticotrophic* hormone (ACTH) hypersecretion). Hyperthyroidism due to hypersecretion of thyroid stimulating hormone is extremely rare. Sometimes impaired vision (compression of optic chiasma by suprasellar extension of a pituitary adenoma) is the first sign of a pituitary tumour. The recurrence rate is higher than for sporadic tumours.

The differential diagnosis of a pituitary lesion should include ectopic secretion from pancreatic tumours inducing acromegaly (ectopic GHRH) or Cushing's syndrome (ectopic ACTH or corticotrophin releasing hormone (CRH)).

Other clinical manifestations

Neuroendocrine carcinoid-like tumours of the duodenum have been reported with high prevalence and they can secrete serotonin, somatostatin and gastrin (causing ZES). **Carcinoid tumours** may occur in the thymus and lung. **Thyroid neoplasia** (adenomas or differentiated carcinomas) are identified with increased frequency.

Adrenocortical adenomas and/or **macronodular hyperplasia** are discovered in one third of MEN1 patients radiologically or at autopsy (comparing with 10% of the general population), the majority being hormonally silent and without an aggressive course.[13] The presence of adrenal lesions seems to correlate with the extent of pancreatic disease: a CT/ultrasonographic analysis of a large Tasmanian MEN1 kindred identified adrenal disease in 75% of patients with pancreatic lesions and in 100% of those with pancreatic lesions and hepatic metastases, whereas none of the patients without pancreatic lesions had adrenal abnormalities.[14] The pathogenic mechanism for adrenal lesions in MEN1 patients is not understood since there is no hypothalamic-pituitary-adrenal dysfunction and the role of pancreatic hormonal hypersecretion is still hypothetical (i.e. similar to Cushing syndrome secondary to excess secretion of gastrin-inhibitory polypeptide).

Lipomas are more common than in the general population. **Pinealomas** and **impaired fertility** have been reported.

Screening for MEN1 syndrome

Presymptomatic detection and identification of gene carriers should be the screening strategy. Prospective screening studies in affected families have lowered the age of detectable onset to the mid-teens and most patients are detected before 25 years, but there is still no clearly demonstrated reduction in mortality by early diagnosis (in contrast to the effects on survival after screening for MEN2 syndrome). A consensus regarding the optimal and cost-effective MEN1 screening programme design is still lacking.

Genetic screening

DNA-based methods are now employed to distinguish gene carriers in MEN1 families since the risk estimated for carrying the defective gene is greater than 99.5%.[15] Non-carriers are excluded from repeated biochemical testing whereas gene carriers are subjected to annual biochemical investigation from the onset of adolescence (above 10–15 years of age). Identification of gene-carrier status at an early age makes it possible for family members to make informed decisions regarding childbearing.

The MEN1 gene itself has not been isolated, direct mutation analysis is not possible and the diagnosis relies on demonstrating the presence/absence of the allele 11q13 (MEN1 locus) identified in at least two affected members of the same family. A panel of flanking polymorphic DNA markers that segregates with MEN1 in a given family are used for linkage analysis and restriction fragment length polymorphism to identify gene carriers with great accuracy (for a review see reference 16).

Biochemical screening

Measurement of serum calcium (ionised or total corrected for albumin), PTH, prolactin and basal serum gastrin are performed every 3 years. Because an optimal interval between screening investigations has not been identified, some groups recommend annual investigations. More extensive screening is recommended by other groups (Table 4.1,)[10] but compliance is greater if screening tests are kept simple and regular. On the other hand serum gastrin, prolactin and calcitonin are needless screening determinations in patients undergoing surgery for primary hyperparathyroidism with no symptoms of MEN syndromes.[17]

Biochemical evaluation of individual tumours

Hyperparathyroidism is diagnosed using the same criteria as in those with sporadic disease, with hypercalcaemia accompanied by elevated/non-suppressed plasma PTH.

Basal gastrin levels as a sole marker would reveal only 20% of these lesions at the time of diagnosis. On the other hand, increased basal levels are not normally found in MEN1 microadenomas and should

Table 4.1 *Biochemical screening profile for MEN1 patients*

Test	Comments
Plasma calcium (ionised/albumin corrected)	Measuring PTH with ionised plasma calcium allows earlier detection than albumin-corrected plasma calcium levels
PTH	Biterminal assays for intact PTH
Prolactin	
Gastrin	Consider stimulation tests
Glucose	
IGFI	
Insulin	Fasting up to 3 days and consider stimulation tests
Proinsulin	
Glucagon	
Pancreatic polypeptide	
Meal test with PP and gastrin measurements	PP elevation twice the ref. range after a test meal indicates the necessity for surveillance of tumour development

be regarded as an indicator of a large pancreatic tumour (with a 50% risk of malignancy) or a duodenal carcinoid. Responses of serum gastrin and PP levels to a meal stimulation test are advocated to improve the sensitivity of the diagnosis; a 560 kcal meal rich in carbohydrates and low in proteins is recommended.[18] A meal-stimulated response twice the normal basal values for gastrin and exceeding by two standard deviations the mean serum PP levels in a control group should lead to enhanced observation and additional investigation. Exaggerated serum gastrin responses appear in approximately one half of patients and serum PP in all patients with verified pancreatic tumours. This test is described as being equally useful in the diagnosis of gastrinomas, PPomas, VIPomas, somatostatinomas, glucagonomas and non-functional pancreatic tumours.

In patients suspected of having an insulinoma, blood samples for glucose, insulin and proinsulin levels should be obtained during episodes of symptomatic hypoglycaemia. Hypoglycaemia and hyper-insulinaemia (and high C peptide levels, to exclude factitious hypoglycaemia) during symptomatic episodes and an elevated ratio of serum proinsulin to insulin are diagnostic. Simultaneous measurement of plasma glucose and insulin levels during a fasting period (up to 72 h) is widely used as a 'provocative' test. A rapid calcium infusion

(2 mg kg^{-1} min^{-1}) is also a potent insulin secretagogue in patients with insulinoma.[19]

Extended investigations including chromogranins, human chorionic gonadotropin subunits, VIP, calcitonin, ACTH, somatostatin and serotonin should be reserved for patients with positive radiology but normal/equivocal elevated routine screening markers. After surgery for pancreatic tumours it is important to include these markers in the follow-up criteria since relapse or liver metastases could produce hormones different from those secreted by the initial tumour.

Pituitary tumours are most readily diagnosed by prolactin and somatomedin C determinations and pituitary imaging (MRI) every 5 years. Since pancreatic tumours can be the source of ectopic GHRH or CRH/ACTH secretion, plasma levels of releasing hormones should also be measured in patients with acromegaly or Cushing's syndrome.

Radiological screening

Imaging studies for parathyroid tumours are not worthwhile unless HPT recurs and repeated surgery is anticipated (see Chapter 1).

Pancreatic tumours are not easy to localise. A multicentric study[20] found that none of the localising techniques have reassuring accuracy rates in most centres: computed tomography (CT) scanning (33.3%), ultrasonography (39.2%) and arteriography (61.6%) being less sensitive than the more invasive percutaneous transhepatic portography (88.7%). In recent years endoscopic and intraoperative ultrasound became very reliable/efficient (Fig. 4.2) but peroperative palpation sometimes remains the only method to unmask some of these pancreatic tumours.

Figure 4.2
Endoscopic ultrasound image of a pancreatic gastrinoma. The transducer is located in the stomach and is scanning the pancreas through the posterior gastric wall, demonstrating a 7 mm neuroendocrine tumour in the pancreatic body (between marks). (Courtesy of Dr S Norton, Bristol Royal Infirmary)

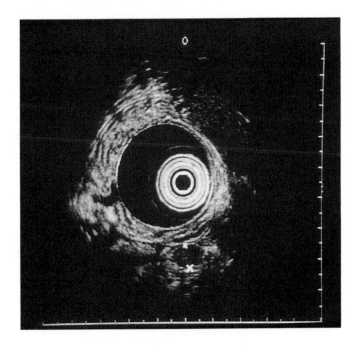

It is suggested that all patients with biochemically proven pancreatic tumours should have adrenal imaging because of the frequent association of the two lesions.

Other techniques

- Intraoperative pancreatic ultrasound.
- Portal venous sampling for pancreatic tumours. Sequential injection of secretin into the coeliac axis with subsequent hepatic vein sampling for gastrin has been reported to localise pancreatic gastrinomas better than angiography alone and to have less morbidity than transhepatic portal venous sampling.[21]
- Selective arterial catheterisation with calcium injection (as an insulin secretagogue) may be helpful for localising insulinomas.[22] Percutaneous transhepatic selective venous sampling of insulin for insulinomas is no longer considered to be necessary.
- Intraoperative selective intra-arterial secretin test with rapid radioimmunoassay for gastrin may be useful to determine whether an operation for Zollinger–Ellison syndrome was curative.[23] If the rapid test is not available, fasting gastrin levels of less than 100 pg ml^{-1} or an increase to less than 200 pg ml^{-1} after a secretin test is used as a biochemical test for cure.

Management options

Parathyroid tumours

Hyperparathyroidism in MEN1 patients begins in a subtle/non-agressive fashion and early surgical treatment is not required. However, some advocate early parathyroidectomy because hypercalcaemia is progressive and potentiates the pancreatic (and possibly the pituitary) disease.[21] All parathyroid tissue should be located and removed because the incidence of recurrent hyperfunction of a parathyroid remnant (if subtotal parathyroidectomy is performed) can exceed 50%. Therefore total parathyroidectomy plus autogenous grafting in the forearm is preferred. Several weeks might be required until the graft functions sufficiently to maintain normocalcaemia and the immediately postoperative hypoparathyroidism is corrected with oral calcitriol and calcium supplements. Parathyroid tissue from MEN1 patients should be cryopreserved for genetic testing or further autotransplantation (if the first failed).

Pancreatic tumours

The objective in all patients is to detect and excise tumours before any malignant potential is declared by hepatic metastases. Surgical treatment can be life-saving for patients with some tumours (insulinoma, VIPoma) and can eliminate the need for expensive daily drug therapy (gastrinoma). Patients with functional hormonal syndromes have one or more discrete tumours rather than islet-cell hyperplasia and microadenomatosis and therefore can be effectively treated by tumour excision without the need of extensive pancreatectomy.

Gastrinomas

The development of efficient antisecretory drugs (as omeprazole) allows effective medical management of ZES without the need for total gastrectomy for acute complications of peptic ulcer disease or unremitting symptoms. The disadvantages of medical therapy include life-long dependency, the possible progression of localised malignancy to lymph nodes and liver and the possible development of multiple enterochromaffin-like tumours, especially within the stomach.[24]

Enucleation should be attempted for lesions in the pancreatic head or duodenum. Distal pancreatectomy is performed for gastrinomas in the tail and body of the pancreas. Total pancreatectomy is reserved for patients with family members who have demonstrated aggressive tumour behaviour. Other surgical strategies include:

- Duodenotomy and palpation of the wall circumferentially from the pylorus to the third part. Small gastrinomas (<0.5 cm) are locally excised and larger gastrinomas are excised with a full thickness margin of duodenal wall;
- Excision of peripancreatic lymph nodes, including those along the common bile duct and within the porta hepatis medial to the coeliac axis;
- Full mobilisation of the head and uncinate process and enucleation of palpable or ultrasonically identified pancreatic tumour;
- Distal pancreatectomy (neck, body and tail), preserving the spleen when feasible.

Recurrent and/or metastatic disease occurs in 50% of patients.[25] Symptomatic therapy includes H_2 blockers, proton pump inhibitory drugs and octreotide. Partial hepatectomy and hepatic transplantation are palliative options in patients with hepatic involvement.

Insulinomas

Enucleation of the insulinoma is the best option. Blind 'subtotal pancreatectomy' is not advisable. Inoperable metastatic insulinomas or recurrent disease can be treated with diazoxide and chemotherapy (streptozocin, dacarbazine and 5-fluorouracil). Octreotide is very effective in blocking pancreatic secretion and reduces the incidence of postoperative complications.

Pituitary tumours

Hypophysectomy plus external beam radiation may be curative for pituitary tumours but medical treatment is extremely efficient for prolactinomas (bromocriptine) and can be considered for acromegaly.

Other tumours

Carcinoids can usually be totally excised. Octreotide has been successfully used but interferon and palliative chemotherapy (metothrexate, cyclophosphamide, streptozocin, 5-fluoroaracil) have still an unproved efficiency.

Current areas of research

Cloning of the suppressor gene involved in the pathogenesis on MEN1 syndrome is a high priority. It will offer a more certain identification of familial patients and may help elucidate the simultaneous tumorigenesis in different endocrine glands. Characterisation of the protein encoded by this putative tumour-suppressor gene will increase the understanding of its role in cellular regulation.

MEN2 syndrome

Multiple endocrine neoplasia type 2 (MEN2) is an autosomal dominant syndrome with incomplete penetrance and varying expression. The thyroid, parathyroid and adrenal glands exhibit hyperplasia or tumours, which can be associated with a diversity of extraendocrine features. Three different forms of MEN2 are identified.

1. *MEN2A* refers to patients with medullary thyroid carcinoma (MTC) associated with phaeochromocytoma (in 50% of patients) and HPT (in 15–30% of patients). This association was first recognised by Sipple in 1961.[26]
2. *MEN2B* is the association of MTC, phaeochromocytomas, a general (not absolute) lack of parathyroid disease and a specific phenotype consisting of marfanoid body habitus, mucosal neuromas and intestinal ganglioneuromatosis. It accounts for approximately 5% of all cases of MEN2.
3. *MTC-only syndrome or familial MTC* (FMTC) refers to patients having inherited MTC without other endocrinopathy.

Aetiology

MEN2 is a familial cancer syndrome arising from a mutation in chromosome 10 (region 10p11.2-q11.2). Based on the frequent allele losses on several other chromosomes it was suggested that several genes contribute to tumour development in MEN2: an initiating locus on chromosome 10 and additional loci on chromosomes 1p, 3p, 9q, 13q, 17 and 22q.[27]

Recent studies demonstrated that germ line point mutations in the RET proto-oncogene segregate with the disease phenotype in MEN2 and FMTC.[28,29] Multiple mutations have been described and are currently being collected by a RET mutation consortium for confirmation of a predicted genotype–phenotype correlation.[30]

The RET proto-oncogene is located on chromosome 10 (region 10q11.2) and encodes a cell-surface glycoprotein related to the family of receptor tyrosine kinases that is expressed in derivates of neural-crest cells and whose ligand is still unknown (for a review see ref. 31). Alterations in one of its three functional domains are implicated in the development of MTC and rearranged versions of RET have also been described in up to 30% of papillary thyroid carcinomas.[32]

Point mutations affecting RET-extracellular domain (codon 609, 611, 618, 620 in exon 10 and 634 in exon 11) are found in 97% of patients with MEN2A and 96% of patients with isolated familial MTC. The catalytic core region of the tyrosine kinase domain is affected in almost all MEN2B patients due to changing of a highly conserved methionine (Met^{918}Thr, in exon 16). Mutations within the intracellular domain of RET (Glu^{768}Asp in exon 13 and Leu^{804}Val in exon 14) have been identified in a FMTC family.

A challenging issue concerns the relationship between genetic mechanisms for MEN2 and Hirschsprung's disease. A point mutation in the RET gene (Cys^{618}Ser) was described in two large unrelated MEN2A kindreds in which Hirschsprung's disease cosegregated.[33] It is suggested that specific mutations in cysteine codons 618 and 620 not only result in MEN2A or FMTC but can also predispose to Hirschsprung's disease with low penetrance.[34]

Mechanisms

C cells of the thyroid, adrenal medullary cells and cells of the autonomic plexus and ganglia of the alimentary tract all arise from the neural crest. A molecular abnormality affecting cells of this lineage could, therefore, readily account for all the dominant features of MEN2. The RET proto-oncogene is normally expressed in C cells, chromaffin and parathyroid cells.[35] Expression of an activated RET receptor in these cell types results in initiation of transformation but it seems likely that these mutations represent only the first step in the oncogenetic pathway.

The incidence of each RET gene mutation varies. In families with MEN2A and FMTC, 80–90% of patients have a mutated codon 634; mutations of codon 620 account for 6–8% of cases and less than 5% of patients have mutations in other codons. When codon 634 is affected, mutation of a single base changes a highly conserved cysteine (encoded by TGC sequence) to another amino acid (arginine (CGC), serine (AGC), tyrosine (TAC), phenylalanine (TTC), tryptophan (TGG)) with major functional implications.

RET is a proto-oncogene, which means that a single activating mutation of only one allele should be sufficient to cause neoplastic transformation. All RET gene mutations identified result in oncogenic activity of the RET protein. Mutations affecting the five cysteine residues of the extracellular domain (i.e. codon 634) activate the RET receptor and cause receptor monomers to dimerize, thereby mimicking the effects caused by the binding of a ligand to the receptor and inducing enhanced phosphorylation and constitutive activation of the tyrosine-kinase domain.

In MEN2B families, a single mutation in exon 16 of RET proto-oncogene (Met[918]Thr) is present in 95% of patients.[36] Codon 918 is part of the encoding for the pocket that recognizes the substrate for the receptor tyrosine-kinase; the mutated receptor is not only constitutively activated but also causes enhanced phosphorylation of a different set of substrate proteins (such as *c-src* and *c-abl*) resulting in cellular transformation. Although it is rare, the absence of this particular mutation of the RET proto-oncogene does not always exclude the diagnosis of MEN2B and in such families routine biochemical screening for medullary thyroid carcinoma and phaeochromocytoma must be maintained for all individuals at genetic risk.[37] Some patients with MEN2B occur 'de novo'[38] and the high incidence of newly discovered mutations could be due to the low reproductive rates of MEN2B patients (increased mortality, low marriage rates, impotence due to neurological problems).

Further evidence for the role of RET mutations in tumorigenesis was obtained by transfecting cell lines with the MEN2A (Cys[634]Arg) and MEN2B (Met[918]Thr) RET constructs. The Ret-MEN2A and Ret-MEN2B proteins are constitutively phosphorylated and their *in vitro* kinase activity is significantly higher than that of the wild-type protein.[39]

The mechanism for development of hyperparathyroidism in MEN2A is not obvious. It is not caused by increased levels of calcitonin since it is not associated with sporadic MTC or MEN2B syndromes. The role of RET in parathyroid development and pathogenesis of hyperparathyroidism remains unclear.

Presentation

MEN2 is inherited as an autosomal dominant trait and men and women are equally affected. Because of a near complete penetrance of the MEN2 gene, all gene carriers are likely to be affected. Clinical expression of each individual component of the syndrome in affected families is variable and not all the components of the syndrome must be present in each member of one family. Changes in the glands appear to be causally and temporally independent of each other and the time-lag between the development of each component of the syndrome varies. The first clinical manifestation of disease may occur during the second or even later decades. Once the diagnosis of an endocrine tumour known to be associated with MEN2 is achieved in a young patient, this should stimulate a search for other tumours in the patient and family because if diagnosed early, all MEN2 lesions are treatable and curable.

Clinical presentation of multiple endocrine neoplasia type 2A

Medullary thyroid carcinoma (MTC)

This is the most common manifestation and the hallmark of MEN2A. It will develop in 90% of gene carriers during life and approximately 20–25% of patients with metastasis will die of the disease.

MTC originates from the thyroid parafollicular cells (C-cells), which synthesise, store and secrete calcitonin. These cells derive from the embryonic neuroectoderm and are more numerous in the lateral upper two thirds of the thyroid (the usual location for MTC). In hereditary MTC, tumours are multicentric and bilateral and occur in a background of diffuse or nodular C-cell hyperplasia – the first abnormality observed in the thyroid gland of MEN2 patients, especially in screen-detected disease.

The age distribution depends on the method of detection, but the age at diagnosis of familial MTC (third decade for MEN2A and second decade for the MEN2B) is earlier than that for sporadic MTC or phaeochromocytoma (see Fig. 4.3). Figure 4.3 shows the percentage of cases not yet diagnosed as a function of age in 30 patients with MEN2 syndrome and 20 patients with sporadic, non-familial phaeochromocytoma. This time-course of diagnosis suggests that MTC appears before phaeochromocytoma but it has not been demonstrated whether

Figure 4.3 *Age and the diagnostic evolution of MTC and phaeochromocytoma in familial patients.*

From Endocrine Surgery, *IDA Johnston, NE Thompson (eds.), Butterworths International Medical Reviews, 1983, pp. 189–202.*

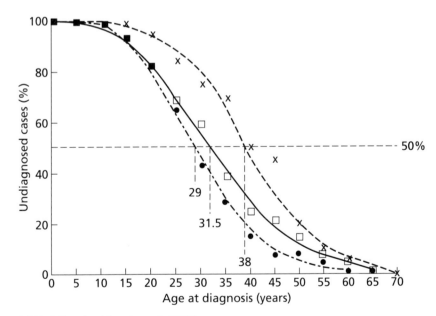

(●) Medullary thyroid carcinoma in MEN2;
(□) Phaeochromocytoma in MEN2;
(X) Sporadic, non-familial phaeochromocytoma

these data reflect a different biological expression of each tumour or are affected by our ability to screen/detect each tumour (i.e. the calcitonin provocation test may be a more incisive/accurate test than urinary cathecholamines).

Clinically apparent cases are identified when a unilateral or bilateral nodule or thyroid mass is found incidentally during a routine examination. A fine-needle biopsy shows characteristic changes for MTC, which can be confirmed by immunocytochemical staining for calcitonin. Metastases to cervical lymph nodes are present in half the patients with a palpable nodule, but distant metastases (lung, liver, bone) occur only late in the course of disease.

Diarrhoea is relatively common in patients with widespread tumours but can also be present at the time of first presentation. The causative humoural factor has not been identified.

Other peptides are secreted by tumoural C-cells, including CGRP (calcitonin-gene related peptide), chromogranin A, somatostatin, ACTH, CRH. Their clinical significance is not well understood apart from the possibility of developing Cushing's syndrome due to ACTH/CRH excess.

Phaeochromocytoma

Phaeochromocytoma was the cause of death of the first patient reported in Sipple's original description of MEN2. As a result of regular family screening, diffuse and nodular hyperplasia of the adrenal medulla are now diagnosed and recognised as precursors of phaeochromocytomas. The symptoms are subtle and may include intermittent headaches, palpitations and nervousness whereas paroxysmal hypertension is rather uncommon. Although the clinical presentation appears not to be severe, this is still a life-threatening condition.

Phaeochromocytomas in MEN2A patients are frequently bilateral but if unilateral it is usually associated with diffuse/nodular enlargement of the other side. Bilateral involvement of the adrenals varies between families and there is asynchronous tumour development. The frequency of malignant forms varies between kindreds but is rare.

Although often presenting later than MTC, phaeochromocytoma needs to be excluded before any operation on a patient known to have RET mutations.

Hyperparathyroidism

Hypercalcaemia and an elevated serum parathyroid hormone level occur in 10–25% of MEN2A patients. If symptomatic, the clinical presentation does not differ from sporadic cases (see Chapter 1) The median age at diagnosis is about 38 years but it is characterised by mild hypercalcaemia which is usually asymptomatic (85% of patients).[40] Generalised but asymmetric parathyroid hyperplasia is the most common histological abnormality.

Cutaneous lichen amyloidosis
Bilateral or unilateral pruritic and lichenoid skin lesions located over
the upper portion of the back have been described in five families
with MEN2A and are considered to be a variant of this syndrome.
It is due to deposition of amyloid at the dermis–epidermis interface
in the affected areas. Because in most patients it precedes the development of MTC, it could serve as a phenotypic marker of MEN2A.
The molecular mechanism is not established.

Clinical presentation of MEN2B syndrome

Distinctive clinical features are pathognomonic for MEN2B syndrome
and usually recognised in early life, making it possible to diagnose
MTC by identification of the phenotype.

Marfanoid habitus can be identified in up to 90% of patients.
It consists of a tall slender body, high arched palate and long
extremities. Arachnodactyly, joint laxity and skeletal deformities
(pes cavus, slipped femoral capital epiphysis, kyphosis, scoliosis,
lordosis) are less frequent. A minority of patients have peripheral
neuropathy, xerophthalmia, xerostomia, facial hyperhidrosis and
dental abnormalities. In contrast with true Marfan's syndrome,
no MEN2B patients have been reported to have ectopia lentis or
aortic abnormalities.

Ganglioneuroma phenotype is also evident in most MEN2B
patients. Neuromas of the anterior one third of the tongue are most
characteristic, but can also be identified on the lips, buccal mucosa,
conjunctiva and eyelids.

Mucosal neuromas of the ocular tissue can be demonstrated by slit
lamp examination and prominent corneal nerves, thickened eyelids
and subconjunctival neuromas can be demonstrated.

Gastrointestinal (GI) symptoms occur in 90% of patients and are a
major feature of the syndrome. Marked hypertrophy of nerve fibres
and an increased number of ganglion cells are present throughout
the GI tract and this diffuse intestinal ganglioneuromatosis causes
colonic motility dysfunction. Severe chronic constipation and diarrhoea, abdominal distension and crampy abdominal pain appear
early in life and precede detection of endocrine disease. Megacolon
and severe colonic diverticulosis are reported.[41]

Although the colonic pathology in MEN2B (ganglioneuromatosis) is
different from that in Hirschsprung's disease (aganglionosis), it is of
great interest that both diseases are related to similar genetic abnormalities in the intracellular tyrosine kinase domain of the RET
proto-oncogene.

Medullary thyroid carcinoma (MTC) in patients with MEN2B
presents at a younger age, as early as the first year of life and the
mean age at diagnosis is 16 years. It is associated with more extensive disease within the thyroid gland, has a higher incidence of
metastatic disease (which remains the main cause of death of patients
with MEN2B) and is much less amenable to surgical cure.[42]

It appears that the aggressiveness of MTC covers a spectrum decreasing from the most severe forms in MEN2B, to sporadic MEN2A to pure familial cases. However, some studies suggest that the natural course of MTC in MEN2B is comparable to that seen in MEN2A and that the major reason for difference in prognosis results from the earlier age of development of MTC in MEN2B.

Phaeochromocytoma occurs later than MTC but 50% of patients after 25 years of age will also have phaeochromocytomas. Its real incidence depends on the duration and intensity of follow-up. Often there are bilateral tumours or adrenal medullary hyperplasia.

Hyperparathyroidism is less common than in MEN2A.

Other associated problems related to health also occur with MEN2B syndrome. The threat of cancer at an early age, the trauma of multiple surgical procedures, the persistent GI symptoms, the skeletal and phenotypic abnormalities have disruptive effects on the psychological well-being and quality of life of patient and family.

Investigative techniques

Clinical examination is the best method of identifying the pathognomonic signs of the MEN2B syndrome. For patients with MEN2A, annual assessment for phaeochromocytoma includes a careful history plus physical examination (supine and erect blood pressure). Thickening of corneal nerves was suggested as a useful screening test for MEN2A but there is no relationship between prominent nerves and either the evolution of the disease or the occurrence of phaeochromocytomas.[43]

Screening for MEN2A and MEN2B syndromes

The need for screening programmes is evident since the penetrance of the gene is incomplete and a negative family history in a patient presenting with MTC or phaeochromocytoma is not a reliable exclusion of familial disease. If a high index of suspicion is maintained, new families with MEN2A are discovered regularly. At least 10% of consecutive, unselected, sporadic MTC are in fact familial and bilateral phaeochromocytomas should certainly prompt screening.

Genetic screening

The initial use of molecular linkage techniques could prove the primary genetic defect in the centromeric region of chromosome 10 with up to 95% accuracy when DNA extracted from two affected patients was compared with DNA from family members. The recent identification of point mutations of the RET proto-oncogene allows identification of gene carriers with 100% certainty in such families. Mutations are present in approx. 97% of MEN2A families[34] and in more than 93% of MEN2B families.[30] Identification of a mutation in a family enables certain determination of members who carry the

Table 4.2 *Methodologies for detection of a single nucleotide mutation of the RET proto-oncogene*[45]

Technique	Principle	Advantages	Disadvantages
Direct DNA sequencing	The Codons in exon 11 (634) and 10 (609, 611, 618, 620) are sequenced from both alleles of RET gene	The only methodology capable of identifying previously non-reported mutations	Technically complex Not easily automatised
Restriction enzyme analysis	80% of reported mutations create or destroy a restriction site. Gel electrophoresis is used to prove that the mutant allele is digested differently by one of a multitude of restriction enzymes available.	Can be used as a sole technique to identify a mutation in a family with a known DNA sequence abnormality	
Single-strand conformational polymorphism analysis	A single nucleotide change results in a conformational change that alters DNA mobility on a non-denaturing polyacrylamide gel	Simple, cost-effective method to identify patients with sequence abnormalities	Does not identify a specific mutation
Denaturating gradient gel electrophoresis analysis	The DNA denaturation is sequence-dependent; therefore, a single nucleotide change will generate a specific denaturation pattern		Uncertainty regarding the specificity of the result
Allele-specific oligonucleotide hybridization analysis	Oligonucleotides containing a normal codon 634 sequence or four mutant codons identified are dotted and immobilised on a membrane. Only perfectly matched DNA sequence from the PCR amplification will hybridise with a probe.	Simple and rapid to perform Ability to identify specifically the causative mutation Useful for screening of families in which a specific mutation has been identified by other techniques	It makes it necessary to synthesise and dot oligonucleotides with all possible mutations A previously undetected or unreported mutation will be missed

mutations and those who do not. Non-carriers are discharged from further regular biochemical screening tests, their risk being no greater than the normal population.

Genetic screening allows early identification of children at risk before any biochemical abnormality becomes evident[44] and allows total thyroidectomy to be recommended for gene-carrier children prior to the age of four.

Genetic DNA is extracted from peripheral blood white cells of at least one affected family member and from those at risk. Millions of DNA copies of a selected portion of RET proto-oncogene are made by polymerase chain reaction (PCR) starting from small fragments that are complementary to the RET gene (oligonucleotide primers) in the region of interest (exons 10, 11, 13, 16). The amplified DNA serves as the starting material for subsequent mutational analysis techniques. At least five methods are currently available to identify RET mutations[45] and some details about each of them are summarised in Table 4.2.

Although very rare, there are recognised sources of error in genetic testing: sample mix-up (can occur as frequent as 5%), contamination with DNA from patients with known RET mutations during laboratory evaluation, failure to amplify or copy both RET-alleles (resulting in the possibility of a false negative result if only the normal allele is included in the analysis). To minimise the impact of such errors on patient care, each analysis can be repeated (whether positive or negative) in a different laboratory on a sample obtained independently.

Biochemical screening

Before DNA-based predictive testing was available, all clinically unaffected first degree relatives were screened annually for MTC, phaeochromocytomas and hyperparathyroidism, from the age of 6 to the age of 35, by measuring pentagastrin-stimulated levels of calcitonin, 24-hour excretion of catecholamines and serum levels of calcium and parathyroid hormone.

Basal levels of calcitonin are not elevated in the early subclinical stages of MTC (premalignant C-cell hyperplasia and microscopic carcinoma) but these patients have an abnormal increase of calcitonin levels during stimulation tests with two secretagogues – calcium and pentagastrin. Because by the age of 30 nearly all gene carriers (95%) have a positive test[46] (Fig. 4.4) and because life-long annual testing is associated with low compliance and high costs, the calcitonin screening is stopped in adulthood.

Serum calcitonin levels in response to stimulation with pentagastrin (bolus injection of $0.5\ \mu g\ kg^{-1}$ body weight) are measured at 0, 1, 2, 5 and 10 minutes postinjection. A 1-minute calcium infusion ($2\ mg\ kg^{-1}$ body weight) can be associated with the pentagastrin injection. Because normal subjects also have detectable basal calcitonin levels and a response to provocative tests (higher in men than in women), interpretation of the results should be adapted to individual labora-

Figure 4.4
Age at which clinical evidence of MEN2A is detected by examination or biochemical screening in MEN2A gene carriers.

Adapted from Reference 46.

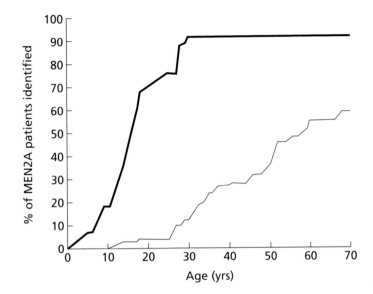

tories. C-cell hyperplasia (as seen occasionally adjacent to benign or follicular thyroid tumours and in Hashimoto's thyroiditis) can cause a false positive pentagastrin test. As with many other screening tests, overlap between normal and early abnormal tests can exist and family members with borderline values should be retested after 3–6 months.

Because there is considerable overlap between pentagastrin tests results in individuals who are RET mutation positive and those who are RET mutation negative, a coupling of pentagastrin test results and RET proto-oncogene analysis on all individuals at risk of developing MEN2A or FMTC appeared to be necessary for the decision to proceed with thyroidectomy.[47] However, the increasing specificity and accuracy of genetic testing makes it sufficient in modern practice.

The importance of early diagnosis is apparent. C-cell hyperplasia was encountered in children as young as 1.5 years old and MTC was documented in a child at 2.8 years of age in MEN2B. If the only evidence of MTC is a minimally increased (over basal values) peripheral plasma calcitonin level (between 250 and 1000 pg ml^{-1}) following provocative testing, the chance of curing the patient (postoperative stimulated plasma calcitonin level < 200 pg ml^{-1}) by total thyroidectomy is approximately 95%. Even if the preoperative stimulated plasma calcitonin level is between 1000 and 5000 pg ml^{-1}, surgery is curative in approximately 90% of patients. Conversely, when the preoperative stimulated plasma calcitonin level exceeds 10 000 pg ml^{-1}, the cure rate falls to 40%.[48]

Urinary catecholamine and metanephrine levels have sensitivity and specificity for diagnosis of phaeochromocytoma. In contrast with sporadic cases, a predominance of adrenaline over noradrenaline secretion can be documented. Because most tumours are evaluated while still small, repeated measurements are necessary to uncover the abnormal secretion of catecholamines, preferably in days when suggestive symptoms are present. Even if the urinary catecholamine values are within the normal range, any operation on a patient with proven RET mutation should be considered to carry the risk of a possible phaeochromocytoma. Pharmacological provocative tests are potentially hazardous and therefore frequently avoided, but physical exercise coupled with the calculation of adrenaline/dopamine ratio has been proposed as an alternative stimulation test for patients with MEN2.

Annual serum calcium is sufficient to exclude hyperparathyroidism in patients with MEN2. If elevated, measurement of intact PTH level is indicated.

Radiological screening

Localisation of MTC recurrence can be determined using radionuclide scanning with [201]Thallium, ^{99m}Tc-DMSA, ^{99m}Tc-sestamibi, ^{131}I-meta-iodobenzylguanidine (MIBG), CT and MRI. Radiolabelled monoclonal antibodies and labelled somatostatin receptors are being evaluated.

Imaging of the adrenals using [123]I- or ^{131}I-MIBG has a very good sensitivity (up to 100%) and detects unilateral or bilateral phaeochromocytomas but should not be used as a screening test (either at diagnosis or during follow-up).[49] CT scanning and T2-weighted MR images are important options in the balance between sensitivity, specificity, radiation exposure and cost.

Management options

A comparison between a screening approach or pentagastrin testing provides convincing cost-efficiency contrasts. Genetic testing currently costs approximately $250 per sample (possibly twice as much if the test is repeated) and needs to be carried out once only. A pentagastrin test with four calcitonin measurements costs $500 per test and needs repeating annually. Considering that biochemical testing will start at age 6 years and a mean age of 10 years for conversion of the pentagastrin test in a gene-carrier child, at least $2000 will be spent to identify a gene carrier. The costs will be much higher for non-carriers tested from age 6 to 35 years.[50]

MTC

The application of genetic screening to the management of hereditary MTC is advantageous because early thyroidectomy might be curative for MTC, is well tolerated and has no significant long-term impact on quality of life.

Long-term follow-up studies of families screened biochemically in which a decision for thyroidectomy relied on abnormal calcitonin levels (basal or stimulated) reported a 85% and higher 15–20-year cure rate. The ability to determine gene-carrier status in affected families provides an opportunity to improve this cure-rate. Two paradigms for clinical management of children with confirmed RET mutations have recently evolved. The first is to perform pentagastrin testing only in children with RET mutations and to perform total thyroidectomy at the time the test converts to abnormal (a similar approach as the previous screening protocols). The second is to perform total thyroidectomy at between 5 and 7 years of age in all children with RET mutations.[51] The 50% of family members without RET mutations are excluded from further screening in both paradigms. Most would favour the second paradigm because almost half the thyroidectomy specimens from RET-positive children with a normal pentagastrin test have microscopic MTC.[52] Up to 50% of children who convert from a normal to an abnormal pentagastrin test are found to have microscopic MTC.

Because surgery of MTC in the preclinical phase has a high probability of curing these patients, genetic screening soon after birth and total thyroidectomy in gene carriers as early as possible should improve the prognosis.[53] Metastases of MTC have been described within the first year of life and this is considered a supplementary reason to perform thyroidectomy as soon as possible (ideally in the first year of life) in children clinically suspected for MEN2B and confirmed by a codon 918 mutation analysis.[54] High incidence of lymph node metastases at the time of first operation for clinically apparent MTC oblige complete total thyroidectomy with routine dissection of the central compartment, removal of lymph nodes in the lateral neck compartment and upper mediastinum, but radical neck dissection does not give an improvement in long-term outcome.

Screening for MTC recurrence relies on calcitonin determination and debulking of macroscopic recurrence is still the best treatment option. None of the chemotherapeutic regimens has proved effective. Doxorubicin is the most effective single agent, but only 30% of patients will have partial responses. Palliative radiotherapy is used for bone pain and octreotide for symptomatic treatment.

Phaeochromocytomas

Because this is a generally late manifestation of MEN2 and is rarely associated with malignant transformation, annual or biannual biochemical screening for individual with RET mutations should suffice. If the diagnosis of phaeochromocytoma is made, surgery is performed 2–3 weeks after alpha receptor blockade. Bilateral adrenalectomy need not be carried out if one adrenal is normal but continued surveillance is required.

Hyperparathyroidism

The parathyroid disease is of secondary importance during neck exploration for MTC. Resection of enlarged parathyroid glands is sufficient for patients with no family history of hyperparathyroidism and a more aggressive approach is reserved for patients with a strong family history of parathyroid involvement.

Research interests in MEN2 syndromes

Apart from a major impact of genetic diagnosis on the management of the MEN2 syndrome, genotype–phenotype correlation studies in patients with identified RET mutations could define the RET signal transduction pathway and its role in the development of neural crest derivatives. Understanding the functions of the RET proto-oncogene and its complex involvement in development and oncogenesis may allow new approaches to treatment which might reverse or prevent tumour formation.

Familial medullary thyroid carcinoma (FMTC)

The occurrence of MTC with a familial inheritance but without the other endocrine or phenotype manifestations of MEN2A or 2B has been reported. In an evaluation of 213 patients from 15 kindreds with familial MTC, 41 such patients were identified.[55] There were no differences in the peak stimulated plasma calcitonin levels at the time of diagnosis or the incidence of regional lymph node metastases when compared with MEN2A subjects but the mean age at diagnosis was significantly higher in these patients than in patients with MEN2A (43.1 years versus 21.1 years), suggesting that MTC developed at a later age or grew more slowly. Its course is more benign than that of MEN2A or MEN2B and the prognosis is good.

In addition to RET mutations common with the MEN2A syndrome, germ-line mutations in exons 13 ($Glu^{768}Asp$) and 14 ($Val^{804}Leu$) of the RET proto-oncogene (involving the tyrosine kinase domain of RET) have been described recently in FMTC families.[56] Both mutations segregate with the disease in these four FMTC families and support the idea that FMTC is a condition different from MEN2A.

A unique kindred manifesting MTC and corneal nerve thickening without other aspects of the MEN syndrome has been described.[57] Of 11 family members spanning four generations seven have corneal nerve thickening and DNA sequence analysis for RET proto-oncogene showed that none of the affected individuals have mutations characteristic for MEN2A or MEN2B families. Linkage analysis showed cosegregation of alleles with the presence of both corneal nerve thickening and MTC/C-cell hyperplasia. This kindred appears to represent a true clinical overlap syndrome whose genetic basis may be distinct from the other syndromes.

Familial papillary carcinoma of the thyroid

Papillary carcinoma of the thyroid is usually sporadic, but occasionally may be familial. In an analysis of 226 consecutive patients with papillary carcinoma, 3.5–6.2% of patients were identified to have another affected relative and in a French series, seven out of 53 papillary carcinomas (13%) were considered to be familial. It was suggested that when two or more persons in a family have papillary carcinoma, all first- and second-degree relatives should have clinical evaluation.[58] Because familial papillary carcinoma is often multifocal, total thyroidectomy is recommended.[59] Because some of the affected patients might be diagnosed as having only a nodular goitre, thyroidectomy should be performed if a family history of papillary carcinoma is certain.

Gardner's syndrome (familial adenomatous polyposis) appears to be associated with a higher risk of thyroid carcinomas. This is an autosomal dominant syndrome consisting of multiple adenomatous polyps frequently in conjunction with osteomas, epidermoid cysts, desmoid tumours, retinal pigmentation and, more rarely, with adenomas in the upper gastrointestinal tract and pancreas and hepatoblastomas. Some have reported about 160 times enhancement of risk for thyroid cancer in young female patients when compared with normal subjects. Up to 90% of lesions were papillary carcinomas, the rest being follicular neoplasms. It predominates in woman (approx. 1:16 male: female ratio), appears at a relatively young age (twenties), and is frequently multicentric, with relatively low aggressiveness but with a significant risk of recurrence. These data suggest that close clinical observation for thyroid neoplasia is important in patients who have a personal or family history of familial adenomatous polyposis. It is unknown whether patients with PTC should have earlier or more frequent examinations for stool blood or sigmoidoscopy than the general population or what effect on clinical outcome such tests could have.

Cowden's syndrome is characterised by multiple mucocutaneous hamartomas, keratoses on hands, feet and mouth and fibrocystic disease of the breast. In a review of Cowden's syndrome, 8/26 patients had thyroid carcinoma (most commonly well differentiated) but little is known about the pathological characteristics and outcome of the thyroid lesion in these patients.

Familial hyperparathyroidism syndromes

MEN syndromes have been already discussed.

Familial isolated hyperparathyroidism (FIHP) is a rare heritable autosomal dominant disorder characterised by hypercalcaemia, inappropriately high PTH levels, and isolated parathyroid tumours with no evidence of hyperfunction of any other endocrine tissues which occur as a genetically and clinically distinct entity. More than 30 kindreds, mostly small, have been reported to display primary hyperparathyroidism only, with no evidence of other associated endocrinopathies.

A study of 19 family members, across four generations, from a large kindred, using DNA markers for MEN1 and MEN2A genes and two polymorphic markers for the prepro-PTH gene, has shown no linkage between FIHP and the MEN1 and MEN2A. In one individual, a parathyroid carcinoma was found after recurrence of hypercalcaemia. This report supports the concept that FIHP is a distinct autosomal dominant syndrome with an increased risk of malignant parathyroid

Table 4.3 *Familial syndromes with parathyroid function*

Dominant disorders	Recessive or uncertain transmission
• Cystic parathyroid adenomas with/without jaw tumours • Familial parathyroid hyperplasia	Parathyroid hyperplasia associated with: • Parathyroid carcinoma • Nephropathy and neural deafness • Colonic neoplasms • Carcinoid tumours of the foregut

transformation.[60] A similar conclusion was supported by the lack of any clinical, biochemical or genetic evidence of MEN syndromes in 37 members of a similar family.[61]

Although the relation with the MEN2 syndrome is still debatable at least in individual patients, it is suggested that isolated familial primary hyperparathyroidism is caused by mutation of a gene located in the MEN1 region on chromosome 11q13, possibly the MEN1 locus.

The association of **hereditary HPT** and **jaw fibroma** is a very rare condition. Jackson *et al.*[62] first described this syndrome and thereafter individual cases have been reported.[63] It associates HPT due to multigland disease and the presence of cementifying and ossifying fibromas of the mandible and/or maxilla (not to include bone lesions normally encountered in HPT, as the 'brown tumours of bone'). This disease is clinically and genetically different from MEN syndromes and appears to result from mutations on the long arm of chromosome 1, where a dominant oncogene (HRPT2) maps in the 1q21–31 region.[64]

Several familial syndromes with parathyroid hyperfunction have been described but some are documented only by individual case reports[65] (see Table 4.3).

Phaeochromo-cytoma as part of other familial diseases

In 10% of patients with phaeochromocytoma, the adrenal tumour is part of a familial disorder (i.e. MEN syndromes, von Recklinghausen disease, Von Hipple Lindau syndrome)

Von Recklinghausen disease is the eponym for type 1 neurofibromatosis (NF1), an autosomal dominant disorder produced by somatic mutations in NF1 gene on chromosome 17. Because of its variable expression, it is estimated that 1 in 3000 people have at least a minor variety of disease, but only 1% of these patients also have a phaeochromocytoma. Two or more of the following clinical criteria are necessary for the NF1 diagnosis and could raise the suspicion of a concomitant phaeochromocytoma:

• six or more café-au-lait spots (larger than 5 mm in prepubertal and 15 mm in postpubertal patients);

- two or more neurofibromas of any type or one plexiform neuro-fibroma;
- freckling in the axillary/inguinal region;
- optic glioma;
- two or more Lish nodules (pigmented hamartomas of the iris);
- distinctive osseous lesions (sphenoid dysplasia or thinning of long bone cortex ± pseudoarthritis);
- a first degree relative with NF1

Patients with type 2 neurofibromatosis do not have phaeochromo-cytomas.

Von Hippel–Lindau syndrome (VHL) includes retinal angio-matosis, haemangioblastoma of the central nervous system, renal cysts and carcinoma, pancreatic cysts, epididymal cystadenoma. In the adrenal glands, VHL may be associated with phaeochromocytomas, which occur more frequently in some families than in others but are quite common in families which have adrenal involvement. They are very rarely malignant (less than 1%).

Patients with VHL are screened yearly for a phaeochromocytoma. Recent data indicate that adrenal tumours are as much as four times more common among people with VHL than previously thought, and that traditional blood and urine tests are inadequate for detection. Clinical examination, ophthalmoscopy, fluorescein angiography and CT of the brain are used to identify other possible lesions. It is antic-ipated that DNA screening for a specific gene on the short arm of chromosome 3 will become available.

Familial primary aldosteronism

Primary aldosteronism can occur in two familial forms.

1. The ACTH-dependent and glucocorticoid-suppressible hyperaldo-steronism is attributed to adrenal hyperplasia since it has not so far been associated with tumours. This form is recognised as familial hyperaldosteronism type I.
2. Familial hyperaldosteronism type II has been only recently recognised: it is not glucocorticoid-suppressible and is frequently associated with aldosterone-producing adenomas.

Primary aldosteronism due to adrenocortical hyperplasia, adenoma, or carcinoma can also occur as part of the MEN syndromes.

The morphology of adrenocortical hyperplasia causing primary aldosteronism ranges from glomerulosa-like (idiopathic hyperplasia of the adrenals, responsive to angiotensin II) to fasciculata-like (glucocorticoid-suppressible hyperaldosteronism, unresponsive to angiotensin II). Both subtypes can be seen in a single family.[66]

Carney syndrome

Bilateral micronodular adrenal hyperplasia (primary pigmented nodular adrenal hyperplasia) is a very rare cause of Cushing's syndrome (1%), which can have a family inheritance as an autosomal dominant disorder or occur sporadically (in children and in adults less than 30 years).

The familial form associates with blue naevi, pigmented lentigines, cutaneous, mammary and atrial myxomas, pituitary somatotroph adenomas and testicular or other tumours (Carney complex).

Autoantibodies that stimulate adrenocortical growth and steroidogenesis are claimed to be involved in the pathogenesis but other autoimmune disorders are not common in these patients or their families.

References

1. Shepherd JJ. Latent familial multiple endocrine neoplasia in Tasmania. Med J Aust 1985; 142: 395–97.
2. Shepherd JJ. The natural history of multiple endocrine neoplasia type 1: highly uncommon or highly unrecognized? Arch Surg 1991; 126: 935–52.
3. Petty EM, Green JS, Marx SJ. Mapping the gene for hereditary hyperparathyroidism and prolactinoma (MEN1 burin) to chromosome 11: evidence for a founder effect in patients from Newfoundland. Am J Hum Genet 1994; 54: 1060–6.
4. Wilkinson S, Teh BT, Davey KR. Cause of death in multiple endocrine neoplasia type 1. Arch Surg 1993; 128: 683–90.
5. Weber G, Friedman E et al. The phospholipase C beta 3 gene located in the MEN1 region shows loss of expression in endocrine tumours. Hum Mol Genet 1994; 3: 1775–81.
6. Beckers A, Abs R, Reyniers E et al. Variable regions of chromosome 11 loss in different pathological tissues of a patient with MEN1 syndrome. J Clin Endocrinol Metab 1994; 79: 1498–502.
7. Marx SJ, Sakaguci K, Green J III et al. Mitogenic activity on parathyroid cells in plasma from members of a large kindred with multiple endocrine neoplasia type 1. J Clin Endocrinol Metab 1988; 67: 149.
8. Friedman E, Sakaguci K et al. Clonality of parathyroid tumours in familial MEN type 1. N Engl J Med 1989; 321: 213–18.
9. Carling T, Rastad J, Ridefelt P et al. Hyperparathyroidism of multiple endocrine neoplasia type 1: candidate gene and parathyroid calcium sensing protein expression. Surgery 1995; 118: 924–31.
10. Skogseid B, Eriksson B et al. Multiple endocrine neoplasia type 1: a 10-year prospective screening study in four kindreds. J Clin Endocrinol Metab 1991; 75: 76–81.
11. Vasen HF, Lamers CB et al. Screening for the multiple endocrine neoplasia syndrome type 1: a study of 11 kindreds in The Netherlands. Arch Intern Med 1989; 149: 2717–22.
12. Thompson NW. Surgical management of MEN1. J Intern Med 1995; 238: 269–80.
13. Skogseid B, Rastad J, Gobl A. Adrenal lesion in multiple endocrine neoplasia type 1. Surgery 1995; 118: 1077–82.
14. Burgess JR, Harle RA, Tucker P et al. Adrenal lesions in a large kindred with multiple endocrine neoplasia type 1. Arch Surg 1996; 131: 699–702.
15. Larsson C, Shepherd J et al. Predictive testing for multiple endocrine neoplasia type 1 using DNA polymorphism. J Clin Invest 1992; 89: 1344–9.
16. Larsson C, Calender A, Grimmond S et al. Molecular tools for presymptomatic testing in multiple endocrine neoplasia type 1. J Intern Med 1995; 238: 239–44.
17. Farndon JR, Geraghty JM, Dilley WG et al. Serum gastrin, calcitonin, and prolactin as markers of multiple endocrine neoplasia syndromes in patients with primary hyperparathyroidism. World J Surg 1987; 11: 253–7.
18. Skogseid B, Rastad J, Oberg K. Multiple endocrine neoplasia type 1 – clinical features

and screening. Endocrine Metab Clin North Am 1994; 27: 1–17.

19. Brunt LM, Dilley WG, Farndon JR. Evaluation of calcium as an insulin secretagogue in patients with insulinoma. Surg Forum 1984; 35: 49–52.

20. Rothmund M, Angelini L, Brunt LM et al. Surgery for benign insulinoma – an international review. World J Surg 1990; 14: 393–9.

21. Fraker DL, Norton JA. Controversy in surgical therapy for APUDomas. Semin Surg Oncol 1993; 9: 437–42.

22. Zeiger MA, Shawker TH, Norton JA. Use of intraoperative ultrasonography to localise islet cell tumours. World J Surg 1993; 17: 448–54.

23. Imamura M, Takahashi K. Use of selective intraarterial secretin injection test to guide surgery in patients with Zollinger–Ellison syndrome. World J Surg 1993; 17: 433–8.

24. Solcia E, Cappela C, Fiocca R et al. Gastric argyrophil carcinoids in patients with Zollinger–Ellison syndrome due to type 1 multiple endocrine neoplasia. Am J Surg Pathol 1990; 14: 503–13.

25. Grama D, Skogseid B et al. Pancreatic tumours in multiple endocrine neoplasia type 1: clinical presentation and surgical treatment. World J Surg 1992; 16: 611–18.

26. Sipple JH. The association of pheochromocytoma with carcinoma of the thyroid gland. Am J Med 1961; 31: 163–6.

27. Mulligan LM, Gardner E, Smith BA et al. Genetic events in tumour initiation and progression in multiple endocrine neoplasia type 2. Genes Chromosomes Cancer 1993; 6: 166–77.

28. Donis-Keller H, Shenshen D, Chi D et al. Mutations in the RET protooncogene are associated with MEN2A and FMTC. Hum Mol Genet 1993; 2: 851–6.

29. Mulligan LM, Kwok JBJ, Healey CS et al. Germline mutations of the RET proto-oncogene in multiple endocrine neoplasia type 2A. Nature 1993; 363: 458–60.

30. Mulligan LM, Marsh DJ et al. Genotype–phenotype correlation in MEN 2: report of the International RET mutations consortium. J Intern Med 1995; 238: 343–6.

31. Pasini B, Ceccherini I, Romeo G. RET mutations in human disease. Trends Genet 1996; 12(4): 138–44.

32. Carlson KM, Dou S, Chi D et al. Single missense mutation in the tyrosine kinase catalytic domain of the RET protooncogene is associated with multiple endocrine neoplasia type 2B. Proc Natl Acad Sci USA 1994; 91: 1579–83.

33. Borst MJ, VanCamp JM, Peacock ML, Decker RA. Mutational analysis of multiple endocrine neoplasia type 2A associated with Hirschsprung's disease. Surgery 1995; 117: 386–91.

34. Mulligan LM, Eng C, Attie T, Lyonnet S et al. Diverse phenotypes associated with exon 10 mutations of the RET proto-oncogene. Hum Mol Genet 1994; 3: 2163–7.

35. Pausova Z, Soliman E, Amizuka N et al. Expression of the RET protooncogene in hyperparathyroid tissues: implications for the pathogenesis of the parathyroid disease in MEN2A. J Bone Mineral Res 1995; 10 (suppl1): 249.

36. Eng C, Mulligan LM, Smith DP et al. Mutation of the RET protooncogene in sporadic medullary thyroid carcinoma. Genes Chromosomes Cancer 1995; 12: 209–12.

37. Toogood AA, Eng C, Smith DP, Ponder BAJ, Shalet SM. No mutation at codon 918 of the RET gene in a family with multiple endocrine neoplasia type 2B. Clinic Endocrinol 1995; 43: 759–62.

38. Carlson KM, Bracamontes J et al. Parent of origin effects in multiple endocrine neoplasia type 2B. Am J Hum Genet 1994; 55: 1076–82.

39. Borrello MG, Smith DP, Pasini B et al. RET activation by germline MEN2A and MEN2B mutations. Oncogene 1995; 11: 2419–27.

40. Raue E, Kraimps JL, Dralle H et al. Primary hyperparathyroidism in multiple endocrine neoplasia type 2A J Intern Med 1995; 238(4): 369–73.

41. O'Riordain DS, O'Brien T, Crotty TB et al. Multiple endocrine neoplasia type 2B: more than an endocrine disorder. Surgery 1995; 118: 936–42.

42. O'Riordain DS, O'Brien T, Hay ID et al. Medullary thyroid carcinoma in multiple endocrine neoplasia type 2A and 2B. Surgery 1994; 116: 1017–23.

43. Dupond JL, De Wazieres B, Fest T et al. Prominent corneal nerves in multiple endocrine neoplasia type 2A: another sign for familial screening? Eur J Intern Med 1995; 6: 177–8.

44. Frilling A, Dralle H, Eng C et al. Presymptomatic DNA screening in families with multiple endocrine neoplasia type 2 and familial medullary thyroid carcinoma. Surgery 1995; 118: 1099–104.

45. Wohllk N, Cote GJ, Evans DB et al. Application of genetic screening information to the management of medullary thyroid carcinoma and multiple endocrine neoplasia type 2. Endocrinol Metab Clin North Am 1996; 25: 1–25.

46. Ponder BA, Ponder MA et al. Risk estimation and screening in families of patients with medullary thyroid carcinoma. Lancet 1988; 1: 397–401.

47. Marsh DJ, McDowall D, Hyland VJ et al. The identification of false positive responses to the pentagastrin stimulation test in RET mutation negative members of MEN 2A families. Clin Endocrinol 1996; 44: 213–20.

48. Wells SA, Dilley WG, Farndon JA et al. Early diagnosis and treatment of medullary thyroid carcinoma. Arch Intern Med 1985; 145: 1248–52.

49. Bonnin F, Lumbroso J, Schlumberger M et al. Interest of MIBG scintigraphy in screening for pheochromocytoma in patients with medullary thyroid carcinoma. Med Nucl 1995; 19: 177–82.

50. Gagel RF, Cote GJ, Martin Bughalo MJG et al. Clinical use of molecular information in the management of multiple endocrine neoplasia type 2A. J Intern Med 1995; 238: 333–41.

51. Wells SA, Chi DD et al. Predictive DNA testing and prophylactic thyroidectomy in patients at risk for multiple endocrine neoplasia type 2. Ann Surg 1994; 220: 237–50.

52. Cote CJ, Wohhlk N, Evans D et al. RET proto-oncogene mutations in multiple endocrine neoplasia type 2 and medullary thyroid carcinoma. Bailliére's Clin Endocrinol Metab 1995; 9: 609–30.

53. Pacini F, Romei C, Miccoli P et al. Early treatment of hereditary medullary thyroid carcinoma after attribution of multiple endocrine neoplasia type 2 gene carrier status by screening for ret gene mutations. Surgery 1995; 118: 1031–5.

54. Samaan NA, Draznin MB, Halpin RE et al. Multiple endocrine syndrome type IIB in early childhood. Cancer 1991; 68: 1832–4.

55. Farndon JR, Leight GS, Dilley WG et al. Familial medullary thyroid carcinoma without associated endocrinopathies: a distinct clinical entity. Br J Surg 1986; 73: 278–81.

56. Bolino A, Schuffenecker I, Luo Y et al. RET mutations in exons 13 and 14 of FMTC patients. Oncogene 1995; 10: 2415–19.

57. Kane LA, Tsai MS, Gharib H et al. Familial medullary thyroid cancer and prominent corneal nerves: clinical and genetic analysis. J Clin Endocrinol Metab 1995; 80: 289–93.

58. Stoffer SS, Van Dyke DL et al. Familial papillary carcinoma of the thyroid. Am J Med Genet 1986; 25: 775–82.

59. Kraimps JL, Fieuzal S, Margerit D et al. Familial papillary thyroid cancers: coincidence or genetic cause. Lyon Chir 1994; 90: 16–18.

60. Wassif WS, Moniz CF, Friedman E et al. Familial isolated hyperparathyroidism: a distinct genetic entity with an increased risk of parathyroid cancer. J Clin Endocrinol Metab 1993; 77: 1485–9.

61. Kassem M, Zhang X, Brask S et al. Familial isolated primary hyperparathyroidism. Clin Endocrinol 1994; 41: 415–20.

62. Jackson CE, Norum RA et al. Hereditary hyperparathyroidism and multiple ossifying jaw fibromas: a clinically and genetically distinct syndrome. Surgery 1970; 108: 1006–13.

63. Inoue H, Miki H, Oshimo K, Tanaka K et al. Familial hyperparathyroidism associated with jaw fibroma: case report and literature review. Clin Endocrinol 1995; 43: 225–9.

64. Szabo J, Heath B, Hill VM et al. Hereditary hyperparathyroidism–jaw tumor syndrome: the endocrine tumor gene HRPT2 maps to chromosome 1q21-31. Am J Hum Genet 1995; 56: 944–50.

65. Mallette LE. Management of hyperparathyroidism in the multiple endocrine neoplasia syndromes and other familial endocrinopathies. Endocrinol Metab Clin North Am 1994; 23: 19–36.

66. Gordon RD, Stowasser M, Klemm SA, Tunny TJ. Primary aldosteronism – some genetic, morphological, and biochemical aspects of subtypes. Steroids 1995; 60: 35–41.

5 Endocrine tumours of the pancreas

Gary R. Peplinski
Jeffrey A. Norton

Introduction

Pancreatic endocrine neoplasms consist predominantly of gastrinomas and insulinomas, but more rare tumours may occur. All these tumours arise from neuroendocrine cells, display characteristic ultrastructural features, and biochemically are amine precursor uptake and decarboxylation cells (APUDomas). Pancreatic endocrine tumours, as a group, are different from most other neoplasms because they commonly produce physiologically uncontrolled levels of hormones, each of which may cause a clinical syndrome. The clinical syndrome identified and the detection of hormone proteins produced allow the classification of pancreatic endocrine tumours into specific types. Potentially life-threatening situations caused by hormone overproduction are a major reason to identify and resect these neoplasms. Some tumours may not secrete any immunohistochemically detectable or clinically relevant peptides and only cause symptoms of mass effect. Except for insulinomas, pancreatic endocrine neoplasms are malignant in a majority of cases.

Insulinoma

Background

In 1927, endogenous hyperinsulinism was first described and was the first syndrome of excessive pancreatic hormone production to be recognised.[1] Hyperinsulinaemia and consequent hypoglycaemia is the major cause of morbidity and potential mortality associated with insulinoma, a neoplasm arising from the pancreatic insulin-producing beta cells. It occurs in one person per million population per year (Table 5.1).[1] The hyperinsulinaemic hypoglycaemia is not well controlled by medical therapy and surgery has remained the cornerstone of treatment over the past 70 years. Insulinomas are unique among pancreatic endocrine tumours because 90% of insulinomas are benign, solitary growths that occur uniformly throughout and almost exclusively within the pancreatic parenchyma, with no evidence of local invasion or locoregional lymph node metastases.[2] The tumour may be

Table 5.1 *Features of endocrine tumours of the pancreas*

Tumour	Incidence (persons/ million/ year)	Hormone secreted	Signs or symptoms	Diagnosis	Location (%) Duo- denum	Location (%) Pan- creas	Malignant (%)	MEN1 (%)
Gastrinoma	0.1–3	Gastrin	Ulcer pain diarrhoea oesophagitis	Fasting serum gastrin > 100 pg ml⁻¹ basal acid output > 15 mEq h⁻¹	38	62	60–90	20
Insulinoma	0.8	Insulin	Hypoglycaemia	Standard fasting test	0	>99	5	4
VIPoma		VIP	Watery diarrhoea hypokalaemia hypochlorhydria	Fasting plasma VIP > 250 pg ml⁻¹	15	85	60	<5
Glucagonoma		Glucagon	Rash weight loss malnutrition diabetes	Fasting plasma glucagon > 500 pg ml⁻¹	0	>99	70	<5
Somatostatinoma		Somatostatin	Diabetes cholelithiasis steatorrhoea	Increased fasting plasma somatostatin level	50	50	70	<5
GRFoma	0.2	GRF	Acromegaly	Increased fasting plasma GRF level	0	100	30	30
ACTHoma		ACTH	Cushing's syndrome	24 h urinary free cortisol > 100 µg plasma ACTH > 50 pg ml⁻¹ no dexamethasone suppression no CRH suppression	0	100	100	<5
PTH-like-oma		PTH-like factor	Hypercalcaemia bone pain	Serum calcium >11 mg 100 ml⁻¹ serum PTH undetectable increased serum PTH-like factor	0	100	100	<5
Neurotensinoma		Neurotensin	Tachycardia hypotension hypokalaemia	Increased fasting plasma neurotensin level	0	100	>80	<5
Nonfunctioning (PP-oma)		Pancreatic polypeptide (PP) neuron-specific enolase GI	Pain bleeding mass	Increased plasma PP level increased neuron-specific enolase level	0	>99	>60	40

as small as 6 mm in diameter and is usually less than 2 cm in size which makes localisation difficult.[3]

Patient presentation

Excessive and physiologically uncontrolled secretion of insulin by the tumour causes periods of acute, symptomatic hypoglycaemia which results in characteristic symptoms. Acute neuroglycopenia induces anxiety, dizziness, obtundation, confusion, unconsciousness, personality changes and seizures.[3] Symptoms commonly occur during early morning hours, when glucose reserves are low after a period of overnight fasting and endogenous insulin overproduction continues. Patients may present when food intake is decreased to reduce weight, as most patients (80%) experience significant weight gain. A majority (60–75%) of patients are women and many have undergone extensive psychiatric evaluation. Potentially life-threatening symptoms may be present for several years before the correct diagnosis is considered.[3] Approximately 5–10% of patients with insulinoma also have MEN1 (Table 5.1). Because insulinoma is rare and neuroglycopenic symptoms are relatively non-specific, a high index of suspicion for insulinoma is necessary when other explanations for these symptoms are not evident. The recognition of symptomatic patients and the liberal use of simple and precise biochemical tests results in accurate diagnosis of insulinoma prior to life-threatening sequelae.

Screening for MEN1

About 5–10% of patients with insulinoma also have multiple endocrine neoplasia type 1 (MEN1). These patients must be recognised because multiple pancreatic tumours nearly always exist, which greatly influences operative management.[4] MEN1 is inherited as an autosomal dominant disease and tumours develop in several endocrine organs. Virtually all patients have four-gland parathyroid hyperplasia, up to 75% develop pancreatic islet cell tumours and pituitary tumours (usually prolactinomas) occur in less than 50% of patients. Functional pancreatic tumours are most commonly gastrinomas, with insulinomas occurring second in frequency.[1] Islet cell tumours of different types may occur simultaneously in a patient with MEN1. Patients may also have thyroid adenomas, adrenocortical tumours, carcinoid tumours and lipomas. Questions should be directed at other possible manifestations of the syndrome and a family history of endocrine tumours. If the clinical history is equivocal or suspicious for MEN1, then the measurement of serum levels of calcium, prolactin, and pancreatic polypeptide may help confirm or exclude MEN1. Screening of other family members for features of MEN1 is indicated when a patient is suspected to have MEN1. The detection of MEN1 will soon be possible by genetic testing, as the gene believed to be responsible for MEN1 has been mapped to the long arm of chromosome 11.[5]

Diagnosis

The classic diagnostic triad, proposed by Whipple in 1935 based on his observations in 32 patients, consists of symptoms of hypoglycaemia during a fast, a concomitant blood glucose level less than 50 mg 100 ml^{-1}, and relief of the hypoglycaemic symptoms after glucose administration.[1] Symptomatic patients suspicious for having an insulinoma may undergo an overnight fast in an outpatient setting, during which time the development of any symptoms are recorded and the serum glucose and insulin levels measured. The development of symptoms during fasting hypoglycaemia strongly suggests an insulinoma.

'Factitious hypoglycaemia', in which exogenous insulin is administered clandestinely, may present with exactly the same symptoms as an insulinoma and may lead to an inappropriate diagnosis.[6] Factitious hypoglycaemia may be suspected more often in a patient with relatives who are diabetic or in a young woman associated with the medical profession, such as a nurse. The diagnosis of insulinoma must be reached (excluding factitious hypoglycaemia) in each patient by using the 72-h supervised standard fasting test in a hospital setting with appropriate biochemical measurements prior to tumour localisation or surgery. Urinary sulphonylurea levels must be measured by gas chromatography-mass spectroscopy and this should be undetectable in patients with insulinoma. Anti-insulin antibodies should not be measurable in those with insulinoma and C-peptide concentrations should be raised in equimolar concentrations with insulin.

Supervised standard fasting test

The standard fasting test is carried out in a hospital setting and includes an examination in which recent memory, calculations and coordination are documented. An intravenous catheter with a heparin lock is inserted and the patient is allowed to drink only non-caloric beverages. Close observation by the nursing staff is necessary. Blood is collected every 6 h for measurement of serum glucose and immunoreactive insulin levels. As the blood glucose level falls below 50 mg/100 ml^{-1}, blood samples are collected more frequently (every hour or less) and the patient is observed more closely. If neuroglycopenic symptoms appear, blood is collected immediately for determination of serum insulin, glucose, C-peptide and proinsulin levels, glucose is administered and the fast is terminated. If a patient remains symptom-free for the entire 72 h, the test is terminated and the above blood levels are measured.

Neuroglycopenic symptoms will manifest in approximately 60% of patients with insulinomas within 24 h after fasting begins,[1] and nearly all patients with insulinomas will have symptoms by 72 h.[7] Approximately 16% of patients with insulinoma will develop symptoms when the blood glucose level is greater than 40 mg 100 ml^{-1}.[3] The blood glucose level eventually decreases below 40 mg 100 ml^{-1} in

Table 5.2 *Standard fasting test results and the differentiation of insulinoma from factitious hypoglycaemia*

Blood measurement	Fasting normal range	Result with insulinoma	Result with factitious hypoglycaemia	Test sensitivity
Glucose	90–150 mg 100 ml^{-1}	<40 mg 100 ml^{-1}	<40 mg 100 ml^{-1}	99%
Immunoreactive insulin (IRI)	<5 μU ml^{-1}	Increased	Increased (usually > 10 μU ml^{-1})	100%
C-peptide	<1.7 ng ml^{-1}	Increased	Normal range	78%
Direct Proinsulin-like Component (PLC)	<0.2 ng ml^{-1}	Increased	Normal range	85%
PLC/total IRI	<25%	Increased	Normal range	87%

approximately 85% of patients with insulinomas during the 72-h fast (Table 5.2, Fig. 5.1). The most definitive diagnostic biochemical test for insulinoma is an inappropriately elevated plasma immunoreactive insulin level above 5 μU ml^{-1} at the time of documented hypoglycaemia and symptoms.[7] The plasma insulin level is usually greater than 10 μU ml^{-1} in most patients (Fig. 5.1).[3] Although prolonged maximal stimulation of insulin secretion in normal subjects does not cause the release of the insulin precursor molecule, proinsulin, some insulinomas secrete proportionately larger amounts of uncleaved proinsulin. Patients with high proinsulin-producing tumours may remain euglycaemic and asymptomatic for longer time periods during the fast because proinsulin is not biologically active. The proinsulin-like component (PLC) is measured at the time of symptomatic hypoglycaemia and termination of the fast. A value greater than 25% or an elevated PLC/total immunoreactive insulin ratio are abnormal and consistent with the diagnosis of insulinoma.[3,7] Some data suggest that an elevated PLC value may be an indication of malignancy[7] but this has not been substantiated by other groups. Hypersecretion of endogenous insulin also results in elevation of the circulating level of C-peptide, a biologically inactive by-product of enzymatic insulin cleavage from the precursor proinsulin molecule. Most patients with insulinomas exhibit C-peptide levels greater than 1.7 ng ml^{-1} (Fig. 5.2).[3]

To exclude factitious hypoglycaemia definitively sulphonylurea levels in the blood from oral hypoglycaemic drugs should be measured. Human antibodies to animal insulin are detectable if the patient is not administering recombinant human insulin. Elevated serum levels of proinsulin or C-peptides during hypoglycaemia effectively excludes the diagnosis of factitious hypoglycaemia because exogenously administered insulin does not contain these proteins and

Figure 5.1 *Serum glucose and insulin levels at the time of development of neuroglycopenic symptoms and termination of the fast in 25 patients with insulinoma. Each number represents a patient. All patients had a serum insulin level >5 μU ml⁻¹, whereas 21 patients had a serum glucose level of <49 mg 100 μl⁻¹. Each patient had an insulinoma resected. Data are from reference 3, with permission.*

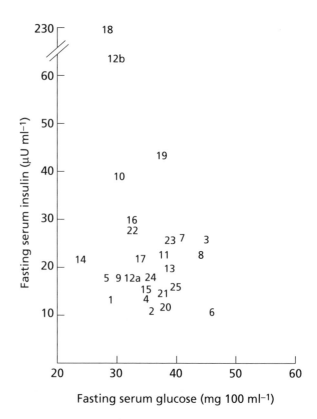

Fasting serum glucose (mg 100 ml⁻¹)

actually suppresses the endogenous production of these substances. Approximately 13–22% of patients with insulinoma, however, do not have elevated serum proinsulin or C-peptide levels and a supervised fast prohibiting exogenous hypoglycaemic administration remains the best test to diagnose insulinoma and conclusively exclude factitious hypoglycaemia. The biochemical parameters measured during the standard fasting test cannot discriminate between patients with MEN1 or sporadic insulinoma.[7]

Nesidioblastosis

Because the surgical managements are different, insulinoma must also be distinguished from nesidioblastosis, a congenital islet cell dysmaturation or malregulation which occurs in infants and causes hyperinsulinaemic hypoglycaemia. Age at the time of presentation is the most important distinguishing factor. Nesidioblastosis occurs most commonly under the age of 18 months. Although the existence of adult nesidioblastosis remains plausible,[8] the diagnosis of nesidioblastosis in an adult should be critically suspect because islet cell hyperplasia may be present in the pancreas of patients with insulinoma and an occult insulinoma may be missed in this situation.[1,9] Biochemical tests (blood glucose, immunoreactive insulin and C-peptide) do not reliably distinguish hyperinsulinaemic hypoglycaemia

Figure 5.2 *Serum C-peptide levels at the time of development of neuro-glycopenic symptoms and termination of the fast in 25 patients with insulinoma. The normal range is provided by the shaded area. 23 of 25 patients had elevated levels. Data are from reference 3, with permission.*

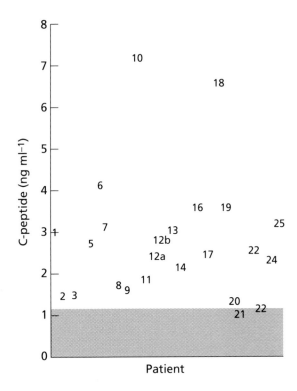

caused by an insulinoma from that attributed to nesidioblastosis. Children symptomatic after age 18 months must be evaluated to exclude an insulinoma, which must be localised and resected as for an adult. Approximately half of infants with nesidioblastosis require a spleen-preserving, near-total pancreatectomy, in which 95% of the pancreas is removed, because this disorder affects the entire pancreas diffusely.[10,11]

Medical management of hypoglycaemia

Medical management should prevent hypoglycaemia so that symptoms and life-threatening sequelae are avoided. In patients with acute hypoglycaemia, blood glucose levels are normalised initially with an intravenous glucose infusion. To prevent hypoglycaemic episodes during diagnosis, tumour localisation and the preoperative period, euglycaemia is maintained by giving frequent feedings of a high carbohydrate diet, including a night feeding. Cornstarch may be added to food for prolonged slow absorption. For patients who continue to become hypoglycaemic between feedings, diazoxide may be added at a dose of 400–600 mg orally each day. Diazoxide inhibits insulin release in approximately 50% of patients with insulinoma. Diazoxide should be discontinued 1 week before surgery to avoid intraoperative hypotension. Calcium channel blockers or phenytoin may also suppress insulin production in some patients. The short-term use of octreotide preoperatively may be beneficial if the patient is not responding well to traditional medical management and surgery is delayed for tumour localisation. Long-term control of hypoglycaemic symptoms with medical management has generally been ineffective but knowledge of the patient's response to medical management is important so that the urgency and potential benefits of surgery can be determined.[12]

Octreotide is a synthetic, long-acting (half life > 100 min) analogue of the naturally occurring hormone somatostatin.[12] Octreotide binds to and activates somatostatin receptors on cells expressing them, inhibiting the secretion of many gastrointestinal peptides. Octreotide may be useful for treating symptoms caused by VIPomas and carcinoid tumours but is not recommended for insulinomas because its efficacy in inhibiting insulin release is unpredictable.[13,14] Similarly, the usefulness of radiolabelled octreotide in imaging insulinomas and in treating metastatic islet cell tumours has been disappointing.[15] The long-term medical management of hypoglycaemia in patients with insulinomas generally is reserved for the few patients (<5%) with un-localised, unresected tumours after thorough preoperative testing and exploratory laparotomy and for patients with metastatic, unresectable malignant insulinoma.[14]

Preoperative tumour localisation

After definitive diagnosis the tumour must be localised and the presence of unresectable metastatic disease excluded. Accurate tumour localisation is the most difficult aspect of management because the tumours are usually very small and solitary.

Non-invasive imaging studies

An initial attempt should be made to localize the tumour and identify metastatic disease using non-invasive tests. The least expensive and invasive imaging modality is transabdominal ultrasonography in which a tumour shows as a sonolucent mass on a background of 'echo dense' normal pancreas. The ability to image the pancreas is severely limited by obesity and overlying bowel gas and the test sensitivity is only 0–25% in most studies (Table 5.3).[3,16–18]

Computed tomography (CT) and magnetic resonance imaging (MRI) (Table 5.3), are able to identify pancreatic tumours as small as 1 cm in diameter. For CT, oral contrast should be administered to differentiate bowel and more clearly define the pancreas, and thin slices of the peripancreatic area at most 5 mm apart should be obtained.[19] The administration of intravenous contrast may cause a blush at the site of some insulinomas due to increased vascularity. The sensitivity of CT for insulinoma ranges between 11 and 40% in most series.[3,16–18,20] MRI may image an islet cell tumour based on increased signal intensity (brightness) on T2-weighted images. The sensitivity of MRI is equivalent to that of CT.[13,16,17]

Table 5.3 *Sensitivities of localisation studies for insulinomas and gastrinomas*

Study	% of tumours localised				
	Insulinoma	Gastrinoma			
		Overall	Pancreas	Duodenum	Liver mets
Preoperative					
Non-invasive					
Transabdominal US	0–25	20–30			14
Abdominal CT	11–40	50	80	35	50
Abdominal MRI	11–43	25			83
Octreoscan	0–50	88			
Invasive					
Endoscopic US	70–90	85	88–100	<5	<5
Selective arteriography	40–70	68		34	86
+ calcium stimulation	88	—	—	—	—
+ secretin injection	—	90–100			
Portal venous sampling	67–100	70–90			
Unlocalised primary tumour	10–20	15			
Intraoperative					
Palpation	65	65	91	60	
Intraoperative US	75–100	83	95	58	
Endoscopic transillumination	—	—	—	70	
Duodenotomy	—	—	—	100	
Unlocalised primary tumour	1	5			

Malignant insulinomas are almost always very large in size (> 4 cm) and are easily imaged by CT or MRI. The extent of bulky metastatic tumour deposits and hepatic metastases are also usually readily identifiable by CT or MRI. Metastases should be identified pre-operatively so that the operative approach can be planned or, if unresectable, unnecessary surgery avoided.

Octreoscan is a relatively new modality which utilises octreotide, a somatostatin analogue, which is labelled with a radioactive tracer and is given intravenously (Table 5.3). The radiolabelled octreotide binds to tumours with somatostatin receptors, causing the tumour to appear as a 'hot spot' on whole-body gamma camera scintigraphy.[21] The scan depends on the ability of a particular islet cell tumour to express somatostatin receptors.[22] Some islet cell tumours like gastrinomas express somatostatin receptors and are nearly always (80%) imaged by labelled octreotide. Less than 50% of insulinomas are imaged by octreoscan[21,22] because they do not consistently express high levels of somatostatin receptors. The octreoscan is not recommended for localising insulinomas. Radioiodinated vasoactive intestinal polypeptide (VIP) scanning[23] may be useful but experience is presently too limited to consistently recommend its use.

Invasive localising procedures

Approximately 50% of patients have small (<2 cm) insulinomas that are not detected by non-invasive imaging tests and a variety of more sensitive invasive tests are used to localise the tumour preoperatively. Endoscopic ultrasonography (EUS) is safe and highly effective when performed by experienced users and may replace other preoperative localisation studies.[24–26] An endoscope is passed into the duodenum and a balloon inflated against the intestinal wall with saline. A 5–10 MHz transducer is used to generate an image of the pancreas through the intestinal and stomach walls. Tumours as small as 2–3 mm in diameter can be identified in the pancreatic head by moving the transducer through the duodenum at the junction of the pancreas. The endoscope must be passed well into the third portion of the duodenum to adequately visualise the uncinate process. Insulinomas in the pancreatic body and tail are imaged by positioning the transducer in the stomach and scanning the posterior wall. Sensitivity for EUS is in the range 70–90% and specificity is near 100% (Table 5.3).[25,27–29]

In patients with negative results after non-invasive imaging studies or EUS, a regional localisation study, either calcium arteriography or portal venous sampling (PVS) may be obtained. These two studies rely on the functional activity of the insulinoma (i.e. excessive insulin production) and not on the capability to image the tumour (i.e. tumour size). The calcium arteriogram appears to be the most informative preoperative test for localising insulinomas. It is replacing PVS as the invasive localising study of choice.[16] Calcium provocation may identify the region of the pancreas containing the tumour (head, body or tail). Arteries that perfuse the pancreatic head (gastroduodenal artery and superior mesenteric artery) and the body/tail (splenic artery) are selectively catheterised sequentially and a small amount of calcium gluconate (0.025 mEq Ca^{2+}/kg body weight) is injected into each artery during different runs. A catheter in the right hepatic vein collects blood for measurement of insulin levels 30–60 s after the calcium injection. Calcium stimulates a marked increase in insulin secretion from the insulinoma. A greater than twofold increase in the hepatic vein insulin level indicates localisation of the tumour to the area of the pancreas perfused by the injected artery (Fig. 5.3). Additionally, injection of contrast may reveal a tumour blush, confirming the location of the insulinoma by direct imaging. It may be necessary to obtain multiple views, including oblique images to evaluate lesions obscured by vessels and bones. This test, therefore, combines the functional advantage of PVS with the more exact localisation capability of an arteriogram. These combined features are especially useful in patients with MEN1, who may have multiple functional islet cell tumours. The reported sensitivity of calcium stimulation is 88% and few false-positive results occur (Table 5.3).[16] The calcium arteriogram may also aid in diagnosis because calcium does not stimulate normal pancreatic beta cells to secrete insulin. It may help exclude factitious causes of hypoglycaemia.

Portal venous sampling (PVS) is performed by measuring insulin concentrations in the portal vein and its tributaries.[25] A catheter is passed through the liver into the portal vein and this may be associated with complications including haemobilia and haemorrhage.[30] It is more costly because approximately 20 blood samples are assayed for insulin. Sensitivity ranges from 67 to 80% (Table 5.3) and there are few false-positives.[3,16–19] Because the calcium angiogram provides similar information, can image the tumour and is less costly and invasive this should replace PVS for invasive localisation.

A small proportion of insulinomas remain unlocalised and are considered occult. When the diagnosis is certain based on the results of the fast, surgical exploration with careful inspection, palpation and intraoperative ultrasound (IOUS) of the pancreas is still indicated. Most of these patients (>90%) will still have an insulinoma identified and removed by experienced surgeons.[1,33]

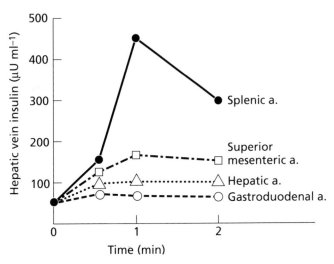

Figure 5.3 *Calcium angiogram in a patient with an insulinoma localised to the pancreatic tail. Intra-arterial calcium was selectively injected into the splenic, superior mesenteric, hepatic and gastroduodenal arteries in four different runs. Blood samples were taken serially from the hepatic vein and insulin levels were measured at 0, 1 and 2 min before and after calcium injection. After injection into the splenic artery, there was a rapid marked rise in hepatic vein insulin levels at 1 and 2 min. This finding localised the insulinoma to the pancreatic tail.*

Operative management

The only curative treatment for patients with insulinoma is surgical resection and surgery should accurately identify and remove all islet cell tumour. Blind pancreatic resection with the hope of including an unidentified insulinoma in the specimen is no longer indicated and intraoperative ultrasonography should be used to identify the tumour and normal pancreatic tissue should be preserved as much as possible. Accurate preoperative localisation correlates with a high probability of identifying the tumour in the same location at surgery and eventual cure. When preoperative localisation studies are inconclusive adequate mobilisation of the pancreas with the use of IOUS results in successful identification and resection of the insulinoma in nearly all patients.

Operative approach

A mechanical bowel preparation is advised. Pneumococcal vaccination is used preoperatively because distal pancreatectomy with splenectomy may be necessary. The prophylactic use of octreotide pre-operatively to reduce complications of pancreatic surgery such as fistulae and pseudocysts may be beneficial, but has not been proven.[31] A standard midline laparotomy or bilateral subcostal incision is recommended to give adequate exposure to the abdomen, which is facilitated by a fixed upper abdominal retractor. The entire abdomen, including regional lymph nodes, is initially inspected for potential metastases, which occur in 10% of sporadic disease. Metastatic insulinoma deposits on the surface of the liver typically appear as firm nodules. IOUS using a 5 MHz transducer may be helpful in identifying deep hepatic metastases.

Suspicious hepatic lesions which are small and peripheral should be excised by wedge resection, and larger or deeper lesions should be biopsied. Samples are sent for immediate frozen-section analysis to exclude tumour. In general, resection of localised tumour metastases is indicated to decrease symptoms associated with hyper-insulinaemia, which may be poorly controlled long-term by medical means. To adequately expose the pancreas, the hepatic and splenic flexures of the colon are mobilised out of the upper abdomen and the gastrocolic ligament is divided to open the lesser sac.

Pancreatic mobilisation

In contradistinction to gastrinomas, virtually all insulinomas are located within the pancreas and are uniformly distributed throughout the entire gland.[3] The head, body and tail of the pancreas must be sufficiently mobilised to permit evaluation of the entire organ. This requires an extended Kocher manoeuvre to adequately lift the head of the pancreas out of the retroperitoneum and division of attachments at the inferior and posterior border of the pancreas to permit evaluation of the posterior body and tail (Fig. 5.4). Because the head of the

Figure 5.4
Operative manoeuvres to identify insulinoma. (a) Kocher manoeuvre with careful palpation of the head of the pancreas. (b) Opening gastrocolic ligament, superior retraction of the stomach, inferior retraction of the transverse colon and careful palpation of the body and tail of the pancreas after incision along the inferior border.

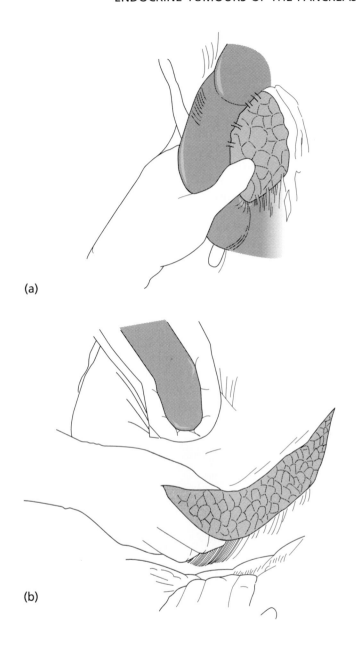

(a)

(b)

pancreas is thick, small tumours which are centrally located may not be easily palpated. The entire pancreatic head must be sufficiently mobilised so that the posterior surface can be adequately examined visually and palpated between the thumb and forefinger. The splenic ligaments may be divided to mobilise completely the spleen out of the retroperitoneum for complete examination and palpation of the pancreatic tail.

Intraoperative manoeuvres to find the insulinoma

Direct inspection of the entire pancreatic surface is carried out first because an insulinoma may appear as a brownish-red purple mass, like a cherry. Most insulinomas are encompassed by pancreatic parenchyma and may not be directly visible. Careful palpation of the pancreas between the thumb and forefinger may identify some insulinomas which feel like a firm, nodular, and discrete mass. Approximately 65% of insulinomas may be identified by the traditional operative manoeuvres of inspection and palpation.[3] Tumours are more difficult to identify when the pancreas is scarred from previous surgery or alcoholism and when tumours arise centrally within the pancreatic head.

IOUS is the best intraoperative method to find and remove insulinoma. IOUS is performed by placing the transducer on the surface of the pancreas, which is covered in a pool of saline to maximise image quality. A 10 or 7.5 MHz real-time probe is used, which has a short focal length and high resolution. An insulinoma appears as a sonolucent mass with distinct margins from the uniform, more echodense parenchyma (Fig. 5.5).

IOUS can localise an occult insulinoma which has not been identified preoperatively[32] and can identify tumours that are not visible or palpable (Fig. 5.5).[3,33] It is particularly helpful in evaluation of the pancreatic head. In conjunction with simultaneous palpation, ultra-

Figure 5.5
Intraoperative ultrasonography of an insulinoma. The insulinoma (arrow) appears sonolucent compared to the more echo dense pancreas. This tumour measures 1 cm in diameter and was not palpable within the pancreatic head.

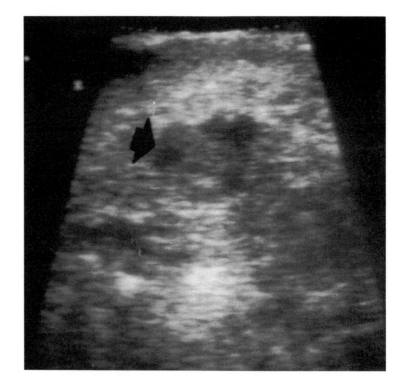

sonography further clarifies lesions.[33] The sensitivity for detecting insulinomas using IOUS is greater than 75%,[18,20] and approaches 100% (Table 5.3).[3,16]

Insulinoma resection

Enucleation means to excise only the adenoma with minimal normal pancreatic tissue and is currently the operation of choice for benign insulinomas. With the use of preoperative localisation and IOUS, blind distal pancreatectomy is no longer advocated. Tumour size, location and surrounding anatomy determine whether enucleation or pancreatic resection is performed. It is important to consider the relationship of the tumour to the pancreatic duct by imaging both structures with IOUS prior to tumour excision. Small tumours which are separated from the pancreatic duct and major vessels by normal pancreas can be safely enucleated (Fig. 5.5). IOUS allows a precise, safe tumour enucleation and helps plan the shortest, most direct route to the tumour while avoiding the pancreatic duct. If a clear margin of normal pancreatic tissue does not exist between the insulinoma and other structures then a distal or subtotal pancreatectomy and splenectomy is advised.[3,32] Ductal injury attempting to resect a tumour in close proximity results in more postoperative morbidity. Evidence of malignancy, such as involvement of peripancreatic lymph nodes or tumour invasion, mandates pancreatic resection and not enucleation.[33] Large tumour size may also be an indication for pancreatic resection. Rarely pancreaticoduodenectomy is indicated if enucleation cannot be performed safely.

Insulinoma and MEN1

Approximately 10% of insulinomas occur in the setting of MEN1 and 20% of patients with MEN1 develop insulinomas. Insulinomas in MEN1 may be multiple and may occur simultaneously diffusely throughout the pancreas.[34] The goal of treatment is to ameliorate the hypoglycaemia by eliminating the source of the hypersecretion of insulin. Difficulty arises in identifying which tumour or tumours produces the excessive insulin but this is usually a dominant, large tumour (> 3 cm) readily identified on abdominal CT.[35] An invasive regional localisation test such as the calcium arteriogram or PVS is indicated to determine if the imaged tumour is responsible for the excessive secretion of insulin. Other small islet cell tumours may also be identified but these are most likely clinically insignificant. If the insulinoma(s) arises within the body or tail of the pancreas, then a subtotal or distal pancreatectomy is indicated because multiple other islet cell tumours are frequently present.[36] A tumour that arises in the head of the pancreas is enucleated, if possible, or alternatively resected by pancreaticoduodenectomy.

Table 5.4 *Results of recent series for insulinoma and localised gastrinoma*

Series	n	Tumour found (%)	Initial remission (%)
Insulinoma			
Pasieka et al.[80]	45	100	100
Doherty et al.[3]	25	96	96
Grant et al.[20]	36	100	97
Gastrinoma			
Mignon et al.[81]	125	81	26
Norton et al.[41]	73	77	58[a]
Howard et al.[58]	11	91	82
Thompson et al.[56]	5	100	100

[a] 5-year disease-free survival was decreased to 30%.

Outcome

Most patients with insulinoma are cured of hypoglycaemia and return to a normal, fully functional life style. Appropriate localisation of sporadic insulinoma and surgical resection of all adenomatous tissue results in a cure rate of greater than 95%.[3,20] Virtually all patients with benign, sporadic insulinomas are cured of their disease and have a normal long-term survival (Table 5.4).[37] Symptoms resolve postoperatively and the fasting serum level of glucose normalises.[3] Although successful resection of the tumour(s) responsible for hyperinsulinism renders most MEN1 patients asymptomatic postoperatively,[35] persistent or recurrent hypoglycaemia due to a missed insulinoma or metastatic disease from the original tumour may develop.[1]

In general, pancreatic surgery for insulinoma should have an associated morbidity rate less than 20% and a mortality rate approaching 0%.[1] Potential complications include fistula, pseudocyst, pancreatitis and abscess. Octreotide reduces the amount of pancreatic drainage[12] and may reduce complications when given preoperatively and postoperatively.[31,38] The use of IOUS decreases complications from ductal injury.

Gastrinoma

Background

Each year, approximately 0.1–3 persons per million population develop gastrinoma, the second most common pancreatic endocrine tumour (Table 5.1).[39] The clinical features of this tumour were first described by Zollinger and Ellison in 1955.[40] Because of awareness of Zollinger–Ellison syndrome (ZES) and the widespread availability of accurate immunoassays to measure serum levels of gastrin, gastrinoma is increasingly diagnosed and treated at an early stage.

Patient presentation

The gastrinoma secretes excessive amounts of gastrin, which may cause epigastric abdominal pain, diarrhoea and oesophagitis. The most common sign is peptic ulcer disease. Diarrhoea, caused by gastrin induced acid hypersecretion and increased bowel motility, is the second most common symptom and may be the only manifestation of ZES in 20% of patients. Oesophagitis with or without stricture occurs with more severe forms of the syndrome. Approximately 20% of patients with ZES will have it as part of MEN1[1] and this syndrome must always be excluded. A significant family history of ulcers, peptic ulceration occurring at a young age, and peptic ulcers in association with hyperparathyroidism and/or nephrolithiasis are all suspicious for MEN1. These patients may have multiple subcutaneous lipomas.

As a result of increased serum gastrin levels, the gastric chief cells are under constant stimulation to produce acid, which causes peptic ulceration and epigastric abdominal pain in 80% of patients. Approximately 0.1–1% of patients who present with peptic ulcer disease have ZES.[39]

Patients with ZES usually have a solitary ulcer in the proximal duodenum, similar to patients with peptic ulcer disease unrelated to gastrinoma and 'typical' ulceration does not exclude ZES. All patients with peptic ulcer disease severe enough to require surgery should be screened preoperatively for gastrinoma by obtaining a fasting serum gastrin level. Recurrent ulceration after appropriate medical treatment, after acid-reducing surgical procedures or peptic ulceration in multiple locations or unusual locations such as distal duodenum or jejunum are all suspicious for ZES. Patients with ZES may present with a perforated ulcer, which may occur in the jejunum. Not all patients with ZES have peptic ulcer disease and 20% of patients with ZES have no evidence of peptic ulceration at the time of presentation.[41]

Diagnosis

The evaluation of a patient suspicious for having ZES begins by obtaining a fasting serum level of gastrin (Fig. 5.6). Hypergastrinaemia occurs in almost all patients with ZES and is defined as a serum gastrin level greater than 100 pg ml^{-1}.[42] A normal fasting serum gastrin level effectively excludes ZES. Antacid medications may cause a false positive elevation in serum gastrin level and those medicines should be withheld for at least three days before measurement of the serum gastrin level.

Achlorhydria is a common cause of hypergastrinaemia and gastric acid secretion is measured to exclude this condition (Fig. 5.6). A basal acid output (BAO) greater than 15 mEq h^{-1} (greater than 5 mEq h^{-1} in patients who have undergone previous acid-reducing operations) is abnormal and occurs in 98% of patients with ZES. Measurement of

Figure 5.6
Flow diagram for the diagnosis and evaluation of patients with suspected Zollinger–Ellison syndrome (gastrinoma).

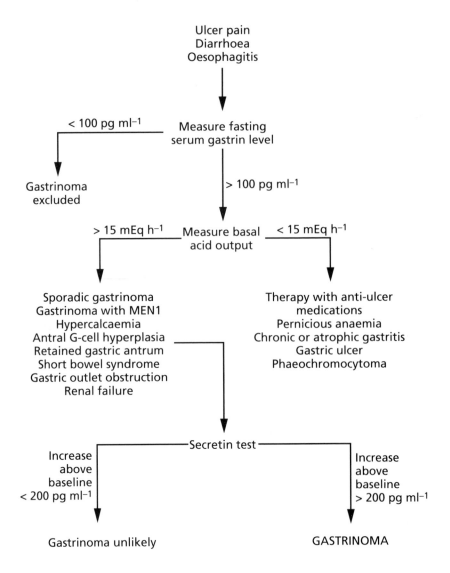

gastric pH is a simpler but less accurate indicator of gastric acid hyper-secretion. A gastric pH greater than 3 essentially excludes ZES whereas a pH less than or equal to 2 is consistent with ZES.

An extremely elevated fasting serum gastrin level (greater than 1000 pg ml^{-1}) and abnormally elevated BAO establish the diagnosis of ZES. Many patients with ZES have gastric acid hypersecretion and minimally elevated fasting serum gastrin levels (100–1000 pg ml^{-1}). For these patients the secretin stimulation test is the provocative test of choice.[1] The secretin test is carried out after an overnight fast, 2 U kg^{-1} intravenous injection of secretin is administered and blood samples are collected immediately before and at 2, 5, 10 and 15 min after secretin. A 200 pg ml^{-1} increase of gastrin above baseline levels is diagnostic of ZES. The test sensitivity is not 100% and approximately 15% of patients with gastrinoma may have a negative secretin test.

Medical control of gastric acid hypersecretion

The management of patients with gastrinoma consists of two phases: to control the symptoms associated with acid hypersecretion and to remove the tumour which is potentially malignant and life-threatening. The development of H_2-receptor antagonists and Na^+-K^+-ATPase inhibitors has made medical control of gastric acid hypersecretion possible in all patients. Patients with ZES typically require 2–5 times the usual dose of anti-ulcer medications to keep the BAO < 15 mEq h^{-1}. Omeprazole at 20–40 mg p.o. twice a day will usually control acid hypersecretion. ZES patients who have reflux oesophagitis or who have had prior operations to reduce acid secretion such as subtotal gastrectomy should have the acid output maintained at < 5 mEq h^{-1}. If acid hypersecretion is controlled, epigastric discomfort resolves and ulcers heal in virtually all patients[40,43,44] Because of the recent advances in the medical treatment of peptic ulcer disease, total gastrectomy is not indicated in patients with gastrinoma.

Adequate medical control of gastric acid hypersecretion with resolution of symptoms and decreased ulcerogenic complications has resulted in increased concern about the potential malignancy of the primary tumour. The most important determinant of long-term survival in patients with ZES is the growth of the primary tumour and its metastatic spread.[44] Tumour progression accounts for the majority of deaths when patients were followed long term.[44] Development of liver metastases is associated with subsequent death from tumour and surgical resection of the primary can reduce the incidence of liver metastases. In a recent study, hepatic metastases developed in only 3% of patients with gastrinoma treated by surgical excision of the primary compared with 23% managed without surgery.[45] The current goal of surgery has shifted from controlling gastric acid hypersecretion to resection of the primary tumour and localised metastatic disease.

Preoperative tumour localisation

In contradistinction to insulinoma, gastrinoma is malignant in 60–90% of patients.[2] Duodenal gastrinomas as small as 2 mm in diameter may have associated regional lymph node metastases.[46] All patients with ZES should undergo preoperative testing to localise the tumour and to define the extent of disease so that appropriate surgical treatment can be undertaken.

Non-invasive tumour localising studies

Initial tumour localisation studies should be non-invasive, attempt to image the primary tumour and adequately assess the liver for metastases. As with localising insulinoma, abdominal ultrasonography has a low sensitivity of only 20–30% for gastrinoma (Table 5.3). Abdominal CT detects approximately 50% of gastrinomas overall, but sensitivity depends greatly on tumour size, tumour location and the presence of metastases.[47] Gastrinomas greater than 3 cm in diameter are reliably detected by CT whereas tumours less than 1 cm in size are seldom imaged by CT.

Primary gastrinomas which arise within the pancreas are identified much more reliably than those in extrapancreatic, extrahepatic locations (80% v. 35%). CT scanning identifies 50% of liver metastases. Abdominal MRI has a low sensitivity (25%) in localising primary gastrinomas, but best shows hepatic metastases (Table 5.3). Gastrinoma metastases in the liver appear bright on dynamic T2-weighted images and have a ring enhancement with gadolinium administration.[48] MRI is especially useful for differentiating hepatic gastrinoma metastases from haemangiomas.

Recent studies indicate that octreoscans may significantly improve the preoperative localisation of gastrinomas.[49] Approximately 80% of primary tumours can be identified and the true extent of metastatic disease is delineated more accurately than CT or MRI. Octreoscan is now the non-invasive imaging modality of choice for gastrinomas.

Invasive tumour localising modalities

Although non-invasive imaging studies are important as initial tests to exclude gross hepatic metastases and unresectable disease, these studies may fail to image the primary gastrinoma. Invasive modalities may be useful to accurately localise the primary tumour prior to surgery.

EUS has a reported sensitivity of 85% for detecting gastrinomas and a specificity of 95% (Table 5.3).[25,28,29] Tumours in the pancreas as small as 2–3 mm may be imaged. Duodenal gastrinomas can be visualised as a submucosal mass with the instrument (Fig. 5.7). The ability to detect duodenal wall gastrinomas directly has been disappointing and liver metastases are not reliably imaged.

Previously the best imaging modality to localise a primary gastrinoma was selective angiography. Angiograms are obtained by selectively catheterising gastroduodenal, hepatic, superior mesenteric and splenic arteries. A hypervascular tumour 'blush' is characteristically observed in the location of the gastrinoma (Fig. 5.8b). Sensitivity is 68% overall for extrahepatic gastrinomas and 86% for hepatic metastases, but only 34% for duodenal gastrinomas (Table 5.3).[50,51] Tumours less than 1–2 cm in size are less reliably detected. Selective arterial secretin injection (SASI) during the angiogram and collection of blood

Figure 5.7 *View of a duodenal wall gastrinoma through an endoscope. The tumour appears as a small submucosal mass which was biopsied and confirmed to be a gastrinoma.*

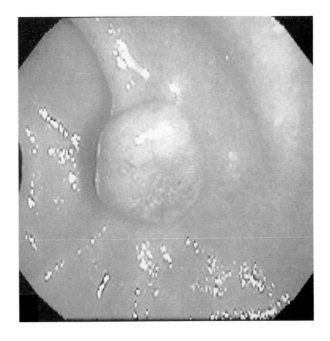

samples from a hepatic vein as well as a peripheral vein for measurement of the gastrin level increases the sensitivity for localising the primary tumour to 90–100% with a specificity of virtually 100% (Fig. 5.8a).[52] Injection of secretin into the artery supplying the gastrinoma causes a rise in the hepatic vein gastrin level by more than 80 pg ml^{-1} in 40 s. The gastrinoma can, thus, be localised to either the pancreatic head, body/tail or the liver. Gastrinomas have been found only in the gastroduodenal artery injection and, therefore, occult tumours are usually in the gastrinoma triangle. PVS for gastrin is similar and provides regional localisation with similar sensitivity to the SASI test. Neither study is particularly useful in ZES patients because gradients are nearly always found in the gastrinoma triangle.

Surgery for tumour eradication

If preoperative imaging studies reveal no evidence of unresectable metastatic disease, then patients with sporadic gastrinoma and acceptable risks should undergo abdominal exploration for tumour resection.

Operative approach

Mechanical bowel preparation and pneumococcal vaccination are required preoperatively. The prophylactic use of octreotide may reduce complications from pancreatic surgery.[31] The surgeon should be prepared for hepatic resection in the event that unsuspected liver metastases are identified intraoperatively. An upper abdominal

Figure 5.8 *Secretin angiogram in patient with Zollinger–Ellison syndrome and gastrinoma localised to the duodenum. (a) Results of secretin injection of selective arteries that perfuse the pancreas and duodenum. Gastrin levels were measured in the hepatic vein before and at intervals after secretin injection. When secretin was injected into the gastroduodenal artery a gastrinoma was visualised in the wall of the duodenum as a blush (b, arrow) and the hepatic vein gastrin levels were most elevated (a).*

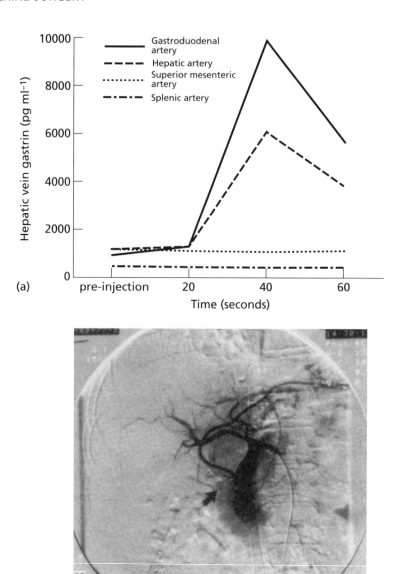

incision that provides adequate exposure for exploration of the entire pancreas, regional lymph nodes and liver is necessary. The abdomen is initially inspected for metastases with particular attention to possible ectopic sites of tumour such as the ovaries, jejunum and omentum. The entire surface of the liver is then palpated for metastatic lesions. Metastases typically appear tan in colour and feel firm. Deep hepatic metastases may be identified by using IOUS with a 5 MHz transducer.

All suspicious hepatic lesions must be either excised or biopsied to exclude malignant gastrinoma. In general, liver metastases which are not identified preoperatively by abdominal MRI or octreoscan are small and potentially resectable at the time of operation. Similarly, hilar and peripancreatic regional lymph nodes are carefully evaluated for metastatic disease.

Intraoperative manoeuvres to find the primary gastrinoma

Successful intraoperative gastrinoma localisation and resection may be extremely challenging because tumours only 2 mm in size may be in the wall of the duodenum. There is also a high rate of associated lymph node metastases and a possible occurrence of primary gastrinomas within lymph nodes with no other identifiable primary tumour.[53] The initial finding of a single involved lymph node may, therefore, represent a primary tumour or metastatic disease from a very small, unlocalised primary tumour. Preoperative studies, like octreoscan, accurately localise the primary gastrinoma and metastases and greatly facilitate the operative management allowing a surgical approach directed to the area containing the tumour. Intraoperative localisation is still necessary because 20–40% of patients in whom the tumour is not apparent using preoperative studies will still have tumour identified at surgery.

Successful tumour identification requires knowledge of where primary gastrinomas arise. The so-called 'gastrinoma triangle' bounded by the neck and body of the pancreas medially, the junction of the cystic and common bile ducts superiorly, and the second and third portions of the duodenum inferiorly, will contain more than 80% of primary gastrinomas.[54] The head of the pancreas and duodenum are first exposed by mobilising the hepatic flexure of the colon out of the upper abdomen and dividing the gastrocolic ligament to open the lesser sac. A Kocher manoeuvre is performed to lift the head of the pancreas out of the retroperitoneum. The entire pancreatic surface is carefully examined visually and palpated between the thumb and forefinger (Fig. 5.4). IOUS is very useful for localising intrapancreatic gastrinomas (Table 5.3). The body and tail of the pancreas may be mobilised and similarly examined after dividing inferior and posterior pancreatic attachments in order to find the few gastrinomas which may arise in the distal pancreas.

Primary gastrinomas have increasingly been recognised as occurring in extrapancreatic locations.[54-56] IOUS is poor at detecting tumours that arise within the duodenum (Table 5.3) and the surgeon must rely more on inspection, palpation and duodenotomy to find these tumours.[33] In 30–40% of patients, the gastrinoma is located in the submucosa of the duodenum. Duodenal gastrinomas are usually very small, less than 6 mm in size, and are difficult to palpate. Endoscopic transillumination of the duodenum may be a useful

Figure 5.9
Density of duodenal gastrinomas found at surgery and method of operative identification. Gastrinomas within the wall of the duodenum are most common in the first portion (D1) and decrease in density moving distally (D3). Duodenotomy is able to find tumours missed by the two other methods.

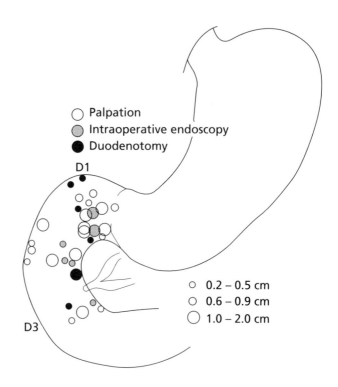

technique for visualising small duodenal tumours and guiding precise tumour enucleation.[57] The gastrinoma appears as a dark, opaque shadow surrounded by the semitransparent red glow of the duodenal wall. If the tumour is not localised by endoscopic transillumination of the duodenum, then duodenotomy is recommended. Duodenotomy to directly inspect and explore the duodenal mucosa will identify duodenal gastrinomas missed by all other means. Duodenal wall gastrinomas are in greatest density more proximally in the duodenum (Fig. 5.9). Tumours are detected most frequently by duodenectomy, followed by intraoperative endoscopy with transillumination and least frequently by palpation (Fig. 5.9). Regional lymph nodes should be systematically sampled as lymph node metastases may be inapparent at exploration and will be found in 55% of patients with duodenal tumours. Gastrinomas can be found by an experienced surgeon in 80–90% of patients with the increased awareness of duodenal lesions (Table 5.4).[56,58]

Approximately 5–24% of gastrinomas are found in extrapancreatic, extraintestinal lymph nodes only with no apparent primary pancreatic or duodenal tumour.[59–62] Whether these lymph node gastrinomas represent primary tumours or metastases from occult pancreatic or intestinal primary tumours is controversial. Primary tumours as small as 2 mm may have associated lymph node metastases[46] and are easily missed intraoperatively without meticulous exploration. There are at least six reported patients without previous gastric or pancreatic resections who appear to be biochemically cured after the sole excision of only lymph nodes containing gastrinoma.[61-63] Peripancreatic lymph nodes from patients undergoing Whipple resection for non-endocrine tumour may contain cells that stain positive for neuroendocrine markers, giving a plausible explanation for lymph node primary gastrinoma.[53] It is reasonable to conclude the operation if careful exploration, including examination of the duodenum with duodenotomy, does not reveal a primary tumour and all involved lymph nodes have been resected.

Tumour resection

As described for insulinoma, tumour enucleation remains the procedure of choice for resecting sporadic gastrinomas. Tumours that arise within the pancreas that are not near the pancreatic duct or major vessels, are safely enucleated. Large pancreatic tumours with vital structures in close proximity must be removed by pancreatic resection. Duodenal gastrinomas may be precisely enucleated using endoscopic transillumination of the duodenum.[57] As much of the duodenal wall as possible is preserved to allow a non-constricting closure. Special attention is paid to avoid the ampulla of Vater. Involved regional lymph nodes are also excised. Although a majority of gastrinomas are malignant, performing a more radical pancreatic resection that includes regional lymph nodes, such as pancreatico-duodenectomy, is currently not indicated for small tumours which are easily enucleated because of the slow progression of disease and symptomatic relief with medical treatment.

The presence of lymph node metastases at the time of operation should not discourage an aggressive surgical approach to remove all gross tumour. Gastrinoma is associated with lymph node involvement in 50–80% of patients and unlike many other types of cancer, lymph node involvement alone without hepatic or distant metastases does not appear to influence survival for gastrinoma.[2,64] Resection of all apparent tumour to eradicate disease increases disease-free survival and may extend overall survival. The development of hepatic and distant metastatic disease, which occurs in 25–90% of patients with gastrinoma, is clearly the most common cause of morbidity and mortality associated with tumour.[41,51,64,65]

Gastrinoma and MEN1

Parathyroidectomy should be performed first in patients with MEN1, primary hyperparathyroidism and ZES because normalisation of the serum level of calcium usually results in a marked decrease in serum gastrin level, allowing better medical control of the symptoms of ZES.[66] Whether or not patients should undergo abdominal exploration is controversial. Earlier surgical series suggest that resecting gastrinoma does not cure MEN1 patients of ZES. More recent studies show that aggressive surgical approaches, wherein the portion of the pancreas producing excess gastrin is resected may result in normalisation of serum gastrin levels.[67] Most gastrinomas in patients with MEN1 are currently thought to be malignant.[35] Only 3% of patients without hepatic metastases who undergo resection of the gastrinoma eventually develop liver metastases as compared to 23% of similar patients who are managed medically over a similar time period.[45] Hepatic metastases are associated with decreased survival from ZES.[64] All patients with MEN-1 and ZES should undergo SASI to determine the pancreatic region of the tumour-secreting gastrin and then undergo surgery to resect the primary tumour and metastases. Tumours that are at least 3 cm in size usually have lymph node metastases.[68] Preoperative abdominal CT is necessary to identify hepatic metastases and plan surgical resection. Octreoscan is also useful in determining the true extent of disease. In patients with MEN1, 70% of gastrinomas are found within the duodenum and approximately 50% of patients may have multiple duodenal tumours.[68] Some advocate performing routine duodenotomy and peripancreatic lymph node sampling whenever a duodenal gastrinoma is found in an MEN1 patient, as well as enucleation of palpable tumours in the pancreas.[67] Others report discouraging results despite similar procedures.[35]

Outcome

The overall survival for patients with sporadic gastrinoma not metastatic to the liver is > 90% at 5 years and > 85% at 10 years (Table 5.4). An immediate postoperative cure rate of 60% can be obtained if all tumour is identified and resected, and over 50% of these patients will remain free of disease at 5 years follow-up.[41] Patients with liver metastases at presentation have an overall survival of only 20–38%.[64]

Other rare endocrine tumours of the pancreas

Other pancreatic endocrine tumours include vasoactive intestinal peptide (VIP)-oma, glucagonoma, somatostatinoma, growth hormone releasing factor (GRF)-oma, adrenocorticotropic hormone (ACTH)-oma, parathyroid hormone (PTH)-like-oma, neurotensinoma, and non-functional islet cell tumour or pancreatic peptide (PP)-oma (Table 5.1).[69] These neoplasms occur in less than 0.2 persons per million per year. In general, these tumours resemble gastrinoma in that all are associated with a high incidence of malignancy. Each of these tumours can also arise in association with MEN1, including GRFoma and PP-oma. The hormones, symptoms and signs, diagnostic tests, sites of occurrence, proportions malignant and frequency of associated MEN1 for each tumour are given in Table 5.1.

PP-omas produce pancreatic polypeptide and neuron-specific enolase which have no clinically appreciable biologically active function and, therefore, patients do not present with a typical hormonal syndrome. Symptoms arise because of a mass effect and include abdominal pain, gastrointestinal bleeding, and obstruction. Diagnosis may only be made after palpation of an abdominal mass or incidental identification of a pancreatic mass on imaging studies. Malignant spread to lymph nodes or liver is common and related to tumour size (>50% for tumours > 3 cm).

For all of these tumours, preoperative abdominal CT is necessary in attempting to localise the primary tumour and to exclude liver metastases.[68] The goals of surgical treatment are to control symptoms caused by excessive hormone production and to potentially cure or decrease disease bulk. The only potentially curative treatment for malignant endocrine tumours is surgical resection.[70–74] Patients with extensive bilobar hepatic metastases are not candidates for surgery and symptoms may respond to chemotherapy, α-interferon or octreotide.[70]

Occult pancreatic endocrine tumours

An 'occult' islet cell tumour is an unlocalised tumour by non-operative tests that occurs in a patient with a definitively diagnosed clinical hormonal syndrome, such as fasting hyperinsulinaemic hypoglycaemia or ZES. The tumour is biochemically proven but its anatomic site remains unclear. Approximately 10–20% of insulinomas and 15% of gastrinomas are occult. Patients with insulinoma should undergo a regional localisation study like the calcium angiogram preoperatively in an attempt to localise the tumour to a specific anatomic area (Fig. 5.3). Patients with occult gastrinomas need not undergo a regional localisation study as these tumours are nearly always in the duodenum within the gastrinoma triangle. Exploratory laparotomy is then the last resort to identify the location of the tumour and resect it. Surgery should not be performed in patients with insulinoma unless IOUS is available, given its advantages in finding small tumours within the pancreas (Fig. 5.5).[1] Surgery in patients with occult gastrinoma should focus on the duodenum including transillumination and duodenotomy (Fig. 5.9).

Abdominal exploration by an experienced pancreatic endocrine surgeon, knowledge of the sites of occurrence of specific tumours, and the use of IOUS results in identification and removal of the tumour in all but a few patients. In the rare instance that a tumour remains unlocalised and unresected after thorough exploration, the decision whether or not to perform a pancreatectomy depends on the particular patient's response to medical management and the results of the preoperative regional localisation study. Pancreatic resection is not indicated if the patient's hormonal syndrome can be well controlled by medical management. When medical management is unsatisfactory, the only alternative is to perform a pancreatectomy based on the regional localisation data. 'Blind' pancreatectomy is never indicated.

Malignant pancreatic endocrine tumours

Background

With improvements in the medical management of syndromes of hormonal excess, growth and metastatic spread of primary islet cell tumours has increasingly become more problematic. Except for insulinomas, which are malignant in only 5–10%, greater than 60% of pancreatic endocrine tumours overall are malignant.[70,73,74] Data concerning the management of these patients is mainly derived from experience with malignant gastrinomas, which occur more commonly as compared to other more obscure pancreatic neuroendocrine tumours.

No diagnostic histological criteria from examination of tumour biopsies or resected primary tumours exist to define malignancy for pancreatic endocrine tumours. Malignancy is definitively established with surgical exploration and histological evidence of tumour remote from the primary lesion, usually in peripancreatic lymph nodes or the liver. Recurrence of tumour at a location distant from a resected primary tumour site also definitively indicates malignancy. Gross invasion of blood vessels, surrounding tissues, or adjacent organs usually suggests a malignant tumour.[71] IOUS showing a pancreatic tumour with indistinct margins may imply local invasion and malignancy.[32] Vary large tumours (>5 cm) have an increased risk of being cancerous.[2] Tumour DNA ploidy and tumoural growth fraction determined by flow cytometry may provide an indication of biological behaviour of some of these tumours. Because islet cell tumours generally grow slowly, metastases may not become evident until years after the initial primary tumour resection.

Evaluation of metastatic disease

Evaluation of a patient with a malignant neuroendocrine tumour begins by assessing the extent of disease using radiological imaging studies. Octreoscan appears to be the single best imaging study to select patients for aggressive surgery to remove metastatic disease.[1] If the tumour binds this isotope, then disease anywhere in the body can be identified. Miliary or extensive bilobar hepatic disease and distant metastases are considered inoperable and, if identified preoperatively, can prevent unnecessary surgery. CT or MRI may identify disease in the chest and abdomen. Specific complaints of bone pain are elicited and, if present, evaluated with bone scan and radiographs.

Malignant primary insulinomas are relatively large, approximately 6 cm, and can usually be readily detected by non-invasive imaging studies.[33] Gastrinomas may metastasise to regional lymph nodes when only millimetres in size. Duodenal primary gastrinomas have been found to have a higher incidence of lymph node metastases (55%) than pancreatic gastrinomas (22%) some suggest that rare gastrinomas to the left of the superior mesenteric artery in the pancreatic tail are always malignant and more commonly produce liver metastases. If multiple insulinomas or gastrinomas are found in a patient, then MEN1 should be suspected.

Surgical management

Pancreatic neuroendocrine carcinomas have a better prognosis than adenocarcinoma of the exocrine pancreas and are often managed with aggressive surgical resection.[49] Surgery is undertaken to decrease tumour bulk so that hormonal syndromes are more effectively controlled by medical management, to relieve symptoms of mass effect, and/or to eliminate cancerous tissue and improve disease-free or overall survival. Preoperative staging studies are important to exclude patients from surgery who would not benefit from resection.

Limited metastases as well as the primary tumour should be resected to adequately debulk tumour to eliminate the hormonal syndrome.[75] Incomplete tumour resection may not improve the ability to control the hormonal syndrome medically. For medically fit patients with metastatic insulinoma in whom hypoglycaemia is poorly controlled by medical management, tumour debulking may control symptoms for prolonged time periods, even in the setting of distant metastases.[41] Approximately 50% of patients with metastatic insulinoma undergoing resection have complete biochemical remission.[76]

Although treatment is generally palliative and not curative, for patients with locally advanced tumours and limited metastatic disease, surgery may be the only therapy that effectively ameliorates life-threatening symptoms and increases survival because these tumours are generally indolent, slow-growing neoplasms.[76,77] Limited regional metastatic disease can often be successfully resected and may be curative if no liver metastases are present.[75] Complete resection of localised or regional nodal metastases with negative margins at the initial surgery provides the highest probability of cure.[1] Although disease-free survival is prolonged in a majority of patients, most eventually develop recurrent tumour.

Approximately 30% of patients with metastatic insulinoma can undergo complete resection of tumour.[76,77] Median survival is increased from 11 months, in patients with metastatic insulinoma who cannot undergo resection, to 4 years in those in whom tumour debulking is possible.[64] Palliative re-resection of recurrent tumour extends median survival from 11–19 months to 4 years.[78] Surgery may also be the most effective treatment for patients with metastatic gastrinoma if most or all of the tumour can be resected.[1] Aggressive resection of liver metastases of gastrinoma, considered resectable by preoperative imaging studies, improves 5-year survival from 28% in patients with inoperable metastases to 79%.[75] Patients with solitary, localised metastatic disease benefit most. Recurrence of disease in more than one lobe of the liver may be treated by hepatic arterial embolisation or orthotopic liver transplant. Patients may also have symptoms such as obstruction secondary to mass effect from the size or location of the tumour or gastrointestinal bleeding from direct tumour invasion into adjacent bowel which are effectively eliminated by resection of the tumour.[75] Pain secondary to neural invasion may be effectively palliated by percutaneous coeliac axis nerve block.

Figure 5.10 *Use of octreotide in a patient with metastatic VIPoma. The patient had voluminous diarrhoea (5–6 kg day⁻¹) and hypokalaemia (serum K=3 mmol l⁻¹) and required large potassium supplements. Following the initiation of octreotide 100 µg BID, the diarrhoea ceased, the patient gained weight and the serum levels of bicarbonate and potassium normalised.*

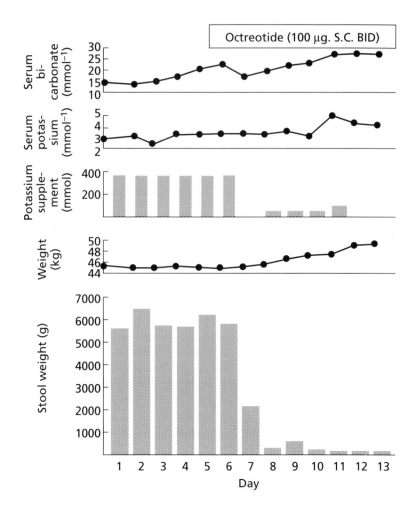

Non-surgical management

Symptoms from extensive metastases may respond to chemotherapy or octreotide, but these treatments are not curative.[1] Combination chemotherapy with streptozocin and 5-fluorouracil is the most effective regimen for metastatic insulinoma, producing at least a partial response in 60% of patients. Doxorubicin may also be used. Patients with metastatic gastrinoma are treated with streptozotocin, doxorubicin, and/or 5-fluorouracil. α-interferon may also provide partial responses. Treatment with octreotide results in unpredictable responses, causing decreased tumour growth in some patients and having no effect in others.[65,69,79] Octreotide may ameliorate symptoms especially in patients with malignant VIPoma (Fig. 5.10) and when symptoms are adequately controlled, patients can live comfortably and productively for many years with metastatic disease.

References

1. Norton JA. Neuroendocrine tumors of the pancreas and duodenum. Curr Prob Surg 1994; 31: 77–164.
2. Peplinski GR, Norton JA. Gastrointestinal endocrine cancers and nodal metastases: biological significance and therapeutic implications. Surg Oncol Clin North Am 1996; 5: 159–71.
3. Doherty GM, Doppman JL, Shawker TH et al. Results of a prospective strategy to diagnose, localize and resect insulinomas. Surgery 1991; 110: 989–97.
4. Thompson NW, Lloyd RV, Nishiyama RH et al. MEN I pancreas: a histological and immunohistochemical study. World J Surg 1984; 8: 561–74.
5. Nakamura Y, Larsson C, Julier C et al. Localization of the genetic defect in multiple endocrine neoplasia type 1 within a small region of chromosome 11. Am J Hum Genet 1989; 44: 751–5.
6. Grunberger G, Weiner JL, Silverman R, Taylor S, Gorden P. Factitious hypoglycemia due to surreptitious administration of insulin: diagnosis, treatment and long-term follow-up. Ann Intern Med 1988; 108: 252–7.
7. Gorden P, Skarulis MC, Roach P et al. Plasma proinsulin-like component in insulinoma: a 25-year experience. J Clin Endocrinol Metab 1995; 80: 2884–7.
8. Farley DR, van Heerden JA, Myers JL. Adult pancreatic nesidioblastosis: unusual presentations of a rare entity. Arch Surg 1994; 129: 329–32.
9. Goudswaard WB, Houthoff HJ, Koudstaal J, Zwierstra RP. Nesidioblastosis and endocrine hyperplasia of the pancreas: a secondary phenomenon. Hum Pathol 1986; 17: 46–54.
10. Thornton PS, Alter CA, Katz LE, Baker L, Stanley CA. Short- and long-term use of octreotide in the treatment of congenital hyperinsulinism. J Pediatr 1993; 123: 637–43.
11. Glaser B, Hirsch HJ, Landau H. Persistent hyperinsulinemic hypoglycemia of infancy: long-term octreotide treatment without pancreatectomy. J Pediatr 1993; 123: 644–50.
12. Gorden P, Comi RJ, Maton PN, Go VLW. Somatostatin and somatostatin analogue (SMS 201-995) in treatment of hormone-secreting tumors of the pituitary and gastrointestinal tract and non-neoplastic diseases of the gut. Ann Intern Med 1989; 110: 35–50.
13. Arnold R, Frank M, Kajdan U. Management of gastroenteropancreatic endocrine tumors: the place of somatostatin analogues. Digestion 1994; 55 Suppl 3: 107–13.
14. von Eyben FE, Grodum E, Gjessing HJ, Hagen C, Nielsen H. Metabolic remission with octreotide in patients with insulinoma. J Intern Med 1994; 235: 245–8.
15. Arnold R, Neuhaus C, Benning R et al. Somatostatin analog sandostatin and inhibition of tumor growth in patients with metastatic endocrine gastroenteropancreatic tumors. World J Surg 1993; 17: 511–19.
16. Doppman JL, Chang R, Fraker DL et al. Localization of insulinomas to regions of the pancreas by intra-arterial stimulation with calcium. Ann Intern Med 1995; 123: 269–73.
17. Vinik AI, Delbridge L, Moattari R, Cho K, Thompson N. Transhepatic portal vein catheterization for localization of insulinomas: a ten-year experience. Surgery 1991; 109: 1–11.
18. Gianello P, Gigot JF, Berthet F et al. Pre- and intraoperative localization of insulinomas: report of 22 observations. World J Surg 1988; 12: 389–97.
19. Fraker DL, Norton JA. Localization and resection of insulinomas and gastrinomas. JAMA 1988; 259: 3601–5.
20. Grant CS, van Heerden J, Charboneau JW, James EM, Reading CC. Insulinoma: the value of intraoperative ultrasonography. Arch Surg 1988; 123: 843–8.
21. Lamberts SW, Bakker WH, Reubi JC, Krenning EP. Somatostatin receptor imaging in the localization of endocrine tumors. N Engl J Med 1990; 323: 1246–9.
22. Lamberts SW, Hofland LJ, van Koetsveld PM et al. Parallel in vivo and in vitro detection of functional somatostatin receptors in human endocrine pancreatic tumors: consequences with regard to diagnosis, localization and therapy. J Clin Endocrinol Metab 1990; 71: 566–74.
23. Virgolini I, Raderer M, Kurtaran A et al. Vasoactive intestinal peptide-receptor imaging for the localization of intestinal adenocarcinomas and endocrine tumors. N Engl J Med 1994; 331: 1116–21.

24. Owens LV, Huth JF, Cance WG. Insulinoma: pitfalls in preoperative localization. Eur J Surg Oncol 1995; 21: 326–8.

25. Thompson NW, Czako PF, Fritts LL et al. Role of endoscopic ultrasonography in the localization of insulinomas and gastrinomas. Surgery 1994; 116: 1131–8.

26. Bottger TC, Junginger T. Is preoperative radiographic localization of islet cell tumors in patients with insulinoma necessary? World J Surg 1993; 17: 427–32.

27. Heyder N. Localization of an insulinoma by ultrasonic endoscopy. N Engl J Med 1985; 312: 860–1.

28. Glover JR, Shorvon PJ, Lees WR. Endoscopic ultrasound for localization of islet cell tumors. Gut 1992; 33: 108–10.

29. Rosch T, Lightdale CJ, Botet JF et al. Localization of pancreatic endocrine tumors by endoscopic ultrasonography. N Engl J Med 1992; 326: 1721–6.

30. Miller DL, Doppman JL, Metz DC, Maton PN, Norton JA, Jensen RT. Zollinger–Ellison syndrome: technique, results, and complications of portal venous sampling. Radiology 1992; 182: 235–41.

31. Buchler M, Friess H, Klempa I et al. Role of octreotide in the prevention of postoperative complications following pancreatic resection. Am J Surg 1992; 163: 125–31.

32. Norton JA, Sigel B, Baker AR et al. Localization of an occult insulinoma by intraoperative ultrasonography. Surgery 1985; 97: 381–4.

33. Norton JA, Cromack DT, Shawker TH et al. Intraoperative ultrasonographic localization of islet cell tumors. Ann Surg 1988; 207: 160–8.

34. Demeure MJ, Klonoff DC, Karam JH, Duh QY, Clark OH. Insulinomas associated with multiple endocrine neoplasia type 1: the need for a different surgical approach. Surgery 1991; 110: 998–1004.

35. Sheppard BC, Norton JA, Doppman JL, Maton PN, Gardner JD, Jensen RT. Management of islet cell tumors in patients with multiple endocrine neoplasia: a prospective study. Surgery 1989; 106: 1108–18.

36. O'Riordain DS, O'Brien T, van Heerden JA, Service FJ, Grant CS. Surgical management of insulinoma associated with multiple endocrine neoplasia type I. World J Surg 1994; 18: 488–93.

37. Service FJ, McMahon MM, O'Brien PC, Ballard DJ. Functioning insulinoma – incidence, recurrence, and long-term survival of patients: a 60-year study. Mayo Clin Proc 1991; 66: 711–19.

38. Lange JR, Steinberg S, Doherty GM et al. A randomized prospective trial of postoperative somatostatin analogue in patients with neuroendocrine tumors of the pancreas. Surgery 1992; 112: 1033–8.

39. Eriksson B, Oberg K, Skogseid B. Neuroendocrine pancreatic tumors: clinical findings in a prospective study of 84 patients. Acta Oncol 1989; 28: 373–7.

40. Zollinger RM, Ellison EH. Primary peptic ulceration of the jejunum associated with islet cell tumors of the pancreas. Ann Surg 1955; 142: 709–28.

41. Norton JA, Doppman JL, Jensen RT. Curative resection in Zollinger–Ellison syndrome: results of a 10 year prospective study. Ann Surg 1992; 215: 8–18.

42. Wolfe MM, Jensen RT. Zollinger–Ellison syndrome, current concepts in diagnosis and management. N Engl J Med 1987; 317: 1200–9.

43. Fox PS, Hofmann JW, DeCosse JJ, Wilson SD. The influence of total gastrectomy on survival in malignant Zollinger–Ellison tumors. Ann Surg 1974; 180: 558–66.

44. Zollinger RM, Ellison EC, O'Dorsio TM, Sparks J. Thirty years' experience with gastrinoma. World J Surg 1984; 8: 427–35.

45. Fraker DL, Norton JA, Alexander HR, Venzon DJ, Jensen RT. Surgery in Zollinger–Ellison syndrome alters the natural history of gastrinoma. Ann Surg 1994; 220: 320–30.

46. Thompson NW, Pasieka J, Fukuuchi A. Duodenal gastrinomas, duodenotomy, and duodenal exploration in the surgical management of Zollinger–Ellison syndrome. World J Surg 1993; 17: 455–62.

47. Wank SA, Doppman HL, Miller DL, et al. Prospective study of the ability of computerized axial tomography to localize gastrinomas in patients with Zollinger–Ellison syndrome. Gastroenterology 1987; 92: 905–12.

48. Semelka RC, Cumming MJ, Shoenut JP et al. Islet cell tumors: comparison of dynamic contrast-enhanced CT and MR imaging with dynamic gadolinium enhancement and fat suppression. Radiology 1993; 186: 799–802.

49. Schirmer WJ, Melvin WS, Rush RM *et al.* ^{111}In-Pentetreotide scanning versus conventional imaging techniques for the localization of gastrinoma. Surgery 1995; 118: 1105–13.

50. Maton PN, Miller DL, Doppman HL *et al.* Role of selective angiography in the management of Zollinger–Ellison syndrome. Gastroenterology 1987; 92: 913–19.

51. Thom AK, Norton JA, Axiotis CA, Jensen RT. Location, incidence and malignant potential of duodenal gastrinomas. Surgery 1991; 110: 1086–93.

52. Imamura M, Takahashi K. Use of selective arterial secretin injection test to guide surgery in patients with Zollinger–Ellison syndrome. World J Surg 1993; 17: 433–8.

53. Perrier ND, Batts KP, Thompson GB *et al.* An immunohistochemical survey for neuroendocrine cells in regional pancreatic lymph nodes – a plausible explanation for primary nodal gastrinomas. Surgery 1995; 118: 957–65.

54. Stabile BE, Morrow DJ, Passaro E. The gastrinoma triangle: operative implications. Am J Surg 1984; 147: 25–31.

55. Pipeleers-Marichal M, Donow C, Heitz PU, Kloppel G. Pathologic aspects of gastrinomas in patients with Zollinger–Ellison syndrome with and without multiple endocrine neoplasia type I. World J Surg 1993; 17: 481–8.

56. Thompson NW, Vinik AI, Eckhauser FE. Microgastrinomas of the duodenum. Ann Surg 1989; 209: 396–404.

57. Frucht H, Norton JA, London JF *et al.* Detection of duodenal gastrinomas by operative endoscopic transillumination, a prospective study. Gastroenterology 1990; 99: 1622–7.

58. Howard TJ, Zinner MJ, Stabile BE, Passaro EJ. Gastrinoma excision for cure. Ann Surg 1990; 211: 9–14.

59. Norton JA. Advances in the management of Zollinger–Ellison syndrome. Adv Surg 1994; 27: 129–59.

60. Wolfe MM, Alexander RW, McGuigan JE. Extrapancreatic, extraintestinal gastrinoma: effective treatment by surgery. N Engl J Med 1982; 306: 1533–6.

61. Norton JA, Doppman JL, Collen MJ *et al.* Prospective study of gastrinoma localization and resection in patients with Zollinger–Ellison syndrome. Ann Surg 1986; 204: 468–79.

62. Bornman PC, Marks IN, Mee AS, Price S. Favourable response to conservative surgery for extra-pancreatic gastrinoma with lymph node metastases. Br J Surg 1987; 74: 198–201.

63. Richardson CT, Peters MN, Feldman M. Treatment of Zollinger–Ellison syndrome with exploratory laparotomy, proximal gastric vagotomy, and H_2-receptor antagonists. Gastroenterology 1985; 89: 357–67.

64. Ellison EC. Forty year appraisal of gastrinoma: back to the future. Ann Surg 1995; 222: 511–21.

65. Norton JA, Sugarbaker PH, Doppman JL *et al.* Aggressive resection of metastatic disease in selected patients with malignant gastrinoma. Ann Surg 1986; 203: 352–9.

66. Norton JA, Cornelius MJ, Doppman JL, Maton PN, Gardner JD, Jensen RT. Effect of parathyroidectomy in patients with hyperparathyroidism, Zollinger–Ellison syndrome, and multiple endocrine neoplasia type 1: a prospective study. Surgery 1987; 102: 958–66.

67. Thompson NW. Surgical treatment of the endocrine pancreas and Zollinger–Ellison syndrome in the MEN1 syndrome. Henry Ford Hosp Med J 1992; 40: 195–8.

68. Macfarlane MP, Fraker DL, Alexander HR, Norton JA, Jensen RT. A prospective study of surgical resection of duodenal and pancreatic gastrinomas in MEN-1. Surgery 1995; 118: 973–9.

69. Carty S, Jensen RT, Norton JA. Prospective study of aggressive resection of metastatic pancreatic endocrine tumors. Surgery 1992; 112: 1024–32.

70. Vinik AI, Strodel WE, Eckhauser FE *et al.* Somatostatinomas, PPomas, neurotensinomas. Semin Oncol 1987; 14:263.

71. Verner JV, Morrison AB. Endocrine pancreatic islet disease with diarrhea: report of a case due to diffuse hyperplasia of no beta islet tissue with a review of 54 additional cases. Arch Intern Med 1974; 1974: 133–492.

72. Capella C, Polak JM, Butta R *et al.* Morphologic patterns and diagnostic criteria of VIP-producing endocrine tumors. A histologic, histochemical, ultrastructural and biochemical study of 32 cases. Cancer 1983; 52: 1860.

73. Caplan PH, Koob L, Abellera RM *et al.* Cure of acromegaly by operative removal of an islet cell tumor of the pancreas. Am J Med 1978; 64: 874.

74. Bresler L, Boissel P, Conroy T, Grosdidier J. Pancreatic islet cell carcinoma with hypercalcemia: complete remission 5 years after surgical excision and chemotherapy. Am J Gastroenterol 1991; 86: 635.

75. Danforth DN, Gorden P, Brennan MF. Metastatic insulin secreting carcinoma of the pancreas. Clinical course and the role of surgery. Surgery 1984; 96: 1027–36.

76. Rothmund M, Stinner B, Arnold R. Endocrine pancreatic carcinoma. Eur J Surg Oncol 1991; 17: 191–9.

77. Modlin IM, Lewis JJ, Ahlman H, Bilchik AJ, Kumar RR. Management of unresectable malignant endocrine tumors of the pancreas. Surg Gynecol Obstet 1993; 176: 507–18.

78. Zogakis TG, Norton JA. Palliative operations for patients with unresectable endocrine neoplasia. Surg Clin North Am 1995; 75: 525–38.

79. Mozell E, Woltering EA, O'Dorisio TM, Fletcher WS, Sinclair AJ, Hill D. Effect of somatostatin analog on peptide release and tumor growth in the Zollinger–Ellison syndrome. Surg Gynecol Obstet 1990; 170: 476–84.

80. Pasieka JH, McLeod MK, Thompson NW, Burney RE. Surgical approach to insulinomas assessing the need for localization. Arch Surg 1992, 127: 442–447.

81. Mignon M, Ruszniewski R, Haffan S, Rigauld D, Rene E, Bonfils S. Current approach to the management of tumoural process in patients with gastrinoma. World J Surg 1986, 10: 702–709.

6 Carcinoid syndrome

Nigel D. S. Bax
H. Frank Woods

Incidence of carcinoid tumours

The symptoms of the carcinoid syndrome are well known but it is extremely unusual for physicians or surgeons to make a diagnosis prior to an appropriate biopsy sample being examined or a laporotomy being performed. In a series of 52 patients in Northern Ireland with abdominal carcinoid tumours the diagnosis was not made pre-operatively on any occasion.[1] Similarly, in just over 120 patients seen in Sheffield over the past 12 years, the diagnosis has not been made before histological diagnosis.

Carcinoid tumours are apparently rare. Ten years ago, reports from Sweden and Northern Ireland put the incidence of metastatic carcinoid tumours at between 0.3 and 0.7 cases per 100 000 of the population per year.[1,2] A similar figure was found more recently in the Trent Region (UK).[3] These rates may be underestimates of the true incidence of the condition since post-mortem studies suggest an incidence two to three times higher.[4,5]

Just under 100 of the patients seen in Sheffield over the past 12 years have come from within 20 miles of the hospital, an area with a population of about 1.6 million. This gives a crude incidence figure of about 0.5 patients/100 000 population/year. These data imply that there may be an underdiagnosis of carcinoid tumours. If the post-mortem data as regards the incidence of the tumour are correct then it might be that there are about 1000 new cases in the United Kingdom each year. Thus, on average, a general practitioner will be likely to see one new case every 30 years. It is not surprising, therefore, that even when a patient presents with flushing and diarrhoea the diagnosis of a carcinoid tumour does not come instantly to mind.

Diagnosis

Clinical history

The diagnosis is difficult to make because of the intermittent nature of the symptoms, especially in the early stages of the condition. The natural history of carcinoid tumours has been well described by Vinik *et al.*[6] who placed special emphasis on the vague abdominal symptoms which often result in a patient being diagnosed as having irritable bowel syndrome (Table 6.1). These symptoms may persist for some years before the diagnosis of a carcinoid tumour is made. Patients may experience symptoms intermittently for up to four to five years before the diagnosis is made[2,7] and in the Sheffield series typical antecedent diagnoses included the irritable bowel syndrome, peptic ulcer disease, gastritis and Crohn's disease. Barium X-ray studies may show what are thought to be typical appearances of Crohn's disease in the terminal ileum with ulcerated mucosa. Carcinoid tumours imitating Crohn's disease has been described previously.[8]

Table 6.1 *History*

Symptom	Character	Differential diagnoses
Abdominal pains	Intermittent Right upper quadrant and right iliac fossa May be a long history Often previous negative investigations	Inflammatory bowel disease Peptic ulcer disease Gallstones Irritable bowel syndrome Neoplasm
Diarrhoea	Intermittent At first occurs in episodes lasting a few days Mainly first thing in the morning May be associated with flushing May occur immediately after eating	Inflammatory bowel disease Irritable bowel syndrome Neoplasm (including endocrine)
Flushing	From barely perceptible to florid Typically affects face and neck Chocolate, alcohol and food may provoke Palpitations and hypotension may occur Telangiectases occur on cheeks and nose Patient may not notice all flushes Mild epiphora and rhinorrhoea	The menopause Emotion Alcohol use Medullary carcinoma of thyroid Mastocytosis

The two symptoms which are reported as occurring ubiquitously in the carcinoid syndrome are flushing and diarrhoea (Table 6.1). Aggregating data from five studies involving about 500 patients showed that at the time of presentation of patients to a tertiary referral centre, a mean of 75% (range 30–94) had flushing and 73% (range 38–86) had diarrhoea.[2,6,7,9,10] Four of these studies reported asthma as a presenting feature in a mean of 15% patients (range 2–23). Three studies reported abdominal pains in a mean of 49% patients (range 25–73), peripheral oedema in a mean of 29% (range 3–66) and pellagra in a mean of 4% (range 0–6). The large ranges may reflect differences in the times at which patients presented to the tertiary referral centres and highlights the difficulties in comparing data from one centre with those from another.

Abdominal pain, diarrhoea and flushing

In 122 consecutive patients with abdominal carcinoid tumours 69% had abdominal pain at the time of diagnosis, 36% had diarrhoea and 29% were flushing (Fig. 6.1a, b, c). Thirty (36%) of the 84 patients with abdominal pain experienced it solely in the epigastrium or right upper quadrant area, with 19 (23%) experiencing it solely in the right lower quadrant. A total of 21 patients (25%) had generalised abdominal pains but only five patients (6%) had pain only on the left side of the abdomen.

In some patients symptoms had been present for many years before the diagnosis was made and it would be difficult to attribute the symptoms in all patients to the presence of a carcinoid tumour. Nevertheless, at the time of diagnosis abdominal pain was both the commonest and most persistent symptom. A common pattern of symptoms was for a patient to have initially a few episodes of abdominal pains, sometimes localised, sometimes colicky in nature, each separated by weeks or even months. The pains became more frequent and by the time of diagnosis most patients had either diarrhoea or flushing or both. A few patients appeared to have none of these symptoms and were usually diagnosed after finding an enlarged liver or other abdominal mass.

Patients with abdominal pain alone had often been investigated with a barium enema, upper alimentary endoscopy, abdominal ultrasonography and blood tests without finding an abnormality. In one series 45% of patients with an abdominal carcinoid tumour presented with intestinal obstruction[1] and data from the 103 patients in the Uppsala series showed that the diagnosis was made more quickly in patients with intestinal obstruction than in those with diarrhoea or flushing.[2]

Many other clinical features occur which include palpitations, bronchial asthma, heart failure, pellagra, other endocrine conditions, weight loss and depression. Although any of these may be associated with the syndrome their presence in isolation in the absence of either

Figure 6.1 *The length of history of (a) abdominal pains, (b) diarrhoea and (c) flushing in 122 patients with abdominal carcinoid tumours.*

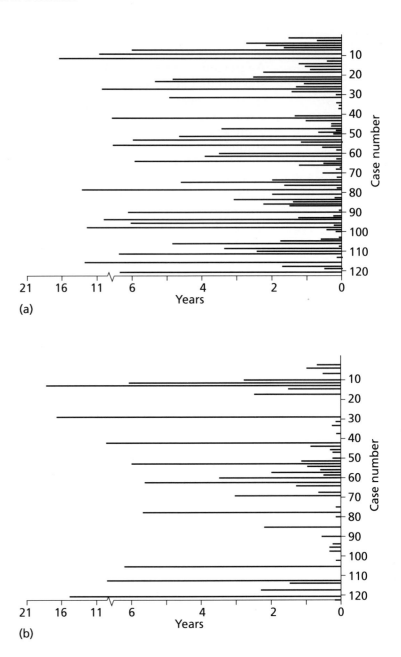

abdominal pain, diarrhoea, wheezing or an abdominal mass should not cause suspicion of a carcinoid tumour.

There is no particular pattern to the diarrhoea except that it tends to occur most commonly immediately on rising in the morning and then tails off as the day progresses. It is unusual to see patients with nocturnal diarrhoea.

The flushing attacks are usually confined to the face and upper chest. They occur spontaneously or may be triggered by drinking alcohol,

Figure 6.1
(continued)

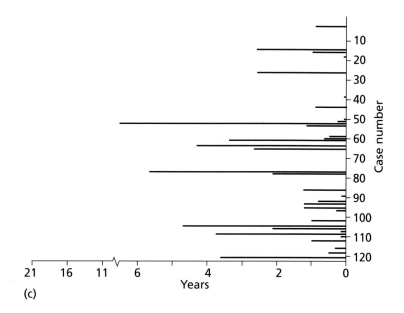

(c)

eating chocolate or occasionally eating hot food or opening the bowels. A flush may be nothing more than a 10–20 s feeling of warmth or mild sweating across the forehead. At the other extreme the whole body may flush for 5–10 min or occasionally longer. The latter type of flush is extremely rare but seen most commonly at the time of induction of anaesthesia and may be associated with rapid changes in the systemic blood pressure and bronchospasm. The most common flushing attack in our patients lasts for between 30 s and 2–3 min and affects only the face, the front of the neck and sometimes the upper chest. It is accompanied, in some, by running of the nose and epiphora. Patients occasionally report concurrent palpitations.

Flushing attacks do not occur until the carcinoid tumour has metastasised. Occasionally, ultrasonography and CT scanning will not reveal any abnormality of the liver in patients who are flushing and the situation may be further confused by a patient with a urinary 5-hydroxyindole acetic acid excretion which is within the reference range. Diagnosis in such extremely rare patients is difficult.

After a few years of flushing there may be a permanent flush across the cheeks and nose. This may vary from mild telangiectasis to a deep ruby or a very dark purple discoloration and, rarely, a blackening of the skin. The flushing attacks in patients with a gastric primary are said to be bright red and patchy,[11] possibly due to the release of histamine. The distinction of colours of flushing is not easy clinically. The presence of a flush of any hue is the important physical sign. Despite flushing that is obvious to others, some patients do not notice that they are flushing, or only notice a few of their attacks. This makes the number of flushes per day a potentially unreliable way of measuring the response to therapy.

Site of the primary tumour

The majority of carcinoid tumours originate in the gastrointestinal tract. Other than from the appendix the main sites of primary tumour have been found to be the jejeno-ileum, rectum and colon.[6] Godwin[12] found approximately 2% of patients had a gastric primary site in a series of nearly 3000. Recently it has been suggested that the stomach may be a far more common site for a primary than had been recognised previously. In a series of 349 neuroendocrine tumours the appendix was the primary site in 30% of patients, colorectum in 16%, stomach in 14% and the small intestine in 9%.[13] Overall, gastric primary carcinoid tumours may represent 10–30% of all carcinoid tumours.[14] There is a particular risk of a gastric carcinoid tumour developing in patients with pernicious anaemia.[15]

Bronchial carcinoids, which account for about 1% of pulmonary tumours and about 10% of all carcinoids, usually present with haemoptysis or pneumonia.

Associated cancers

It had been thought that there was an increased prevalence of other cancers in patients with carcinoid tumours but a recent large population-based study of over 1000 patients showed no overall increased risk of a patient having a second tumour.[16]

Clinical examination (Table 6.2)

There may be no abnormalities on physical examination. Facial telangiectasia may be present as may peripheral oedema and pellagra.[11] The percentage of patients with these signs varies between studies and probably reflects the stage of the disease. Pellagra was seen in two of the 122 patients described above whereas others have found it in 6% of patients.[11]

There may be a mass in the right iliac fossa which is often tender. The mass is usually larger than the primary tumour itself and consists of fibrous tissue which may involve the bowel wall and mesentery. The liver may be enlarged, sometimes with discrete masses palpable on the surface which may be tender. Central abdominal masses may be due to enlargement of lymph nodes. Ascites is rarely detected except in very advanced disease. Jaundice is uncommon, even in the period shortly before death.

Examination of bones for tenderness on percussion or springing may result in pain where secondary deposits are present.

An elevated jugular venous pressure raises the possibility of tricuspid or pulmonary valve disease.

Metastases to the eye are rare but fundoscopy should be performed. In a series of 410 patients with such metastases, carcinoid was responsible in 9 (2.2%).[17] None of the patients had a small bowel primary

Table 6.2 *Clinical examination*

General
  May be normal
  Weight loss
  Peripheral oedema
  Telangiectasia
  Bright eyes (epiphora)

Abdomen
  Mass in right iliac fossa/para-aortic region
  Hepatomegaly
  Ascites
  Rectal mass

Cardiovascular
  Raised JVP
  Tricuspid regurgitation/stenosis
  Pulmonary stenosis

Skin
  Pellagra (rare)
  Peripheral oedema (rare initially)

Bones
  Tender with secondaries

Respiratory
  Wheezing (rare initially)

tumour; seven had a bronchial primary. Decreased vision is the commonest symptom of a choroidal secondary tumour with proptosis and diminished eye movements the commonest symptoms of orbital secondaries. Choroidal carcinoid secondaries are orange in colour on fundoscopy.

Investigations (Table 6.3)

Urine

The most well-known biochemical test is the estimation of the 24 h urinary excretion of 5-hydroxyindoleacetic acid (5-HIAA). Tryptophan is metabolised to 5-hydroxytryptophan (5-HTP) which is rapidly metabolised to 5-hydroxytryptamine (5-HT). Much of the 5-HT is present in platelets with some being metabolised by an intermediate step to 5-HIAA. Although about 85% of carcinoid tumours occur in the gastrointestinal tract[12] the clinical and biochemical behaviour is related to the site of origin within the bowel.

Table 6.3 *Investigations*

Urine	Minimum of two 24 h urines for 5-HIAA estimation
	Quantitative not qualitative assay
	If borderline result repeat urine collection with diet control
	5-HIAA excretion relates to tumour mass and activity
	Some patients produce little or no 5-HIAA excess
	In these, if possible, measure 5-HTP excretion
	Ensure laboratory has acid in urine collection bottle (otherwise 5-HIAA degrades)
Blood	Basic tests may be normal
	↑ alkaline phosphatase and gamma GT – ↓ prognosis
	Alkaline phosphatase and gamma GT may rise quickly in 3–6 months before death
	Plasma chromogranin A ↑ with neuroendocrine tumours
	Estimation of plasma gut peptide concentration of unknown value
	Estimation of plasma serotonin concentration of unknown value
X-rays	Barium follow-through may show terminal ileal distortion/stricture
	Chest X-ray may show consolidation/mass/be normal
	Bone secondaries may be sclerotic (typically seen in vertebrae)
Ultrasonography	Mass lesions in liver
	Occasionally see primary
	Rectal tumours and local spread seen with transrectal views
	Useful for measuring tumour size changes with therapy
CT scan	Mass lesions in liver
	Mesenteric lesions with 'star-burst' appearance
	Poor for seeing primary tumour
^{111}**In-octreotide scintigraphy**	Shows unsuspected lesions
	Not all carcinoid tumours are seen (may not have relevant receptors)
	Shows sites of tumours
	Not specific for carcinoid tumours
	Possible false-negative result
	Expensive
Bone scan	Symptomless patients may have positive scan
	Perform if any bone tenderness or pain
Angiography	Not a routine investigation
	Mesenteric angiography prior to bowel surgery (if possible)
	Hepatic angiography prior to embolisation
Cardiac echocardiography	Perform in all
	Cardiac changes rarely seen until syndrome present for over 3 years

Carcinoid tumours were classified by Williams and Sandler[18] by their site of origin as foregut, midgut and hindgut. Patients with foregut tumours (respiratory tract, stomach, duodenum, jejunum and pancreas) may have relatively small amounts of 5-HIAA in the urine but a marked excess of 5-hydroxytryptophan, possibly because of a relative lack of aromatic amino acid decarboxylase. These tumours are more likely to produce other hormones such as gastrin and ACTH.[19] Bronchial carcinoid tumours may cause Cushing's syndrome due to ectopic ACTH production.[20]

Midgut and hindgut tumours produce relatively more 5-HIAA than 5-HTP but differ from each other in respect of their production of other hormones.[14] The clinical utility of estimating concentrations of various gut and other hormones that might be produced by carcinoid tumours has not been established. The differences in the biological and clinical behaviour of carcinoid tumours from different sites and the differences they exhibit in ultrastructure and immuno-histochemistry[19] show that the term 'carcinoid' covers a large family of neuroendocrine tumours.

The 24 h urinary excretion of 5-HIAA remains the most valuable biochemical screening test for the presence of metastatic carcinoid tumour. The estimation of 5-HIAA concentration in the urine may be qualitative or quantiative. The former method is still being used but this should not continue. A recent quality control exercise showed that where a qualitative method was used 10/25 (40%) of the results were incorrect whereas where a quantitative method was used 2/40 (5%) were incorrect (Forrest, personal communication). The urinary excretion of 5-HIAA is variable and reliance should not be placed on the results from a single 24 h urine collection. Many protocols for diagnosis and follow-up of patients rely on two 24 h urine collections. Food containing large amounts of 5-HT, such as aubergines, avocado pears, bananas and many nuts may cause a slight elevation of the urinary 5-HIAA but this is not thought to be of relevance in most patients.[6]

Imaging

Abdominal ultrasonography may reveal hepatic masses from which a guided biopsy may be taken. In the Shefficial series of patients this has become the commonest method of diagnosis. Previously, the commonest method of diagnosis of gastrointestinal carcinoids was from the histological appearance of tumour taken at laporotomy following the patient presenting with intestinal obstruction. Ultrasonography may reveal primary small bowel carcinoid tumours[21] but computed tomography (CT) of the abdomen may be of less help.[22] The typical CT appearances of carcinoid tumour deposits within the mesentery are of discrete masses with radiating spokes (Fig. 6.2). About 40% of mesenteric masses due to carcinoid contain calcification.[23] Transrectal ultrasonography is of value in staging and following the response to surgery in rectal carcinoids.

Figure 6.2 *A mesenteric secondary carcinoid tumour showing radiating spokes.*

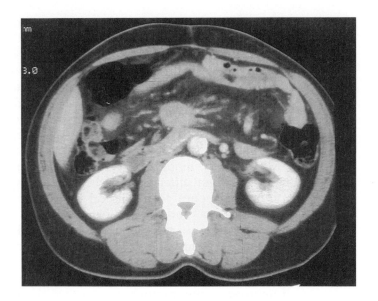

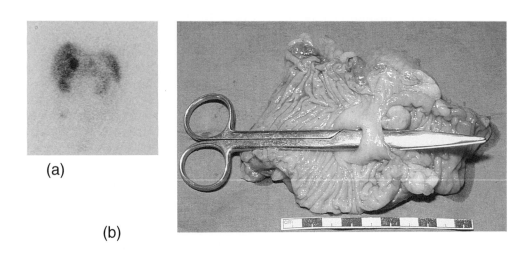

(a)

(b)

Figure 6.3 *An ¹¹¹In-octreotide scan (a) showing increased uptake in the region of the terminal ileum and within the liver, and the operative finding (b) showing the terminal carcinoid. At operation it was possible to remove all hepatic secondary deposits. (b) Courtesy of Professor A. Johnson.*

The scintigraphic localisation of a carcinoid tumour was first described in 1989[24] and since then the Dutch group have reported their experience with this technique in over 1000 patients.[25] The technique relies on attaching a radioligand to a somatostatin analogue which will in turn attach itself to somatostatin receptors which are abundant on the surface of carcinoid tumours. Previously unsuspected carcinoid deposits have been found in over 50% of patients studied using ^{111}In-octreotide (Pentetreotide). An ^{111}In-octreotide scan showing abnormal uptake in the right iliac fossa region together with hepatic secondaries is shown in Fig. 6.3 together with the terminal ileal tumour removed at operation.

Postoperative studies in patients in whom it had been thought that there had been complete removal of tumour showed probable residual tumour in about 30% of patients. A recent study involving 100 patients showed abnormal uptake in 77, true-negative results in 11 patients and false-negative results in 12, when compared with standard imaging techniques.[26] There are at least three different subtypes of somatostatin receptor and octreotide does not bind to all with equal affinity. This might explain the true-negative results. The presence of receptors that bind radiolabelled octreotide might help determine which patients would respond to octreotide therapy. The pentetreotide test is, however, very expensive and it would not seem appropriate to use it in this way. It is far cheaper to give a patient octreotide and see if they respond. The intraoperative use of ^{111}In-octreotide with a hand-held gamma ray detector does not improve tumour localisation.[27]

Whenever possible, mesenteric angiography should be carried out as part of the planning for a resection of a bowel carcinoid mass. The bowel may be tethered down into a mass of fibrous tissue making resection difficult and a knowledge of the vascular supply is of help. Hepatic angiography need not be performed routinely, but is of value in those undergoing embolisation therapy.

Blood tests

There are no basic blood tests that are of any diagnostic assistance. Frequently, the serum alkaline phosphatase and gamma glutamyl transferase are only slightly elevated even in the presence of considerable metastatic disease in the liver. Elevated concentrations of these enzymes have been found to be inversely related to survival.[28] Within the 3–6 months prior to death the concentrations of these enzymes increase to as much as ten times the upper limit of the reference range.

An elevated plasma concentration of chromogranin A is of diagnostic significance suggesting the presence of a neuroendocrine tumour but the test is not widely used at present.[20]

Histopathology

Expert histopathology is essential in establishing the diagnosis. The diagnosis should not be made solely on the basis of whether the cells are argyrophil or argentaffin positive. Foregut carcinoids are argyrophil positive. The entero-chromaffin-like cells that form the major cell-type in gastric carcinoid tumours, are argentaffin negative.[29] Midgut tumours are predominantly argentaffin positive and hindgut tumours typically are non-reactive. Carcinoid tumours look like adenocarcinomas and may be diagnosed as such unless the tissue is examined for neuron-specific enolase and chromogranin.[6] Antibodies raised to the various subtypes of chromogranin have been used for immunohistochemical staining of a range of neuroendocrine tumours but the clinical relevance of subtypes in a tumour is not known.[30]

Treatment

The aim of treatment to relieve the local and distant effects caused by the tumour and its secretions. Optimal control of the carcinoid syndrome results from removal of carcinoid tumour. If this is not possible, then the biological activity of the tumour and sometimes its size, may be diminished by hepatic artery embolisation, drug therapy or radiotherapy. Table 6.4 summarises treatment options.

Surgery

If the patient is fit for surgery then debulking the patient of tumour, or as much of the tumour as possible, provides the best outcome of all available therapies.[31,32] Surgical debulking may greatly diminish the symptoms of the syndrome,[33,34] decreases the urinary 5-HIAA excretion[35] and should be attempted whenever possible.

Table 6.4 *Treatment*

Surgery	Attempt to remove as much tumour as possible Cover operation with octreotide Gives the best long term results
Embolisation of hepatic secondaries	Indicated when surgical removal of tumour not possible Antimicrobial and octreotide cover needed May have pain and fever afterwards
Drugs	Octreotide for patients with the carcinoid syndrome In unresponsive patients consider using interferon Simple therapy such as codeine phosphate may control diarrhoea Somatostatin analogues and interferon are very expensive
Radiotherapy	Decreases pain from bone secondaries Possible value in shrinking tumours

Many patients still present as an acute intestinal problem requiring urgent surgery. Typically, the findings at operation are of a mass, often in the right iliac fossa, which consists of loops of small bowel adherent to each other and the ascending colon. The tumour, which may be no more than 1–2 cm in diameter, forms the nidus of the mass. There may be mesenteric deposits and seedlings in the peritoneum. In addition, secondary deposits are usually seen on the surface of the liver. Faced with such a situation it is not surprising that a diagnosis of inoperable disseminated malignancy is made, a defunctioning procedure is performed and biopsies taken. A few days later the histopathology report raises the possibility of carcinoid. Nearly half the patients in one series were diagnosed as a result of presenting in the above manner.

The survival of patients with operable carcinoid disease is longer than of patients with inoperable disease.[32] In a series of 48 patients all with hepatic metastases, 11 who had surgery alone were alive and apparently tumour free three months later, 6 of the 27 who had been treated with embolisation and octreotide had died and 8 of the 10 treated with octreotide alone had died.[33] These two studies highlight the difficulties in conducting trials of therapy in patients with carcinoid tumours. The numbers in each treatment group were very small and the groups were not well matched as regards the stage of disease.

At any time during surgery, but particularly at the time of induction of anaesthesia, patients may have sudden and marked changes in blood pressure. Hypotension or hypertension can occur at various times, with prolonged and extensive flushing and bronchospasm. These are the features of a carcinoid crisis. There are no indicators as to which patients might react adversely to anaesthesia or surgery. Patients with a greatly elevated urinary 5-HIAA excretion, and thus a presumed large tumour load, appear to be no more likely to have a carcinoid crisis than patients with only minimal elevation. Octreotide therapy has prevented these complications.[36] In patients not already receiving octreotide, treatment is started the day before surgery with a first dose of 50 µg followed 8 h later by 100 µg. This dosage is continued eight hourly thereafter so that by the time a patient is anaesthetised they have received four or five doses. The octreotide is given subcutaneously at this stage. The final preoperative dose is given an hour before induction. Further doses of 10–20 µg may be given intravenously during the operation as the clinical state dictates. Episodes of hypotension caused by the tumour releasing vasoactive peptides responds well to such treatment. Patients who are already receiving octreotide prior to operation continue the therapy and are given a regular dose one hour before induction.

Somatostatin analogues

A chance observation led to the use of somatostatin analogues in the treatment of the carcinoid syndrome. Two patients with medullary carcinoma of the thyroid flushed on receiving pentagastrin and it was thus postulated that gastrin might be the cause of the carcinoid flush. Somatostatin was known to inhibit gastrin release and when given to patients with carcinoid disease it abolished pentagastrin-induced flushing.[37] Gastrin is now known not to be responsible for carcinoid flushing but the serendipity of these early experiments has resulted in the production of a number of somatostatin analogues which have a beneficial effect in the carcinoid syndrome.

A single dose of somatostatin has a very short duration of effect due to its rapid metabolism which makes it of no practical value in controlling carcinoid symptoms. The somatostatin molecule was modified to make it longer acting and by 1986 a study of the effects of this new drug, octreotide, was reported.[38] A review of over 60 published studies has shown that diarrhoea and flushing may be controlled, on average in about 80% of patients. As many as 90% of patients may benefit with appropriate dose titration but few obtain complete relief of symptoms.[39] The initial dosage of octreotide should be 100 µg tds subcutaneously, increasing the dosage by 50–100 µg every 8 h until symptoms are controlled.

A disadvantage of octreotide is that it has to be given a number of times each day by repeated subcutaneous injections. In an attempt to circumvent this problem a number of long-acting somatostatin analogues are being developed which will be administered once a week or at longer intervals.

Octreotide does not appear to cause regression of carcinoid tumours, nor, regrettably, prolong life.

The response to octreotide may diminish with time,[38] but the cause for this is not known. Octreotide therapy is well tolerated although its injection may cause a slight and transient stinging sensation. Many patients complain of smelly motions and this is due to the increase in the fat content of the stools. Occasionally, patients may have worsening of diarrhoea and in some, gallstones and biliary sludge may develop.

Interferon

Oberg and his colleagues administered human leucocyte interferon to a small group of patients with metastatic carcinoid tumour.[40] Symptoms were improved in two-thirds of the patients. A larger study provided evidence of clinical benefit and a decrease in 5-HIAA excretion in about half the patients for a median time of 34 months.[41] Further studies have demonstrated that, overall, the beneficial effects of interferon-2α are similar to, or slightly less marked than octreotide and, like octreotide, there are no data to support it having a significant effect on tumour size. The dosages commonly used vary between 3 and 6 mega units given daily for three or six days of each week. Far higher dosages have been used but it is uncertain that this gives any therapeutic advantage.

Side effects with interferon are more troublesome than with octreotide. The commonest is a feeling of an influenza-like illness a few hours after the injection. Paracetamol 1 g, taken at the time of the injection appears to lessen this problem. Some patients still experience fever, myalgia and fatigue.

The optimal time to use interferon is not known. It is probably best at present to use it in patients who have not responded to treatment with octreotide or in those whose initial response to octreotide has lessened significantly.

There is no evidence to support the use of either octreotide or interferon in the absence of the syndrome. If a patient fails to respond to octreotide having titrated the dosage up to 500 μg tds then it is appropriate to try interferon-2α. The reason for a patient not responding to octreotide therapy might be that the tumour is relatively depleted of receptors to which octreotide may bind. If diarrhoea is the sole problem then codeine phosphate may help and at considerably less expense than octreotide or interferon both of which cost around £10 000 per year per patient. No interferon preparation is currently licensed in the UK for use in the treatment of carcinoid patients.

Cytotoxic therapy and the use of other drugs

There is no evidence to support the use of cytotoxic therapy in patients with carcinoid tumours. Many of the studies using such agents were conducted between 10 and 20 years ago, but more recent studies with agents such as dacarbazine, adriamycin, cisplatin, fluorouracil and streptozotocin have failed to show any significant antitumour effect.

A number of other drugs including ketanserin, cyproheptadine, calcitonin, codeine phosphate, and in the past, methysergide and parachlorophenylalanine, have been used in an attempt to control the symptoms of the disease. None have been compared directly with octreotide or interferon.

Hepatic embolisation

The treatment of obliterating the arterial supply to hepatic secondary carcinoid tumours was first demonstrated in 1977.[42] It is now an established treatment in controlling the symptoms of the carcinoid syndrome and probably is effective because it causes necrosis of the tumour. A number of embolic agents have been used including gelatin sponge, stainless-steel coils, polyvinyl alcohol foam and absolute alcohol (ethanol). More recently a mixture of cyanoacrylate and ethiodised oil has been used.[43] The advantages of the liquid embolising medium over particulate solutions are that they can be administered closer to the tumour. The symptomatic improvement obtained by this therapy appears to be as good as that seen with octreotide treatment with the added advantage that embolisation causes a decrease in the tumour mass within the liver. Cytotoxic drugs have been administered

(a)

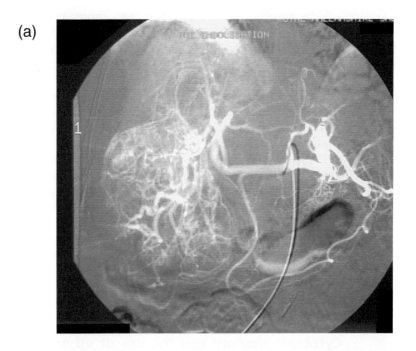

(b)

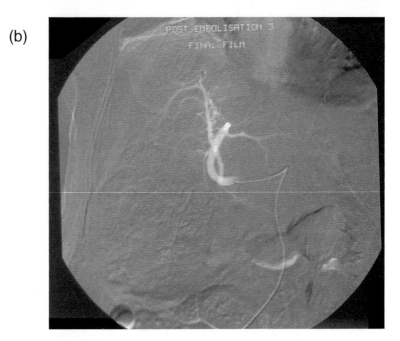

Figure 6.4 *Hepatic angiogram showing a carcinoid tumour (a) before and (b) after injection of absolute alcohol into the artery supplying the tumour. Photo courtesy of Dr P. Gaines.*

with chemoembolising agents but outcome data are sparse. It is not known whether this combination gives any advantage over chemo-embolisation alone. There were more 5-year survivors and a greater degree of biochemical response in patients who received embolisation plus interferon compared with a group who received interferon alone but embolisation was not found to have a statistically significant effect on survival.[44]

Patients should be taking octreotide before embolisation and receive their usual dose one hour before the procedure starts. Metronidazole and cefuroxime should be administered intravenously at the same time and this antimicrobial therapy is continued for one week after the embolisation. Injection of the alcohol causes intense pain in some subjects and pethidine (50–100 mg) is given slowly intravenously a few minutes in advance. Usual post-angiogram observations of the leg, pulse rate, blood pressure and wound site are made on the ward. Some patients become slightly intoxicated and must be warned about this in advance.

Patients may experience pains over the right upper abdomen and lower right chest for three or four days after embolisation. The pain may be pleuritic which will raise the possiblity of a pulmonary embolus. There may be an intermittent pyrexia, probably related to tissue necrosis, which raises concern about an hepatic abscess or septicaemia. The pain usually lasts only a day or two but the pyrexia may persist for a week or slightly longer. A result from an embolisation using absolute alcohol is shown in Figure 6.4?

Radiotherapy

It has long been thought that carcinoid tumours are radioresistant. Radiotherapy is excellent in relieving the pain from bone secondaries. A few recent reports have raised the possibity that secondary deposits in the liver and elsewhere shrink in response to radiotherapy.[45]

Monitoring the response to therapy

A reasonable aim is an 80% or greater decrease in the frequency of flushing and diarrhoea. Relief of pain should also be achieved. A decrease in the urinary 5-HIAA excretion should be seen. Such a decrease is associated with a decrease in the frequency and severity of symptoms but does not appear to be related to changes in tumour growth. Any lessening of the response to therapy is not of predictive value as regards survival. Tumour size may be evaluated by routine scanning techniques but as the tumour is usually slow growing scans do not need to be performed more than at six monthly.

Survival data in relation to carcinoid disease are difficult to interpret because they are based on survival from the time of diagnosis rather than from the time of onset of the disease. With this reservation one might expect that ten years after diagnosis in patients with abdominal carcinoid tumour, 60% with operable disease would be alive, whereas for patients with inoperable disease or hepatic metastases the figures would be 40% and 20%, respectively.[32]

Concluding remarks

The symptoms occurring in patients with metastatic carcinoid tumour were first recognised as conforming to a pattern in the 1950's and were labelled as the carcinoid syndrome.[10,46] A feature of the disease that had been described over 100 years ago[47] and frequently mentioned in the literature until about 1950, was that of abdominal pain. Most reports during the last 30 years have been from tertiary referral centres and by the time a patient is seen they may have had their primary bowel tumour removed, and, therefore, the main cause of pain.

There is an important distinction to make between carcinoid disease and carcinoid syndrome. If the development of the syndrome occurs before making the diagnosis then the opportunity to cure the disease will almost certainly have been lost but this is usually the case in our experience. The challenge is to make the diagnosis in a patient who presents with intermittent abdominal pain. Even in the absence of the syndrome any patient with a long history of small bowel obstruction should be suspected of having a carcinoid tumour.[48]

Acknowledgement

The management of carcinoid tumours requires close liaison between pathologists, clinical chemists, radiologists, surgeons, anaesthetists and clinical oncologists and we thank our colleagues Alan Johnson, Bill Thomas, John Smith, Peter Gaines, Tim Stephenson, Robert Forrest, Charles Reilly, John Peacock, David Radford and Aidan Batchelor for their help and guidance. We thank too, all those other colleagues who have referred patients to us.

References

1. Buchanan KD, Johnston CF, O'Hare MMT *et al.* Neuroendocrine tumours. A European view. Am J Med 1986; 81 (Suppl 6B): 14–22.

2. Norheim I, Oberg K, Theodorsson-Norheim E *et al.* Malignant carcinoid tumours. Ann Surg 1987; 206: 115–25.

3. Woods HF, Bax NDS, Ainsworth I. Abdominal carcinoid tumours in Sheffield. Digestion 1990; 45 (Suppl): 17–22.

4. Berge T, Linell F. Carcinoid tumours. Acta Pathol Microbiol Scand 1976; 84: 322–30.

5. Weil C. Gastroenterohepatic endocrine tumours. Klin Wochenschr 1985; 63: 433–59.

6. Vinik AI, Thompson N, Eckhauser F *et al.* Clinical features of carcinoid syndrome and the use of somatostatin analogue in its management. Acta Oncol 1989; 28: 389–402.

7. Bax NDS, Woods HF, Batchelor A *et al.* The clinical manifestations of carcinoid disease. World J Surg 1996; 20: 142–6.

8. Stark S, Bluth I, Rubenstein S. Carcinoid tumour of the ileum resembling regional ileitis clinically and roentgenologically. Gastroenterology 1961; 40: 813–17.

9. Thorson AH. Studies on carcinoid disease. Acta Med Scand 1958; 161 (Suppl 334).

10. Kahler HJ, Heilmeyer L. Klinik und Pathophysiologie des Karzinoids und Karzinoid syndroms unter Berucksichtigung der Pharmacologie des 5-Hydroxytryptamins. Ergeb Inn Med Kinderheilkol 1961; 16: 292–5.

11. Grahame-Smith DG. The carcinoid syndrome. London: W Heinemann, 1972.

12. Godwin DJ. Carcinoid tumours: an analysis of 2,837 cases. Cancer 1975; 36: 560–9.

13. Hauser H, Wolf G, Uranus S *et al.* Neuroendocrine tumours in various organ systems in a ten-year period. Eur J Surg Oncol 1995; 21: 297–300.

14. Gilligan CJ, Lawton GP, Tang LH *et al.* Gastric carcinoid tumours: the biology and therapy of an enigmatic and controversial lesion. Am J Gastroenterol 1995; 90: 338–52.

15. Sjoblom SM, Sipponen P, Miettinen M *et al.* Gastroscopic screening for gastric carcinoids and carcinoma in pernicious anaemia. Endoscopy 1988; 20: 52–6.

16. Westergaard T, Frisch M, Melbye M. Carcinoid tumours in Denmark 1978–1989 and the risk of subsequent cancers. A population-based study. Cancer 1995; 76: 106–9.

17. Harbour JW, Potter PD, Shields CL *et al.* Uveal metastases from carcinoid tumour. Ophthalmology 1993; 101: 1084–90.

18. Williams ED, Sandler M. The classification of carcinoid tumours. Lancet 1963; i: 238–9.

19. Creutzfeldt W, Stockman F. Carcinoids and carcinoid syndrome. Am J Med 1987; 82: (Suppl 5B): 5–16.

20. Oliaro A, Filosso PL, Casadio C *et al.* Bronchial carcinoid associated with Cushing's syndrome. J Cardiovasc Surg 1995; 36: 511–14.

21. Rioux M, Langis P, Naud F. Sonographic appearance of primary small bowel carcinoid tumour. Abdom Imaging 1995; 20: 37–43.

22. Sugimoto E, Lorelius LE, Ericksson B *et al.* Midgut carcinoid tumours. CT appearance. Acta Radiol 1995; 36: 367–71.

23. Woodard PK, Feldman JM, Paine SS *et al.* Midgut carcinoid tumours: CT findings and biochemical profiles. J Comput Assist Tomograph. 1995; 19: 400–405.

24. Krenning EP, Bakker WH, Breeman WAP *et al.* Localization of endocrine related tumours with radioiodinated analogue of somatostatin. Lancet 1989; i: 242–5.

25. Krenning EP, Kwekkeboom DJ, Bakker WH *et al.* Somatostatin receptor scintigraphy with [^{111}In-DPTA-D Phe 1]- and [^{123}I-Tyr3]-octreotide: the Rotterdam experience with more than 1000 patients. Eur J Nucl Med 1993; 20: 716–31.

26. Kalkner K-M, Janson ET, Nilsson S *et al.* Somatostatin receptor scintigraphy in patients with carcinoid tumours: comparison between radioligand uptake and tumour markers. Cancer Res (Suppl) 1995; 55: 5801s–4s.

27. Ohrvall U, Westlin JE, Nilsson S *et al.* Human biodistribution of [^{111}In]diethylenetriaminepentaacetic acid- (DTPA) -D-[Phe 1]-octreotide and peroperative detection of endocrine tumours. Cancer Res 1995; 55 (23 Suppl): 5794s–800s.

28. Neijt JP, Lacave AJ, Splinter TA *et al.* Mitoxantrone in metastatic apudomas: a phase II study of the EORTC Gastro-Intestinal Cancer Cooperative Group. Br J Cancer 1995; 71: 106–8.

29. Sundler F, Hakanson R. Gastric endocrine cell typing at the light microscopic level. In:

Hakanson R, Sundler F (eds) The stomach as an endocrine organ. Amsterdam: Elsevier Science Publishers, 1991, pp. 9–26.

30. Stridsberg M, Oberg K, Li Q *et al.* Measurements of chromogranin A, chromogranin B (secretogranin I), chromogranin C (secretogranin II), and pancreastatin in plasma and urine from patients with carcinoid tumours and endocrine pancreatic tumours. J. Endocrinol 1995; 144: 49–59.

31. Moertel CG. Karnofsky Memorial Lecture. An odyssey in a land of small tumours. J Clin Oncol 1987; 5: 1502–22.

32. Wangberg B, Getered K, Nilsson O *et al.* Embolisation therapy in the midgut carcinoid syndrome: just tumour ischaemia? Acta Oncol 1993; 32: 251–6.

33. Ahlman H, Schersten T, Tisell LE. Surgical treatment of patients with carcinoid syndrome. Acta Oncol 1989; 28: 403–7.

34. Que FG, Nagorney DM, Batts KP *et al.* Hepatic resection for metastatic neuroendocrine carcinomas. Am J Surg 1995; 169: 36–42.

35. Woods HF, Bax NDS, Smith JARS. Small bowel carcinoid tumours. World J Surg 1985; 9: 921–9.

36. Veall GRQ, Peacock JE, Bax NDS *et al.* Review of the anaesthetic management of 21 patients undergoing laparotomy for carcinoid syndrome. Br J Anaesth 1994; 72: 335–41.

37. Frolich JC, Bloomgarten ZT, Oates JA *et al.* The carcinoid flush: provocation by pentagastrin and inhibition by somatostatin. N Engl J Med 1978; 299: 1055–7.

38. Kvols LK, Moertel CG, O'Connell MJ *et al.* Treatment of the malignant carcinoid syndrome. Evaluation of a long-acting somatostatin analogue. N Engl J Med 1986; 315: 663–6.

39. Harris AG, Redfern JS. Octreotide treatment of carcinoid syndrome: analysis of dose-titration data. Alim Pharm Ther 1995; 9: 387–94.

40. Oberg K, Funa K, Alm G. Effects of leucocyte interferon on clinical symptoms and hormone levels in patients with mid-gut carcinoid tumours and carcinoid syndrome. Lancet 1983; 309: 129–33.

41. Oberg K, Norheim I, Lind E *et al.* Treatment of malignant carcinoid tumours with human leucocyte interferon – long term results. Cancer Treat Rep 1986; 70: 1297–304.

42. Allison DJ, Modlin IM, Jenkins WJ. Treatment of carcinoid liver metastases by hepatic artery embolisation. Lancet 1977; ii: 1323–5.

43. Winkelbauer FW, Niederle B, Pietschmann F *et al.* Hepatic artery embolotherapy of hepatic metastases from carcinoid tumours: value of using a mixture of cyanoacrylate and ethiodized oil. Am J Radiol 1995; 165: 323–7.

44. Jacobsen MB, Hanssen LE, Kolmannskog F *et al.* Interferon-alpha 2b, with or without prior hepatic artery embolization: clinical response and survival in mid-gut carcinoid patients. The Norwegian carcinoid study. Scand J Gastroenterol 1995; 30: 789–96.

45. Chakravarthy A, Abrams RA. Radiation therapy in the management of patients with malignant carcinoid tumours. Cancer 1994; 75: 1386–90.

46. Sjoerdsma A, Weissbach H, Udenfriend S. A clinical, physiologic and biochemical study of patients with malignant carcinoid (argentaffinoma). Am J Med 1956; 20: 520–32.

47. Ransom WB. A case of primary carcinoma of the ileum. Lancet 1890; ii: 1020–3.

48. Stewart WH, Bartlett RM, Bishop HM *et al.* Carcinoid tumours presenting with acute abdominal signs. Ann Surg 1961; 154: 112–20.

7 Developmental abnormalities and benign breast disease

Robert E. Mansel
Hemant Singhal

Introduction Benign breast disease is common with an estimate that over half the female population will, at some time, seek medical attention for a breast problem and approximately one in four women will undergo a breast biopsy. Benign conditions of the breast have been neglected in comparison to cancer, despite the fact that only 6–10% of patients presenting to a breast clinic may have cancer. It is important that the clinician proves that the woman with a breast problem (i.e. lump, tenderness, pain, nipple retraction or discharge) does not have a malignancy.[1]

The multiplicity of terminology for benign breast disease in the past has resulted in some confusion. The situation would be better served by abandoning terminology that implies disease and substituting terms that imply a range of normality and change. The breast is under systemic hormonal influence and it might be expected that the breast would be uniform throughout its substance. This is not usually the case and great variation may exist in one part from another. Both the epithelial and stromal elements in the lobule are under hormonal influence and normality is dependent on a balanced relationship between the two elements. The cyclical changes of heaviness and fullness are not associated with significant histological change, but superimposed on these are the more radical changes of pregnancy and lactation. These changes occurring over a reproductive life of nearly forty years give ample opportunity for minor aberrations to occur.[2]

Aberrations of normal development and involution (ANDI): the concept

The management of benign breast conditions is dependent on the understanding of the normal processes within the breast and the aberrations that lead to clinical presentation. Most benign breast complaints are due to disorders based on the normal process of development, cyclical change and involution. Most benign conditions, therefore, show a predominance in a particular period of reproductive life. It has increasingly become obvious that the concept of fibrocystic disease is quite inadequate in describing benign breast disease since it implies a clinical and histological equivalence that is fallacious. For each disorder, there is a spectrum from normal through mild abnormality (aberration) to disease. The very common occurrence of these benign changes with no clinical correlations has led to the

Table 7.1 *A framework of pathogenesis for the classification of benign breast disorders*

Reproductive period	Normal process	Benign breast disorder	Benign breast disease
Development	Ductal development	Nipple inversion Single duct obstruction	Mammary duct fistula
	Lobular development	Fibroadenoma	Giant fibroadenoma
	Stromal development	Adolescent hypertrophy	(Severest form)
Cyclical change	Hormonal activity	Mastalgia Nodularity Focal Diffuse	(Severest form)
	Epithelial activity	Benign papilloma	
Pregnancy and lactation	Epithelial hyperplasia	Blood-stained nipple discharge	
	Lactation	Galactocele and inappropriate lactation	
Involution	Lobular involution	Cysts and sclerosing adenosis	
	Ductal involution Fibrosis Dilatation	Nipple retraction ⎫ Duct ectasia ⎬	Periductal mastitis with suppuration
	Micro papillomatosis	Simple hyperplasias	Lobular hyperplasias with atypia Duct hyperplasias with atypia Intracystic papilloma

suggestion that they be called aberrations rather than disease.[3] The 'aberrations of normal development and involution' (ANDI) concept has been proposed as a framework for benign breast disorders that is comprehensive, accurate in terminology and based on pathogenesis.[4] This concept encompasses pathogenesis, clinical and histological significance and general principles of management. The concept of ANDI has now been extended to include duct ectasia and duct sclerosis (Table 7.1).

Aetiology of benign breast disease

Epidemiological studies that clarify the aetiology of benign breast disease are few. Results in the literature are often from badly designed studies in selected populations with poorly defined diagnostic groups and biopsy proven benign breast disease leading to a select population with an obvious bias. However, several important factors can be found consistently through case control epidemiological studies, notably that biopsy for benign breast disorders was more common in thin nulliparous women with a family history of breast cancer.[5]

Role of dietary factors

There has been much interest in the role of dietary factors in the aetiology and progression of benign breast disease. Due to its wide consumption and the many biochemical and physiological effects, caffeine has been extensively studied in clinical and experimental studies. To date the data are inconsistent and inconclusive. Deficiency of essential fatty acids in the diet can lead to a deficient production of prostaglandin E_1 which may potentiate the effects of prolactin on the breast. Higher tissue level ratios of saturated to unsaturated fatty acids may lead to similar potentiation of the endocrine response. A high red meat intake with low consumption of fresh vegetables and vitamin A increases the risk of proliferative benign breast disease. Conversely it has been shown that a reduction in fat consumption reduces breast pain.

Endocrine factors such as increased oestrogen, decreased progesterone and increased prolactin have been considered but serum levels of these hormones during the menstrual cycle have not shown any difference between those with mastalgia and those without. Breast pain and cyst formation, however, are seen in the menopausal age group but are rarely seen in the absence of oestrogen. Oestrogen is necessary for the development of these conditions. Although measurement of hormonal profiles for groups of patients may show little variation, it is possible that minor individual variations in hormonal levels and end organ responsiveness may play a role in the aetiology.

The widespread use of the oral contraceptive pill has prompted numerous detailed studies of its effect on breast disease. Most results from large studies have shown a decrease in benign breast disease in long-term pill users. Fewer biopsies for benign breast disease were performed in this group in the large prospective Oxford FPA study. The protective effects seem related to the progesterone component of the pill. Controversy still exists on the effects of the pill on epithelial hyperplasia.

Periductal mastitis is linked to cigarette smoking. Woman who smoke and have periductal mastitis develop more inflammation and recurrence of the disease after corrective surgery is more frequent. This effect may be due to altered oral bacterial flora in smokers leading to breast duct colonisation or direct ischaemic effects of nicotine on breast ducts.

Factors altering hepatic metabolism of oestrogen, with an alteration in the ratio of C2 hydroxylation products (inactive metabolites) to C16 hydroxylation (active metabolities) may play a role. Exercise, intake of vegetables containing indole-3-carbinol both increase C2 hydroxylation whereas smoking increases the active C16 metabolities. These studies emphasise a potentially important pathway for chemo-prevention studies.

Cancer risk

There have been many studies linking histological changes in benign breast biopsies and subsequent risk of breast cancer. In many of these reports there was no attempt to standardise criteria and patient populations were often small. Over the past decade, three groups agreed to use the same definition of benign changes and a unified set of criteria for the diagnosis of these lesions. The separate and combined analysis of cytology, histology and metaplastic features gave a measure of tissue organisation, which was frequently predictive of concurrent cancer and/or future cancer development. In proliferative breast disease, the markers of cancer risk may be classified into histological categories of slightly (1½–2 times), moderately (4–5 times) and markedly (9–10 times) increased risk above the general population. The results from the three groups (Nashville, Nurses Health Study (NHS), and the Breast Cancer Detection Demonstration Project (BCDDP) were similar and showed that if the biopsy revealed proliferative disease without atypia, the subsequent risk was approximately 1.5 times. If the biopsy revealed atypical hyperplasia (AH) the risk was approximately 4.5 times. If the patients with AH had a family history of breast cancer, the subsequent risk approached that of patients with in situ carcinoma (approximately 8–10 times). In patients with AH, the breast cancer risk was much higher in pre- than post-menopausal patients. Although the classification scheme proposed by Page and co-workers is useful in assigning different levels of risk to women with benign breast disease, it has not been universally accepted. A major short-term goal should be to encourage pathologists to apply these criteria in a reproducible manner in daily practice.[6,7]

Diagnosis Significant progress in the assessment of breast complaints and early detection of malignancy has been achieved by improvement of mammographic technique and application of ultrasonography, cytology and stereotactic techniques. Problems in diagnosis are still encountered in patients after surgery, radiation therapy or silicone implants. Ultrasonography has a role as a primary and an ancillary modality in the diagnosis of breast abnormalities. It differentiates cystic from solid abnormalities and thereby guides further interventions.[8] Doppler ultrasonography is useful for certain indications.[9] Newer techniques such as digital luminescence radiography and contrast-enhanced MR imaging are being developed and are likely to be clinically important. MR spectroscopy, positron-emission tomography, transillumination, ductoscopy and biomagnetism offer interesting new aspects for research but the value of CT, thermography and biostereometry is not established.[10-12]

Breast symptoms are appropriately evaluated by a breast-oriented history and by the diagnostic triad ('triple assessment') of clinical breast examination, fine needle aspiration for cytology (FNAC) and breast imaging (mammography or ultrasonography).[13,14] When there is a palpable dominant mass the diagnostic triad yields a reliable clinical diagnosis with a sensitivity of 100%.[13,15] If there is no concordance or if there is any doubt about the diagnosis either on the part of the physician or the patient, a wide bore needle biopsy may obviate the need for open surgical biopsy and allows a definitive histological diagnosis. FNAC is a quick, accurate, cost-effective procedure and is best used at initial discovery of a lesion. Its sensitivity ranges from 90 to 97% in large series.[16,17] A positive result on FNAC is sufficiently accurate to justify one-stage diagnosis and treatment.

All patients over the age of 35 presenting with breast symptoms should have mammography. Patients under 35 can be imaged using ultrasonography. Only the diagnosis of a simple cyst will obviate the need for further evaluation or therapy. Doppler ultrasonography of breast lesions may give further information but this is currently not in routine clinical practice.

Congenital anomalies

Embryonic development

The breast is a distinguishing feature of the class mammalia and is a modified sudoriferous gland developing in the fifth and sixth week of fetal life as two ventral bands of thickened ectoderm ('milk lines'). The bands extend bilaterally from the axilla to the inguinal region and normally paired glands develop in the pectoral area. Each mammary gland develops as an ingrowth of ectodermal tissue into the underlying mesenchyme. During 13 to 20 weeks of intrauterine life each primary bud initiates the outgrowth of 15–20 secondary buds. Epithelial cords develop from these secondary buds and extend into the surrounding mesenchyme. Canalisation of the outgrowths forms lactiferous ducts and their branches. The lactiferous ducts open into epithelial depressions forming the mammary pit. Proliferation of the surrounding mesenchyme causes the mammary pit to elevate forming the nipple.

Absence of the breast or nipple

Amastia or absence of the breast is a rare condition and is presumably due to failure of the milk line to develop. The condition is usually unilateral. An association with the absence of pectoral muscles and syndactly has been described. Unilateral hypoplasia of the breast is seen more commonly than complete absence. Some degree of asymmetry between the breasts is normal with the left usually being slightly larger than the right. True asymmetry between the breasts can be treated by enlarging the smaller breast or reducing or elevating the larger breast or sometimes by using a combination of these procedures. Absence of the nipple or athelia is extremely rare and is usually associated with amastia. Absent nipples can be reconstructed with skin from the inner thigh, labial skin or by nipple sharing.

Supernumerary nipples and accessory nipples

Supernumerary or accessory nipples occur in 1–5% of people and result from the persistence of one or more nests of ectodermal cells in the milk line. Supernumerary nipples or breasts may occur in any size or configuration and are often mistaken for skin papillomas. Axillary breast tissue is usually bilateral and becomes more obvious with pregnancy and lactation. Supernumerary breasts have been reported at other sites including the groin, labia majora, inner sides of thighs and buttocks. Accessory nipples rarely require treatment for other than cosmetic reasons.

Disorders of development

Hypertrophic abnormalities of the breast

Prepubertal breast enlargement in girls in the absence of other signs of sexual maturation is a common occurrence. It is not a reason for investigation unless accompanied by other signs of sexual maturation, when it may be due to hormone secreting ovarian or adrenal tumours. The breasts do not develop synchronously and reassurance should be given and biopsy or excision avoided.

Juvenile hypertrophy of the breast is a relatively rare condition rapidly leading to gigantomastia in peripubertal females. The pathology is limited to the breast, with otherwise normal growth and development.

In adolescent girls the normal development of the breast can occasionally continue with overgrowth of periductal tissue. Proliferation and increased branching of the ducts without lobule formation can lead to juvenile or virginal hypertrophy. Endocrine abnormalities have not been detected as an underlying cause, though a higher rate of infertility has been reported. The nipple and areola may be difficult to recognise as they are stretched when the breasts continue to become pendulous. The weight of the breast results in neck and back pain with indentation of the shoulder skin by the bra straps. Medical treatment with danazol and bromocriptine has been tried but reduction mammoplasty is the treatment of choice. Occasionally the condition recurs when a further resection may be needed. Histology of the resected breast tissue is remarkably normal with a relative increase in the stromal component.

A number of techniques are available for reduction mammoplasty, each aiming to reduce the breast size and correcting the associated ptosis. The nipple and areola are preserved on a de-epithelialised pedicle which may be inferior, superior or centrally based depending on the technique chosen. Alternatively a free graft of the nipple and areola may be used if the desired degree of movement is difficult to achieve with a pedicle technique. Immediate postoperative complications include haematoma, infection and fat necrosis. Scarring of the breast may make subsequent examination and imaging of the breast difficult.

Gynaecomastia

Gynaecomastia is the commonest condition affecting the male breast and is an enlargement of ductal and stromal tissues that is structurally different from the surrounding subcutaneous fat. The condition is entirely benign and usually reversible. It may be physiological as in neonatal, pubertal and senescent hypertrophy which are due to an excess of oestrogens relative to testosterone. Specific causes of gynaecomastia need to be considered in all patients, but many will be idiopathic in apparently healthy men. These include hypogonadism, neoplasms, drugs and systemic diseases (Table 7.2).

The presentation is usually with a tender enlargement of the breast, often unilateral. In non-obese patients nearly 2 cm of subareolar breast tissue is required before the presence of gynaecomastia can be confirmed. Patients may be concerned about the cosmetic appearance, tenderness or pain or the possibility of underlying malignancy. Malignancy should be suspected in patients without a cause for gynaecomastia with an eccentric, hard lump or ulcerating lesions. Investigation with mammography and fine needle aspiration cytology are appropriate.

Treatment

Since most patients have hormonal imbalance or drug-induced disease firm reassurance that this is a benign and self-limiting condition will suffice. Medical therapy is seldom of value except when a specific diagnosis has been established. Discontinuation of causative drugs or improvement in the medical condition leading to gynaecomastia often results in breast regression. Testosterone has been of variable value,

Table 7.2 *Causes of secondary gynaecomastia*

Decreased androgens		
	Reduced production	Congenital anorchia
		Chromosomal abnormalities e.g. Klinefelter's syndrome
		Bilateral cryptorchidism
		Viral orchitis
		Bilateral torsion
		Granulomatous disease
		Renal failure
	Androgen resistance	Testicular feminisation
Increased oestrogens		
	Increased secretion	Testicular tumours
		Carcinoma lung
	Increased peripheral aromatisation	Adrenal disease
		Liver disease
		Starvation re-feeding
		Thyrotoxicosis
Drug induced		
	Antiandrogens	Spironolactone
		Cyproterone
	Oestrogenic activity or bound to oestrogen receptors	Digitalis
		Griseofulvin
		Cannabis
	Disturbance in gonadotrophin control	Phenothiazines
		Reserpine
		Cimetidine
		Methyldopa
		Isoniazid
		Metoclopramide
		Tricyclic antidepressants

but some dramatic results have been reported. Tamoxifen, clomiphene and danazol have been tried in small numbers of patients with a heterogeneous case mix with variable results. Surgical removal of the breast tissue is indicated for failure of medical treatment or where the degree of breast enlargement is a cosmetic or psychological problem. Subcutaneous mastectomy is performed through a periareolar or inframammary incision depending on the extent of tissue to be excised. The nipple is elevated leaving a small amount of adherent breast tissue and subcutaneous fat. Flaps are dissected only a small distance superiorly and inferiorly in a deep subcutaneous plane, so that a good proportion of subcutaneous fat is retained with the flap. This ensures that the deformity of a swelling is not replaced with a hollow. Division of the cone of breast tissue into two or four pieces eases the dissection and subsequent haemostasis.

Fibroadenoma

The tumour appears usually in young women as a rubbery, firm, smooth and mobile mass. These characteristic features make clinical diagnosis easy in most young women but the situation is not so obvious in the older woman where fibrotic changes of involution decrease the mobility of the lump. Calcified fibroadenomas are sometimes found in the elderly, as a hard, discrete but mobile mass and they are readily demonstrated on mammography. Fibroadenomas arise from lobules and are therefore seen predominantly at ages 15–25. Hyperplastic lobules which are histologically identical to fibroadenomas are found in so many breasts, as to be regarded as normal.[18] A full spectrum from hyperplastic lobules to fibroadenoma can be detected, without the continued growth characteristic of neoplasms and can, therefore, be regarded as aberrations of normal development. Fibroadenomas show hormonal dependence similar to the lobules from which they are derived. Lactational changes can be seen in the lobules during pregnancy and changes of involution are evident in the perimenopausal period. Most fibroadenomas are 1–2 cm in size and growth beyond 5 cm is unusual. They may be multiple, especially in Oriental and Negro races.

The clinical diagnosis of fibroadenoma may be incorrect in up to 50% of patients and investigation with ultrasonography and FNAC should be obtained in all patients. Excision of all fibroadenoma is not essential as only a small number increase in size, a majority get smaller and some disappear.[19,20] If clinical and diagnostic investigations confirm the lesion to be a fibroadenoma the patient can be given the choice of observation or excision after reassurance.[21] Excision performed through an incision along Langer's lines is preferred. The histological appearance is characteristically a combination of pale stroma and duct-like structures lined by regular epithelial cells. The risk of cancer within a fibroadenoma is small (1 in 1000 lesions). It is usually lobular carcinoma in situ, as would be expected from the lobular origin of fibroadenomas, and carries an excellent prognosis. Ductal carcinoma is significantly less common and is usually direct infiltration by an adjacent cancer or cancer extending along the duct into the lobules. Treatment is directed by that for the primary cancer and the presence of the fibroadenoma is ignored. Follow-up studies of fibroadenomas treated by observation show that around 30% will reduce in size over 1 year.

Disorders of cyclical change

Mastalgia

Mastalgia is one of the commonest symptoms, affecting up to 70% of woman at some time in their lives. It accounts for approximately 50% of referrals to a specialised breast clinic and is also the most frequent reason for breast-related consultation in general practice. Mastalgia is cyclical in two-thirds of patients, non-cyclical in the rest or pain arising from the chest wall deep to the breast. Premenstrual discomfort and nodularity are so common that they should be considered to be normal. The aetiology of mastalgia remains obscure. Water retention has been suggested as a cause of mastalgia and premenstrual tension and justifies the use of diuretics to help relieve these conditions. Studies with tritiated water comparing the total body water on day 5 and day 25 of the menstrual cycle, however, have failed to show any changes. Some have suggested that psychological factors play a significant role in the causation of mastalgia but there is no scientific basis for this. Increased oestrogen, decreased progesterone and increased prolactin were thought to be likely factors but measurement of serum levels of these hormones through the menstrual cycle have not shown any difference between those with mastalgia and controls. There is some biochemical evidence showing that overstimulation of the breast cells due to interference with ATP degradation by methylxanthine consequent to high caffeine intake may play a role. Deficiency of essential fatty acids in the diet can lead to a deficient production of prostaglandin E_1 which may potentiate the effects of prolactin on the breast.

The most important factors in the evaluation and treatment of breast pain consist of a thorough history, physical, and radiological evaluation. These can be used to reassure the patient that she does not have breast cancer. After exclusion of breast cancer 85% of patients can be discharged from the clinic without specific treatment.[22] In 15% of patients, however, the pain is severe enough to affect lifestyle and warrants therapy and a systematic approach can achieve relief of pain[23] (Fig. 7.1). Therapy may consist of a well-fitting bra, a decrease in dietary fat intake, manipulation to reduce saturated fat or supplement essential fatty acid intake and discontinuance of oral contraceptives or hormone replacement therapy. Those women resistant to these simple measures may experience relief from using gammalinolenic acid as first-line therapy. Treatment with gammalinolenic acid is continued for about 3 months and about 70% of patients with cyclical mastalgia will have a moderate to good response. Danazol or bromocriptine are usually used as second-line agents, both of which are effective treatments but have a much higher incidence of side effects. Danazol is started at a dose of 200 mg daily and continued for at least two menstrual cycles. Those obtaining a response can then be maintained on a dose of 100 mg on alternate days, or 100 mg on days 14 to 28 of the menstrual cycle. About 25% of patients of Danazol experience side effects of weight gain, nausea or oily skin.

Figure 7.1
Principles of mastalgia treatment.

From Peplinski GR, Norton JA. Gastrointestinal endocrine cancers and nodal metastasis: biological significance and therapeutic implications. Surg Oncol Clin North Am 1996; 5: 159–171.

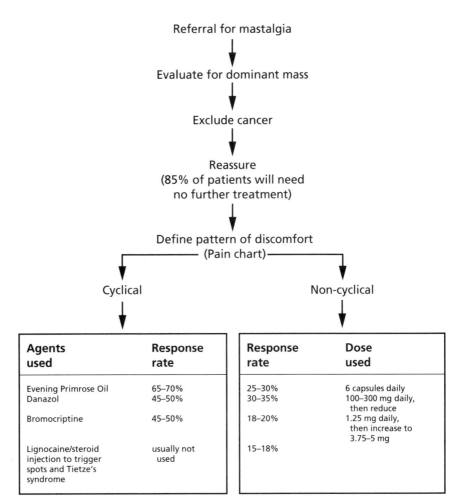

Bromocriptine, a prolactin-lowering drug, is used at a dose of 2.5 mg twice daily but is introduced at 1.25 mg daily for 3–4 days then increased by similar amounts at 3–4 day intervals to achieve the desired dose. By using gammalinolenic acid as first-line therapy and danazol or bromocriptine as second-line agents a clinically useful improvement to pain can be anticipated in 92% of patients with cyclical and 64% with non-cyclical mastalgia. Patients with severe recurrent or refractory mastalgia may require treatment with tamoxifen, goserelin or testosterone, but the short- and long-term adverse effects of these drugs preclude their use as first-line agents. Predicting which treatment will be most efficacious for any particular woman is not easy because presenting features, personal or family history of breast disease, reproductive history are not predictive of success rates.[24,25] The aetiology of cyclical mastalgia is poorly understood but lack of previous breast feeding and low levels of physical exercise have been identified as contributing factors. The consistent finding of an increased prolactin stimulation response, probably due to oestrogen dominance, has led to the use of treatment with prolactin-lowering drugs and antioestrogens. The efficacy and safety in mastalgia of gestrinone (which has androgenic, anti-oestrogenic, and antiprogestagenic properties) and vaginal micronised progesterone have been investigated in recent studies, with gestrinone showing encouraging results.

Chest wall pain is usually self-limiting, but symptomatic relief can often be obtained using steroidal and local anaesthetic injections or non-steroidal anti-inflammatory drugs.

Disorders of involution

Involution changes become obvious by the age of 35. The involution of stroma and epithelium may not occur at the same rate or in an integrated fashion, over the 20-year period of this process. When the stroma involutes faster than the epithelial acini, these remain and form microcysts which are so common as to be regarded a normal part of an involuting breast. Obstruction of the efferent duct leads to macrocyst formation. This concept fits well with the common occurrence of the macrocyst and the fact that they are frequently multiple. Many are not clinically detectable.

In sclerosing adenosis, the complex interrelationship between involution and stromal fibrosis superimposed on the cyclical changes leads to a complex picture of epithelial acini surrounded by fibrous tissue.

Cysts

Cysts are the commonest single abnormality found in patients attending a breast clinic and the majority are a manifestation of ANDI. Less common cystic lesions include galactocoele, oil cysts of fat necrosis, papillary cystadenomas and those associated with necrosis in a phyllodes tumour or carcinoma. Hydatid cysts are very rare. Microcysts may be present in a majority of women, at some time during the process of involution and some will develop clinically detectable macrocysts. Cysts are most frequent between the ages of 38 and 53 years.

If a breast lump is suspected to be a cyst it should be aspirated directly or using ultrasonographic guidance. The cyst fluid has a variable colour from a pale yellow to brown or dark green. The routine cytological examination of cyst fluid is not rewarding and can be potentially misleading. It is mandatory to confirm that the cyst has disappeared after aspiration and that the fluid is not blood stained. If ultrasonography shows a solid component to the cyst this should be investigated as for a solid lesion with FNAC or wide bore needle (WBN) biopsy.

The fluid filling the cysts (breast cyst fluid, BCF) contains unusual amounts of biologically active substances, including hormones and metabolites. Measuring BCF cations (K^+, Na^+) permits classification of cysts into two major subsets (type I and type II), conceivably associated with a difference in the apocrine cells in the lining epitheliums. Type I cysts (high K^+/Na^+ ratio) accumulate huge amounts of dehydroepiandrosterone sulphate, oestrone sulphate, androstane-3α,17β-diol glucuronide, androsterone glucuronide and contain more testosterone and dihydrotestosterone than type II. Conversely, type II cysts (low K^+/Na^+ ratio) contain more progesterone and pregnenolone.[26] The risk of cyst relapse is significantly higher in women with type I cysts or with multiple cysts at presentation.

Various proteins and several polypeptide growth factors including EGF and IGF-I are frequently found in cyst fluid. Biochemical analysis of these components may shed further light on the role of gross cysts in relation to cyst recurrence and the risk of breast cancer. Several reports indicate that patients with macrocysts have a two- to fourfold higher risk of developing cancer.

Epithelial hyperplasia

Epithelial hyperplasia refers to an increase in the number of layers of epithelial cells lining the terminal duct lobular unit. The degree of hyperplasia is graded as mild, moderate and severe. During the premenopausal period mild and moderate changes are common and are known to regress spontaneously. They should be regarded as part of ANDI as they are common and are associated with minimal or non-significant increased risk of breast cancer in the absence of other factors. Dupont and Page have classified epithelial hyperplasia into ductal and lobular based on histological criteria. Atypia within the hyperplasia is important as this leads to increased risk of subsequent cancer. There is no clinical counterpart to this pathology finding within the concept of ANDI. The majority of patients with epithelial hyperplasia are asymptomatic and this is a finding on histology for a biopsy done for other reasons. Epithelial hyperplasia may be seen as an incidental finding in up to 3% of biopsies.

Residual breast tissue

Not all breast tissue involutes at the same rate in all individuals. This may lead to clinical and mammographic asymmetry which may be difficult to differentiate from a carcinoma. Some studies have shown that hormone replacement therapy may enhance the incidence of finding islands of residual breast tissue.

Nipple discharge

A small amount of fluid can be expressed in up to two thirds of all non-lactating women by application of suction to the nipple. This is regarded as physiological. The fluid should never be blood stained and varies in colour from a clear off-white fluid through yellow to dark green. The fluid may come from a single or multiple ducts. Nipple discharge is significant when it occurs spontaneously and is a dominant symptom, but is an uncommon presentation to the breast clinic constituting under 3% of patients.

Serous discharge is characterised by its yellow colour and is often sticky. Blood staining can be minor to produce a serosanguineous discharge or heavily blood stained. This discharge is often due to epithelial hyperplasia in the form of a duct papilloma. The condition is most often benign, but the risk of malignancy increases with age. Duct ectasia may lead to blood stained nipple discharge with ulceration within the ducts. The discharge associated with breast cancer is usually blood stained and associated with a palpable lump. In a minority of patients no cause of the discharge is established even after operations such as major duct excision. A coloured opalescent discharge is seen most often in duct ectasia but can rarely occur with cysts. Milky discharge is on most occasions physiological and can be seen in the neonatal period (witch's milk) due to hormonal stimulation of the neonate breast. It is also seen in pregnancy, lactation and the postlactational period. Mechanical stimulation can lead to a milky discharge. Hyperprolactinaemia produces galactorrhoea and this may be caused by a pituitary tumour and drugs that block or deplete dopamine (e.g. phenothiazines, metoclopramide, domperidone, methyldopa).

Investigation of the discharge should include Haemostix® testing for blood, cytological examination and assessment of the breast with examination and mammography. An algorithm for management is outlined in Fig. 7.2. Surgical excision of the involved duct as a microdochectomy is preferred for a single discharging duct. Total duct excision is the favoured approach for a patient with multiple duct discharge and in patients over the age of 50 with a single duct discharge as the risk of malignancy is higher.

Duct ectasia/periductal mastitis

Periductal mastitis is characterised by mastalgia of a non-cyclical nature, nipple discharge and periareolar inflammation that may be associated with nipple retraction. The formation of mammary fistulae and non-lactating breast abscess is frequently seen. In periductal mastitis the major ducts are not dilated, but are surrounded by an inflammatory response that consists of polymorphs, plasma cells, lymphocytes and granulomas with giant cells and epithelioid cells are usually seen. The aetiology of the inflammation is unknown.

Duct ectasia typically occurs in the perimenopausal or late premenopausal groups. Periductal mastitis and duct ectasia affect the major breast ducts. The dilatation usually affects 3–4 of the ducts within 2–3 cm of the nipple. The reason why these particular segments and only some ducts are affected is unclear. The dilated ducts allow

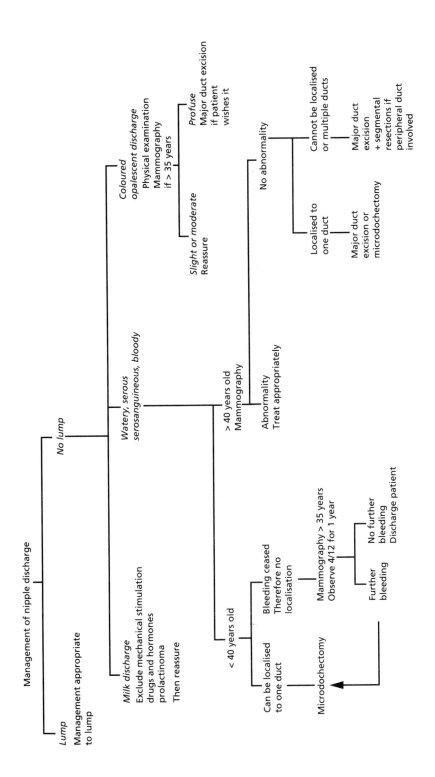

Figure 7.2 *Management of nipple discharge.*

From Peplinski GR, Norton JA. Gastrointestinal endocrine cancers and nodal metastasis: biological significance and therapeutic implications. Surg Oncol Clin North Am 1996; 5: 159–171.

secretions to collect leading to a nipple discharge. The leakage of secretion into the periductal tissue causes an inflammatory response, with infiltration by neutrophils, macrophages and plasma cells. This inflammation leads to periductal fibrosis and nipple retraction. This explanation of pathogenesis, however, does not explain the presence of periductal mastitis in the younger patient with no associated duct ectasia. An alternative theory suggests an autoimmune basis leading to destruction and weakening of the muscle layer with secondary dilatation of the ducts. It is possible that both processes contribute to the clinical picture. The role of bacterial infection in the pathogenesis is controversial but the presence of anaerobic bacteria in the ducts has been confirmed in a number of studies. Infection is more common after biopsy of breasts showing duct ectasia on histology. *Bacteroides* species, together with *Staphylococcus aureus*, *Proteus* and streptococci have been isolated. The presence of bacteria is more usual in the recurrent lesion. The absence of bacteria in many patients and the rapidity of resolution without antibacterial treatment would suggest that the inflammation may be a chemical response to leaked ductal secretion.[1,27]

Management of duct ectasia and periductal mastitis includes antibiotic therapy for the acute inflammatory episode. Ongoing symptoms are best resolved with the operation of total major duct excision. Special care to section and excise all ducts is needed to prevent recurrence of the condition. Free eversion of the nipple is often indicative that all ducts have been sectioned.

Mammary fistula

Mammary fistula is a rare recurrent condition characterised by draining abscesses about the nipple on one or both breasts. Because little is known about the disease, it is often misdiagnosed and inappropriately treated. The clinical and pathological findings are similar to duct ectasia or periductal mastitis, with a swelling or mass at the areola, draining fistula from the subareolar tissue, a chronic thick, pasty discharge from the nipple and pain. Histologic examination reveals keratinising squamous epithelium replacing the lining of one or more lactiferous ducts for a variable distance into the subareolar tissue. Core excision of the fistula and all of the retroareolar fibroglandular tissue and the ductal tissue within the nipple is the usual definitive therapy. Where sepsis is present at the time of excision the wound may be managed by packing.

Benign tumours

Duct papilloma

Benign papillomas of the ducts are very common and should be regarded as aberrations of cyclical change rather than true benign tumours. These lesions may be single or multiple. Symptoms are present usually when major ducts are affected. The most frequent is a finding of nipple discharge that may be blood stained. Treatment consists of microdochectomy, excising the involved duct.

Lipoma

These soft, lobulated and radiolucent lesions are quite common in the breast. A similar soft mass, 'pseudolipoma', can often be found around a carcinoma, caused by indrawing of the adjacent fat by the spiculated tumour. All patients over the age of 35 with a clinical diagnosis of a lipoma should be investigated as for a breast lump with triple assessment.

Mammary hamartomas

Mammary hamartomas are breast disorders currently underestimated and not well recognised. Hamartomas account for 1.2% of benign lesions and 4.8% of benign breast tumours. Clinically they present with a palpable lump, usually painless. Typically, but inconsistently, mammography shows a sharply circumscribed density, separated from adjacent normal breast by a thin radiolucent zone. Macroscopically, hamartomas are slightly larger and softer than fibroadenomas. They are well defined, white/pink and fleshy, with yellow islands of fat tissue. Histologically, hamartomas exhibit 'pushing' borders with pseudoencapsulation and consist of a combination of variable amounts of stromal and epithelial components. Stromal components mainly consist of a prominent fibrohyalin background with small islands of adipose tissue and oedematous changes. Epithelial structures show variable features of benign breast disease. The overall architecture is lobulated. Hamartomas result more from breast dysgenesis than from any tumorous process.

References

1. Hughes LE, Mansel RE, Webster DJT. Benign disorders and diseases of the breast. Concepts and clinical management. London: Baillière Tindall, 1989.
2. Mansel R. Benign breast disease. [review]. Practitioner 1992; 236: 830–4.
3. Love SM, Gelman RS, Silen W. Fibrocystic disease of the breast – a non disease. N Engl J Med 1982; 307: 1010–14.
4. Hughes LE, Mansel RE, Webster DJT. Aberrations of normal development and involution (ANDI): a new perspective on pathogenesis and nomenclature of human breast disorders. Lancet 1987; ii: 1316–19.
5. Bundred NJ. Aetiological factors in benign breast disease. Br J Surg 1994; 81: 788–9.
6. Page DL, Dupont WD. Risk factors for breast cancer in women with proliferative breast disease. N Engl J Med 1985; 312: 146–51.
7. Dupont WD, Parl FF, Hartmann WH et al. Breast cancer risk associated with proliferative breast disease and atypical hyperplasia [see comments]. [review]. Cancer 1993; 71: 1258–65.
8. Jokich PM, Monticciolo DL, Adler YT. Breast ultrasonography. Radiol Clin North Am 1992; 30: 993–1009.
9. Cosgrove DO, Kedar RP, Bamber JC et al. Breast diseases: color Doppler US in differential diagnosis. Radiology 1993; 189: 99–104.
10. Donegan WL. Evaluation of a palpable breast mass. N Engl J Med 1992; 327: 937–42.
11. Jackson VP. The status of mammographically guided fine needle aspiration biopsy of non-palpable breast lesions. Radiol Clin North Am 1992; 30: 155–66.
12. Sickles EA. Management of probably benign breast lesions. Radiol Clin North Am 1995; 33: 1123–30.
13. Kaufman Z, Shpitz B, Shapiro M, Rona R, Lew S, Dinbar A. Triple approach in the diagnosis of dominant breast masses: combined physical examination, mammography, and fine-needle aspiration. J Surg Oncol 1994; 56: 254–7.
14. Bland KI, Love N. Evaluation of common breast masses. Postgrad Med 1992; 92: 95–7.
15. Vetto J, Pommier R, Schmidt W et al. Use of the 'triple test' for palpable breast lesions yields high diagnostic accuracy and cost savings. Am J Surg 1995; 169: 519–22.
16. De Freitas R, Jr, Hamed H, Fentiman I. Fine needle aspiration cytology of palpable breast lesions. Br J Clin Pract 1992; 46: 187–90.
17. Ciatto S, Bonardi R, Cariaggi MP. Performance of fine-needle aspiration cytology of the breast – multicenter study of 23 063 aspirates in ten Italian laboratories. Tumori 1995; 81: 13–17.
18. Parks AG. The microanatomy of the breast. Ann R Coll Surg Engl 1959; 25: 295–311.
19. Wilkinson S, Forrest AP, Rifkind E, Chetty U, Anderson TJ. Natural history of fibroadenoma of the breast. Br J Clin Pract 1988; 67–8.
20. Wilkinson S, Anderson TJ, Rifkind E, Chetty U, Forrest APM. Fibroadenoma of the breast: a follow up of conservative management. Br J Surg 1989; 76: 390–1.
21. Cant PJ, Madden MV, Close PM, Learmouth GM, Hacking EA, Dent DM. Case for conservative management of selected fibroadenomas of the breast. Br J Surg 1987; 74: 857–9.
22. Fentiman IS. Mastalgia mostly merits masterly inactivity [editorial]. Br J Clin Pract 1992; 46: 158
23. Holland PA, Gateley CA. Drug therapy of mastalgia. what are the options? Drugs 1994; 48: 709–16.
24. Gateley CA, Bundred NJ, West RR, Mansel RE. Reproductive factors associated with mastalgia. Cancer Detect Prev 1992; 16: 39–41.
25. Gateley CA, Miers M, Mansel RE, Hughes LE. Drug treatments for mastalgia: 17 years experience in the Cardiff mastalgia clinic. J R Soc Med 1992; 85: 12–15.
26. Miller WR, Dixon JM, Scott WN, Forrest APM. Classification of human cysts according to electrolyte and androgen conjugate composition. Clin Oncol 1983; 9: 227–32.
27. Webb AJ. Mammary duct ectasia–periductal mastitis complex. Br J Surg 1995; 82: 1300–2.

8 Breast screening and screen-detected disease

Mark W. Kissin

Introduction In July 1985 a committee was set up under the chairmanship of Professor Sir Patrick Forrest to consider information available on breast cancer screening by mammography. Their brief was to examine the range of provision for mammographic facilities in the UK, and for the screening of symptomless women and means to implement the screening policy. The Forrest report was published in 1986[1] and the principal conclusion was that the introduction of mass screening by mammography would lead to a reduction in breast cancer deaths and to achieve this, a fundamental change in the back-up services for breast disease would be required. On the basis of these findings UK population breast screening was introduced in 1988 and is now universally available.

There was no evidence that clinical examination, breast ultrasonography, or breast self-examination were effective tools for screening. In contrast, evidence existed in 1985 in the form of randomised control trials and case controlled studies to show that mortality from breast cancer could be reduced in women attending for mammographic screening. The details of the evidence for this are summarised in Table 8.1. Using meta-analysis, for women in the age group 50–74 screening mammography reduces the death rate by 26% regardless of the number of mammographic views per screen, the screening interval, or the duration of follow-up.[2] For younger women aged between 40 and 49 years the most reliable information comes from the Swedish randomised trials which show a 13% reduction in cancer mortality in patients invited for screening. This reduction in mortality only appears after 8 years of follow-up, at a time when the woman is post-menopausal.[3]

The breast screening programme in the UK was modelled on the randomised control trial carried out in the Swedish Two Counties study[4] which screened women aged 40–74 with a screening interval of 24 months for women under 50, and 33 months for those over 50.

Table 8.1 *Evidence for benefit of breast screening*

Study	Date	Age	Study type	Screening interval (months)	Number of views	Clinical exam.	Rounds of mammography	Follow-up year	Outcome (RR)
Edinburgh	1979	45–64	RCT	24	2	✓	4	10	−17%
Malmo	1976	45–69	RCT	18–24	2	✗	6	12	−9% to −14%
2 Counties	1977	40–74	RCT	24–33	1	✗	5–6	12	−36% to −18%
Canada – 1	1980	40–49	RCT	12	2	✓	5	7	+36%
Canada – 2	1980	50–59	RCT	12	2	✓	5	7	−3%
HIP	1963	40–64	RCT	12	2	✓	4	10	−2%
Stockholm	1981	40–64	RCT	28	1	✗	3	8	−29%
Gothenberg	1982	40–59	RCT	18	2	✗	3	7	−14%
DOM	1974	50–64	C-C	26	2	✓	5	12	−48%
Florence	1977	40–70	C-C	30	2	✗	3–7	10	−47%
Nijmegen	1975	35–65	C-C	24	1	✗	4	8	−49%
UK	1979	45–64	C-C	24	1	✓	4	7	−24%

RR, relative risk of death; RCT, randomised controlled trial; C-C, case control study. Negative score confers benefit.

A single mammographic view was taken and clinical breast examination was not used.

In this chapter the screening process, changes in surgical practice mandated by screen-detected disease and the success of the programme are examined.

The screening process

Organisation of service

The process of screening is undertaken under the supervision of 90 screening centres. The size and location of these vary from region to region and are a mixture of fixed and mobile units. A standard so called 'Forrest' unit was designed to screen a population of 41 000 women in the target age group of 50–64 years. Sophisticated computer networks have been developed, in conjunction with general practitioner lists to ensure women in the target age group are identified and receive an invitation for screening. For screening to be successful over 70% of the target population must accept their invitation. Where individual GP practices or screening centres start to fall below this level of acceptance, extra publicity campaigns are mounted to improve the uptake. The levels of uptake are lower in inner city conurbations and in more remote areas of the country. There may be special requirements when screening ethnic minorities. The screening centres are staffed by health care professionals who are trained and well motivated in the screening process. This team works together with clear screening protocols, agreed patterns of referral, built in quality assurance programmes, and continuing audit and education. The first phase of the breast screening project was concerned mainly with development of the screening centres, recruitment of trained staff, and setting standards to assess the whole process. The second phase was one of consolidation and learning as the first round of screening became complete. The third and current phase involves the development of end points, resetting standards, and defining treatment outcomes. Six training units were set up around the country to educate members of screening teams with the screening process and then to carry out

Figure 8.1 *The screening process. QA, quality assurance.*

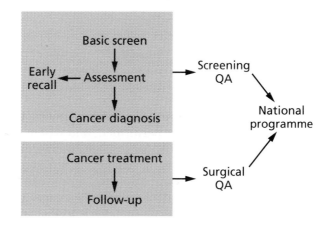

continuing medical education (Edinburgh, Guildford, King's College Hospital, Manchester, Nottingham and Cardiff). The organisation of the screening process is summarised in Fig. 8.1, and the current standards for radiological and surgical quality assurance are discussed on pp. 233–4.

The basic screen

Women at first screening have two view mammography on each breast. Initially single view mammography in the 45° oblique plane was carried out, but subsequent trials have shown two views to be superior and one is also taken in the craniocaudal position (Fig. 8.2). Physical examination is not carried out but a questionnaire is filled in by the women and details of any symptoms noted for the benefit of the radiological team who are reading the mammograms. Women who are unable to keep their initial appointment for screening are able to take up the offer of screening for up to six months after their initial invitation. Screens are repeated every three years up to the age of 64 with a single oblique view. Women are invited practice by practice and some are brought into the screening programme aged at 50 (or just under), 51 or 52. After the age of 64 women no longer receive an invitation but are eligible for screening mammography on demand. Relatively few numbers of women over the age of 65 routinely partake of this service, only 20 042 in 1995.[5] Their reasons for attending are varied and include women who have already been through the screening process who have fallen over the upper age limit for invitations. At the end of any screening day the mobile units return the films to the central base where the films are processed and read by a radiologist with a specialist interest in breast imaging. Quality assurance standards ensure expertise in mammographic interpretation. In many units double reading is now carried out. Communication of the result to the patient should occur within two weeks.

Assessment

Women are recalled for assessment for two reasons. A technical recall occurs when the mammographic films fail to reach standard quality features, due to errors in exposure, developing or positioning (Fig. 8.2). Women with a true radiological abnormality are recalled for clinical assessment. This process includes further standard or specialised radiological views of the breast including magnification and paddle compression views. Clinical examination and ultrasonography are performed, and where necessary needle aspiration cytology for palpable lumps, and image guided cytology for impalpable ones undertaken. The precise arrangements of each assessment centre varies from region to region. Many include a surgeon as part of the assessment team. The purpose of the assessment is to return the majority of women back to the normal screening process. A relatively

Figure 8.2
Technical problems, two view versus one view, interval cancer. Mammograms from 58-year-old woman with a left-sided cancer. (a) 45° oblique view 1995 showed no specific abnormality. At that stage a single view was taken. The star indicates the pectoralis major muscle and for technical reasons this muscle should come down further towards the back of the plate. The lower inner quadrant is not adequately imaged. (b) 45° oblique view 1996 when presenting with interval lump in lower inner quadrant. Arrow shows an edge of a lesion again not well visualised. (c) Craniocaudal view with obvious tumour (arrowed) in most medial aspect of breast.

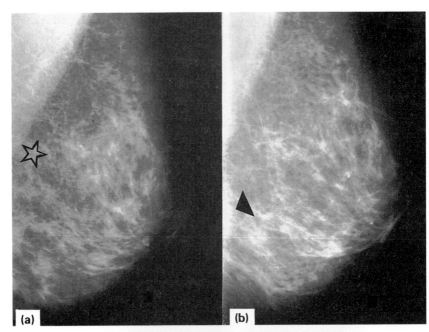

(a) (b)

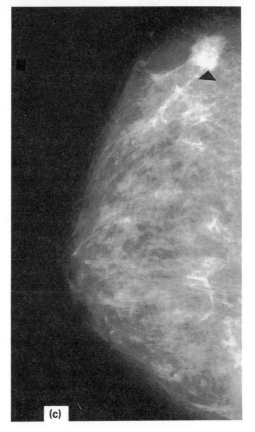

(c)

small number are put onto early recall where the degree of abnormality is not sufficient to warrant an intervention. In women found to have a definitive abnormality the purpose of the assessment clinic is to make a positive diagnosis. This should reduce the number of surgical procedures required for diagnosis alone and make use of surgical time more efficient.

Cost

The cost of a basic screen for an individual client was £12 in 1986 but the cost of the whole project is expensive in health care terms. In 1986 the capital cost at the outset of the screening project was estimated at £31 000 000 with an estimated £18 000 000 annual running cost. The cost of a quality of life adjusted year gained by screening was estimated at £3310. This translates to similar cost of the benefits of kidney transplantation. In 1992 the Humberside screening service found that the cost of each cancer detected was £5533 with an average cost of £32 per woman screened.[6] In 1996 the national running costs had risen to £25 000 000. Some of the mammographic equipment now needs replacing and with 'Baby Boom' patients born in 1945–1955 coming into the screening age many centres will require another mobile screening van. Economics of breast screening has been kept under close scrutiny by a research facility at Brunel University. The average total personal cost incurred to a woman as a result of attending for screening was £11.17, and for assessment £41.21. These costs include travel to screening and loss of earnings. The average resource cost per invitation for screening is £2.00–£11.00, for the actual basic screen itself £5.00–£14.00 on a static unit and £8.00–£12.00 on a mobile unit, and attendance at an assessment clinic £33.00–£58.00.

Trials

The research and development aspect of the breast screening project set up three trials to answer specific questions regarding the screening process. Trials in the screening methodology are considered here and those concerning therapeutic options are discussed below.

One versus two view mammography

A randomised controlled trial was set up between nine breast screening centres in England (West London, Brighton, Worthing, North London, Liverpool, Reading, Winchester, Leeds and Southampton), where 40 163 women being screened were randomised to have one view, two view, or two view mammography in which one view was read by one reader and both views were read by another. In addition to detecting 24% more cancers, two view mammography was associated with a 15% lower recall rate. The cost of two view screening was higher, being £26.46 compared with £22.00 per examination, but the average cost per cancer detected was similar, being £5330 versus £5310.

The trial concluded that two view mammography is medically more effective than one view.[7] The National Co-ordinating Committee for the Breast Screening Project, therefore, changed the organisation of services so that the basic screen now always consists of two views rather than one although subsequent rounds involve just the 45° oblique view (Fig. 8.2).

One versus three year screening interval

The interval of screening trial involves 100 000 women randomised between mammograms on a yearly basis with those having the ordinary three yearly cycles. Patients have been recruited from Cardiff, Epping, Gateshead, Newcastle and Nottingham. No data have yet been published, but the results will have a direct interface with the interval cancer rate (see below).

The Forties Trial

The most controversial trial was the 'Forties trial' in which 65 000 women aged 40 or 41 were invited to have two-view mammography carried out in eight rounds on an annual basis. The cancer detection rate and outcomes in this group were then compared to 135 000 controls. Guildford and Edinburgh were chosen as pilot sites for this study and 27 other centres have subsequently contributed patients. As yet there are no published data on the progress of this trial, but it does pose many problems. Screening in this age group demands the very highest quality of mammography as the breasts in these premenopausal women tend to be denser. In addition, the natural incidence of cancer in this age group is lower and therefore the cancer detection rate will be smaller. The 1995 Review detailed 53 000 women screened, with 156 cancers being detected at a rate of 2.9/1000. This is approximately half the rate found in the 50–64-year-old group. Overview statistics show that screening at this age is not translated into benefits for people attending until they move into their postmenopausal phase. The cost for increased extra year of life saved by screening in this age group will be considerably more than in the National Screening Project.

Screening the older woman

At the present time the screening process stops at age 64, despite the fact that the incidence of breast cancer continues to rise as women get older. The cut off age limit has caused concern with pressure groups for the elderly and has brought criticism of an ageist stance being taken by the screening programme. In order to determine whether screening in the over 65s will be cost effective, pilot studies are now being undertaken in Brighton and Wakefield. Preliminary evidence suggests a cancer detection rate of 12/1000 which is twice that in the 50–64-year-old group.

Changes in practice

Pathology

In general terms the same pathological entities found in symptomatic patients are also found by the screening process but the so-called 'lead-time' effect means that there is a shift in prognostic features to the better end of the spectrum, for example, for infiltrating duct cancers the Nottingham Prognostic Index will be lower. There is also an increased number of non-invasive cancers and special types of cancer which might not have any significant biological potential and these account for so called 'lag-time' bias.

Radial scars

Radial scars or complex sclerosing lesions are one of the commonest benign entities found by the screening process. The radiological features that distinguish them from stellate cancer is the presence of long radicules radiating from a central core. Characteristically they are seen better on one mammographic view than another. They are almost always asymptomatic and sometimes the mammographic features are alarming. The difficulty surrounding these lesions is that some are associated with serious underlying pathological conditions. In a series of 43 radial scars 35% were associated with cancer and a further 12% with atypical ductal hyperplasia. When cancer was present it was either ductal carcinoma *in situ* (DCIS), tubular cancer or infiltrating duct cancer which was grade 1 and node negative.[8] It is difficult to know whether these are cancers in evolution or involution. As there is no reliable mammographic or cytological sign to distinguish benign from more aggressive types of radial scar it is current national recommendation that all should be removed. An example of a radial scar taken from the 'Forties trial' is shown in Fig. 8.3. In the year ending March 1996, 143 patients from South Thames West had benign breast excision biopsies and 29 (20%) of these were radial scars.

Axillary lymph nodes

A key component to prognosis is the pathological status of axillary lymph nodes removed by sampling or clearance. It is one of the three fundamental components of the Nottingham Prognostic Index. Node positivity in symptomatic breast cancers ranges from 25–55% but in screen-detected disease the rate is much lower at 15–25%.[9] The current recommendation from the quality assurance programme is that lymph nodes should be removed but not for patients with DCIS alone. Despite this recommendation there is considerable variation in axillary lymph node surgery among surgeons dealing with screen detected disease (Fig. 8.4). A similar pattern is seen in other regions. In the first year of the Avon screening project, for example, 46 invasive cancers were treated, but lymph node dissection was only carried out in 27. As 40% of these were positive, patient selection is being carried out, probably on the basis that for cancers less than 10 mm in size or of grade 1 when node positivity will be very low.[10] Failure to remove nodes may

Figure 8.3
Complex sclerosing lesion (radial scar) detected in the prevalent round of the Forties trial. Craniocaudal views showing dense left breast with arrowed spiculated densities in right breast. Histology showed radiating ducts with florid epithelial hyperplasia but no atypia.

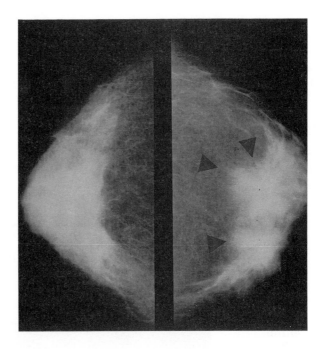

lead to a false sense of security and under utilisation of appropriate adjuvant strategy. The Manchester group found that in the prevalent round very small cancers are very unlikely to be associated with positive nodes and, therefore, a lymph node procedure could theoretically be omitted. Interestingly they have found that the lymph node positivity rate is considerably higher in incident screened cancers than those from the first round. In the year ending 1996, audit data from South Thames West Region showed that there were 391 invasive cancers; 313 (80%) had a lymph node procedure and out of these 82 were associated with positive nodes (26%). Of those patients with positive nodes, 65% had one, two or three positive nodes, 20% had four to nine positive nodes, and 15% had more than 10 positive nodes.

DCIS

In symptomatic practice DCIS accounts for 4% of all cancers but in screen-detected patients it accounts for up to 20%. The increase in the numbers of non-invasive cancers had led to a reclassification of this pathological entity according to cell type and necrosis, rather than morphological features. An example of screen-detected DCIS is shown in Fig. 8.5. When DCIS is widespread, the treatment of choice is mastectomy which usually comes as a shock to the patient as she has no symptoms. These women should be offered immediate breast reconstruction whenever possible. When DCIS is more localised initial surgical treatment of choice is wide local excision made possible by the technique of needle localisation biopsy (see below). Having obtained local control there are no clear guidelines as to the

Figure 8.4
Lymph node procedures by surgeons in the South Thames West Region. Solid bars, node procedures on invasive cancers = 231; open bars, total invasive cancers = 327.

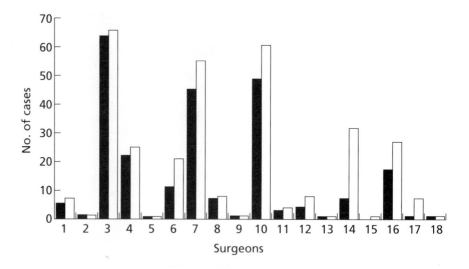

Figure 8.5
DCIS magnification views of a central area in the left breast. The appearances show typical calcifications without density in a 65-year-old woman. This was her second invitation for screening and she was asymptomatic and the calcification had been absent 3 years previously. Histology showed a 10 mm zone of large cell comedo DCIS with secure margins. Adjuvant treatment with tamoxifen as part of DCIS trial.

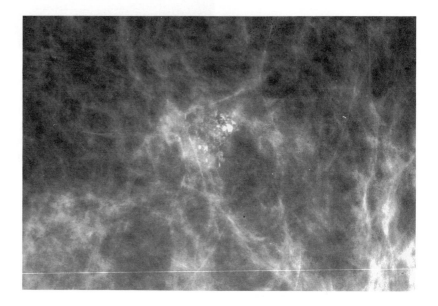

most efficacious adjuvant therapy. Trials after local surgery are currently in progress in the UK and America (see below). DCIS is almost always impalpable and the diagnosis depends on the image guided procedures.

Special types
Special types of breast cancer are found with much greater frequency in screened populations and include tubular, tubular mixed, cribriform, mucoid and papillary cancers as well as ductal carcinoma of no specific type grade 1. The quality assurance target is that these should

account for more than 30% of all invasive cancers detected and it is expected that more than 50% of invasive cancers will be less than 15 mm in diameter.

Techniques for diagnosis

In symptomatic breast clinic diagnosis of cancer is established by triple analysis involving clinical examination, mammography and fine needle aspiration cytology (FNAC). These can be supplemented by ultrasonography and information during aspiration on the texture of the underlying lesion.[11] These tests can be conducted as a one-stop process with the advantage that the patient can be counselled and have a care plan formulated at the initial visit.[12] Up to 70% of abnormalities detected by breast screening may be impalpable and newer techniques have to be utilised to make a diagnosis.

FNAC

Until 1994 the usual method of obtaining a diagnosis from an impalpable lesion involved image guided cytology using stereotactic mammography. An alternative method is ultrasound-guided sampling. A computerised device is added to a conventional mammographic unit and this calculates the depth and precise position of the impalpable lesion. Using a 21 gauge needle, cytology samples are taken by a series of passes in a single plane.[13] The inadequacy rate of this technique depends on the number of passes and varies from 0 to 26%. The sensitivity is 61% (range 55–80%), specificity 72% (range 56–80%), false negative rate 14% (range 0–19.5%) and the positive predictive

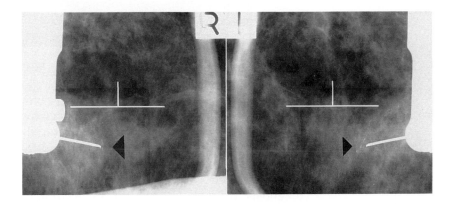

Figure 8.6
Stereotactic FNA biopsy. Arrow shows zone of micro-calcification without density with right and left parallax images showing the needle within the zone of interest.

Figure 8.7

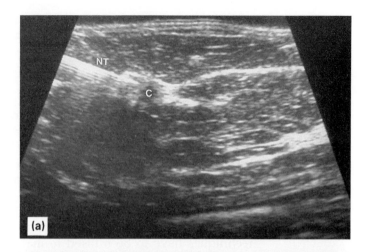

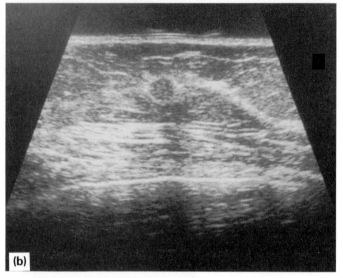

value 99%.[14] An example of a stereotactic biopsy is shown in Fig. 8.6. This technique has a high sensitivity, specificity and diagnostic accuracy with low morbidity. The main complications are vasovagal attacks and haematoma formation. The cytological analysis lends itself to a one-stop process with diagnosis on the same day. The main problem relates to the inadequacy rate and the impossibility of differentiating between invasive cancer and DCIS. The technique requires an experienced cytologist as part of the breast care team to give a diagnosis of malignancy and to accurately grade the cytological appearances.[15] Ultrasound-guided FNAC is quicker and easier to perform and is also more comfortable for the patient. It enables real time positioning of the needle so that sampling error can be reduced (Fig. 8.7). The method is not practical for some impalpable lesions which are not seen ultrasonographically, especially those including microcalcification alone and architectural disturbance.

Figure 8.7 *Ultrasound-guided FNA biopsy and localisation; 60-year-old woman without breast symptoms. (a) Ultrasound-guided FNA biopsy needle tip (NT) shown in real-time within cancer (C). (b) Ultrasound image prior to excision. (c) Specimen radiograph showing adequate margin of resection. The histology showed an 8 mm infiltrating duct cancer grade 1 (subscore 3), negative nodes and no DCIS or vascular invasion. Prognostic index score 2.2, no further adjuvant therapy.*

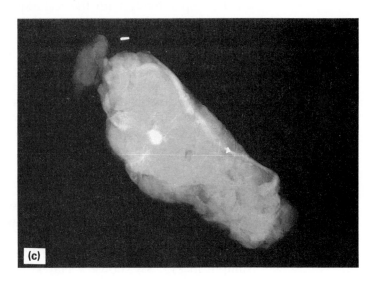

Core biopsy

Stereotactic core biopsy has been available since 1994 as a means of improving the preoperative diagnostic rate of cancer. Local anaesthetic is used to infiltrate around the core placement site. For optimal results five passes are made using a 14 gauge needle fired from an automated biopsy gun. An increased false negative rate and a comparable inadequacy rate may indicate learning curve effects.[16] Others with a well-established stereotactic programme[17] have seen preoperative diagnosis rise from 72% to 90% leading to a 64% reduction in the need for diagnostic open biopsy. In addition the preoperative detection of DCIS rose from 39% to 82% which led to improved management of operating lists and surgical decisions. The current recommendation for each screening centre is to use either a stereotactic FNA or core biopsy according to facilities available. Both techniques complement each other and when used in conjunction can help reduce the need for unnecessary procedures. A more recent advance has been the introduction of core biopsies taken using a prone table and digital mammography. The Swansea team reported a 98% positive predictive value using ultrasound-guided cores with a considerable reduction in the need for open diagnostic biopsy.[18]

New surgical procedures

As the screening process moves from the prevalent (first screen) to the incident rounds (subsequent screens) more of the abnormalities detected will be asymptomatic and impalpable. The diagnosis is established preoperatively with the techniques described above. With the exception of the few patients who choose to have mastectomy or are advised to have mastectomy because of multifocality, the majority of screen-detected cancers are suitable for a breast conserving surgical procedure. The technique of needle localisation permits the two primary aims of breast conserving surgery: satisfactory tumour control and good cosmetic appearance. Having removed relatively small pieces of breast tissue containing impalpable abnormalities the surgeon is responsible for orientating the specimen for accurate pathological assessment.

Needle localisation biopsy

This technique requires close co-operation between surgeon and radiologist. A needle is placed into the breast under ultrasound or X-ray control using a stereotactic machine or, more usually, a grid system. A variety of different needles with fixation devices can be used. An example in Fig. 8.8 shows a Hawkins 2 needle, which has a hook which flicks into position after accurate placement at the target. The needle has to combine durability so that the surgeon can find it when inside the breast and good fixation to withstand displacement. Needles are usually put in from a superior or lateral aspect of the breast. It is not always necessary to follow the pathway of the needle at surgery. It is possible to calculate the position of the target and plan to intercept the needle close to it.[19] The aim of needle localisation biopsy is to remove a ball of tissue with the needle tip and target at its centre. When done for diagnostic purposes, the weight of the specimen should not exceed 20 g and the time taken for specimen check radiography to be back in theatre should not exceed 10 min.[20] If the procedure is being done for therapeutic reasons then a much larger weight of tissue is usually excised to give a minimum of 10–15 mm margin in all directions where possible. Should specimen radiography show one of the margins is too close, further tissue should be taken immediately. The use of two planar specimen radiography facilitates this imaging process. If the diagnosis of cancer has not been previously established, the use of frozen section is discouraged, particularly if the target is microcalcification alone. The operative procedure should be covered by a single injection of antibiotics to discourage wound infection, and the procedure can be done as a day case unless it is combined with a lymph node procedure. More than 80% of marker wires should be within 10 mm of the target in any one plane, and 95% of impalpable lesions should be correctly removed at the first localisation biopsy. Better images are obtained for specimen radiography by X-raying the specimen on the mammographic unit in the X-ray department. This also allows compression to be used which gives magnified images of the target and the margins of safety. The factors involved with successful needle localisation have been analysed in 152 patients.[21] A favourable outcome for the patient (need for re-excision and the number of operations) was directly related to the experience of the surgeon and the size of the target lesion.

One-stage surgery

A primary aim of the screening service is to reduce the number of unnecessary biopsies to a minimum. The increased use of preoperative cytology and core biopsy means the majority of patients with impalpable cancers will have a positive diagnosis prior to first surgical intervention. If the target is microcalcification alone, then there is a strong possibility that this represents non-invasive disease and a day case procedure can be undertaken. Only if subsequent definitive histology shows the presence of invasion are lymph nodes required at a second surgical procedure. A second surgical procedure will also be required if the margins are less than 5 mm. When the diagnosis of cancer is established in an impalpable lesion with features of either asymmetric density, spiculate density or a complex lesion is found then a one-stage surgical procedure involving removal of cancer and lymph nodes can be carried out. Quality assurance guidelines suggest that in 90% of patients where a preoperative diagnosis is established, no further surgery should be required for incomplete excision. Once the learning curve has been negotiated all centres should report improved usage of one-stage surgery. The Avon screening service reported a 77% inadequate surgical clearance rate out of 114 localisation biopsies, but in only 19% of these had a preoperative diagnosis of cancer been established.[22] Increasing the use of preoperative diagnostic techniques will decrease the need for re-operation but problems will persist with DCIS where radiographs underestimate the extent of microscopic change.

Care of the specimen

It is a surgeon's responsibility to ensure the correct orientation of the specimen for pathology studies. A variety of systems have been devised to ensure this. The safest is placement of metal clips in a set pattern.[23] This aids identification of margins during the operation and subsequent orientation for the pathologist. A series of ligatures can be placed in set directions and these can be colour coded or of different lengths according to the margin. Other systems utilise pinning the specimen on a template or board. Specimens should be sent as quickly as possible to the pathology department where the margins are marked with India ink or organically coloured gelatins.[24] This shows up on subsequent histology slides and means accurate margin estimation can be made.

Figure 8.8
Needle localisation biopsy. (a) Hawkins 2 needle inserted from above with needle tip close to microcalcifications (arrowed). Calcifications were new on second screen having been absent three years previously. Stereotactic cytology was positive for cancer. (b) Specimen radiograph confirming excision of calcifications (arrowed). Note ligaclips used to orientate specimen. Histology showed 10 mm zone of large cell comedo DCIS with 5 mm margins. Patient was randomised to receive tamoxifen as part of DCIS trial.

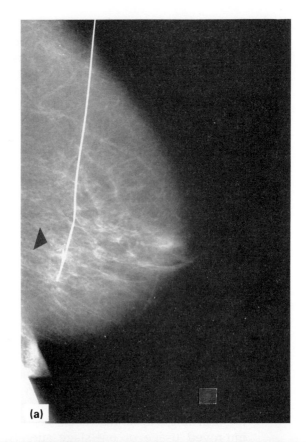

(a)

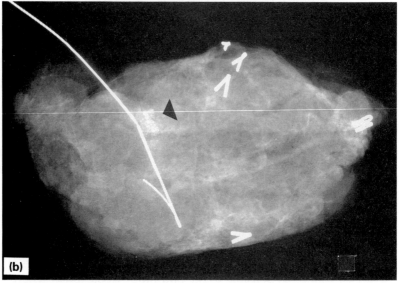

(b)

Pathology report

The minimum data set includes the type of cancer, maximum diameter, grade, the presence of DCIS, the presence of vascular invasion and lymph node status. This in turn provides all the information required to construct a prognostic index and to plan therapy. The pathologist is responsible for filling out the details on an audit form submitted to the quality assurance team on every tumour. In the same way the surgeon is responsible for filling out details of the surgical procedure and other quality objectives.

Therapeutic trials

DCIS trial

This trial, set up in 1990, addresses the use of adjuvant strategies following the complete local excision of a small focus of DCIS. Patients are randomised on a two by two factorial basis comparing surgery alone against the addition of either tamoxifen or radiotherapy, or tamoxifen and radiotherapy. By April 1996, 1100 patients had been randomised, the vast majority coming from this country and one tenth coming from Australasia. One of the key issues not addressed by this trial has been the width of safety required after local excision. Preliminary data from the NSABP DCIS trial (B-17) suggest that the addition of radiotherapy to local surgery significantly reduced the number of local recurrences.[25] Although the UK DCIS has accrued according to target, a vast number of patients with DCIS are treated outside the context of the trial without any specific scientific basis.

BASO 2

A similar randomisation on a two by two factorial basis exists for good prognosis cancers found by the screening programme. These include the various special types of cancer and duct cancers not otherwise stated (NOS) which are grade 1, node negative and smaller than 20 mm in maximum dimension. The outcome of this trial will help to decide whether radiotherapy can be safely withheld to certain good prognosis groups with a significant reduction in the cost of treating each individual cancer. Unlike the DCIS trial it is recommended that the patients entering BASO 2 have a 1 cm margin of clearance around the cancer. Fifty units are now entering patients throughout the UK and by September 1996, 421 had been entered into the study out of a total of 1200 planned for the trial.

Outcomes of the programme

Two undoubted strengths of the screening programme are the quality assurance measures that have been put in place and the enthusiasm of the staff. Through these it is possible to get results of the screening process and to record the treatments being carried out. Initially only surrogate measures of breast cancer mortality can be produced in the form of prognostic index measurement. The Nottingham Prognostic Index divides patients into good, medium and poor prognosis groups according to a scoring system.[26] This has been validated in groups of patients from 1983 to 1987 and 1988 to 1992. A score of less than 3.4 represents an excellent prognosis with a 10-year survival prospect of more than 85%, whereas a prognostic score greater than 5.4 is associated with a poor prognosis with a 10-year survival prospect of below 20%. In a symptomatic group of patients, 34% were in the good group, 52% in the moderate group and 14% in the poor prognostic group. In contrast, during the first 4 years of screening 1988 to 1992, 71% of patients are in a good prognostic score group, 25% in the moderate one and only 4% in the poor one. This shift may be evidence of breast screening obtaining its expected targets. It might represent a lead time bias. These figures apply only for invasive disease. The Nottingham figures also show an increase in non-invasive disease from 4% up to 1987, 7% in symptomatic patients up to 1992, to 24% in screen-detected patients up to 1992. Some of these patients with non-invasive disease may have progressed to invasion.

Quality assurance (QA) programme

The QA guidelines for surgeons in breast cancer screening was first published in 1992 and revised in 1996. It became the first guideline document in the UK for any aspects of surgery and the first in the world for breast cancer screening.[20] The quality criteria are set for four main domains which are: the general performance of the unit, biopsy rates, treatment profiles and waiting times. The general performance quality criteria are largely dependent on the radiological aspects of the screening process and assessment and are not surgeon dependent. Biopsy quality objectives are very much surgeon dependent with the help of the cytologist and radiologist. Technical aspects are under scrutiny here. The treatment-related objectives are fairly loose without many specific targets. The waiting time objectives are perhaps the most contentious. It may not be possible to admit 90% of patients with screen-detected cancers within three weeks of informing the patient that surgical treatment is required because of resource limitation. If waiting time between diagnosis and therapeutic intervention and from decision to operate for diagnosis and admission were to lengthen considerably then it is suggested that the screening process should be halted. Problems in waiting times, discussed through the QA programme at a national level allow pressure to be exerted on hospitals to allow more beds and operating lists to ensure the backlog is cleared.

Each of the 17 old regions of health care in the UK have a QA team which includes a representative of each of the healthcare specialties involved in screening (surgeon, radiologist, cytologist, histologist, specialist breast nurse, radiographer, programme manager, office worker and physicist). The QA team should meet at least twice a year to discuss regional and national issues and to examine whether screening QA targets are being met.

QA inspections

Crude assessment of performance of each region is easily obtained and can be broken down according to each screening centre. Considerable variation in performance may be noted. Data from one screening centre can be broken down to see whether any members of that team are performing outside guidelines. The QA team inspects each of the screening centres on an annual basis. Problems such as lack of machines, space, or personnel can be identified as well as poor practice which needs correction.

Avoiding mistakes

Errors in the screening process occur and it is the job of the QA team to identify these, examine what has gone wrong, take corrective action and ensure that similar events are avoided. In radiology there is always a balance between sensitivity and specificity which means a trade off between an acceptably low recall rate and an acceptably low missed cancer rate. The latter may declare as interval cancers and it is therefore important for surgeons involved with screening to flag any interval cancer back to the radiological QA team.

Once a patient comes to surgery, it is the surgeon's responsibility to try and make sure that all the evidence for diagnosis of cancer is concordant. Postoperative checks that mammographically identified lesions (impalpable) have been totally removed must occur. This can be by specimen radiography or, if doubts remain, early check mammography.

Changes in practice

The quality assurance programme can produce worthwhile changes in practice at local and national levels. An example at local level would be the correction of surgical practice to that which ensured that all women who required nodal surgery received it. Some surgeons might compromise on this aspect of care.

As far as national surgical standards are concerned, the targets set in 1996 become more stringent than those set in 1992. In the old guidelines the re-operation rate was supposed to be less than 30% but is now less than 10%; the preoperative diagnostic rate was more than 60% but is now more than 70%, and the special type of cancer rate was more than 20% and is now more than 30%. Radiological changes in standards have included the change from one view to two view mammography on the first screen, a move from a less than 7% recall rate to less than 5% for the prevalent round and a change from 5% to 3% in the incident round, and an increase in the cancer detection rate from 50 to 55 per 10 000 women. For the prevalent round the new target is 3.6 invasive cancers per 1000 women screened and 4.0% is the corresponding figure for the incident round. Tumours of less than 15 mm diameter are now expected to account for at least 50% of invasive cancers and the expected rate of DCIS now falls between 10 and 20%.

National results

The only national results available are those for screening related events rather than treatment related ones. Results from 1990 to 1995 are summarised in Tables 8.2 and 8.3.[26] The number of women invited in 1994–1995 was 1 507 000 and this is close to capacity. The uptake for screening has now increased to 77% and the rise of 5% over the last 2 years has meant a decreased ability to maintain throughput, accounting for the decrease in the total number of women screened. The recall rate has continued to fall as each team completes the learning curve and this also accounts for the decreased biopsy rate. The latter has also been influenced by the use of stereotactic and ultrasound-guided biopsy techniques. The cancer detection rate and the total number of cancers remain fairly static as has the small cancer detection rate. All these points emphasise that the function of the screening programme has plateaued as the learning curve has been negotiated. As the screening process evolves it is important to distinguish between prevalent and incident rounds. The results from 1994–1995 show a much higher recall rate in the prevalent round, a lower uptake rate, a higher cancer detection rate but a fairly static number of lesions of good prognosis.

Information on treatments for screen-detected lesions is more difficult to compile due to a large number of different computerised systems used to retrieve the data, a relative lack of data managing staff and a general reluctance by surgeons to fill in forms giving details of treatment. In April 1996 the national audit review of treatment failed to obtain core treatment data from a number of regions. Nonetheless information was available on 4141 patients with cancer. The number of surgeons per region dealing with screen-detected disease varied from 16 to 31 and only 13 surgeons saw more than 50 screen-detected cancers per year. Only four of 11 regions were able to reach the QA target of more than 60% having a preoperative diagnosis for cancer. The vast majority of patients had one or two therapeutic operations. The need for a second operation varied between 17 and 39% depending on whether there was invasive or non-invasive disease. Only 1% of patients needed a third therapeutic operation. Lymph node status was unknown in 6–73% of patients and the node positivity rate varied between 14 and 25%.

Table 8.2 *UK national screening results (1990–1995)*

	1990/1	1991/2	1992/3	1993/4	1994/5
Invited (×000s)	996	1443	1612	1610	1507
Uptake	71%	71%	71%	72%	77%
Recall	7%	6%	5%	6%	6%
Biopsy	1%	0.9%	0.8%	0.8%	0.5%
Cancer detection rate/1000	6.2	6.2	5.7	5.5	–
Cancers	4400	6600	6600	6700	6500 (20% DCIS)
Small invasive cancers (<10 mm # <15 mm)	900	1500	1500	1500	# 2660

Table 8.3 *UK national screening results (1994–1995)*

	Prevalent round	Incident round
Uptake	75%	89%
Recall	7%	3.4%
Cancer rate (per 1000)	6	4.3
DCIS	19%	19%
Small invasive cancers (<15 mm)	53%	55%

Of 2517 invasive cancers where treatment options have been recorded, 655 (26%) had a mastectomy and 74% had a breast-preserving procedure. Surgical practice seems to be relatively stable around the country as the mastectomy rate between different regions only varied between 20 and 35%. For cancers measuring 10 mm or less in size the mastectomy rate was still as high as 20% with a range between regions of 8–31%. As the QA standard for the mastectomy rate for small cancers is less than 50%, this target is easily being reached and despite the variation in mastectomy rate region by region, the QA standard for mastectomy rate for women with small cancers could, on the basis of this audit, be tightened up to be less than 30%.

Regional results

The national picture remains incomplete with regard to treatment for screen-detected cancer but any region with an active QA programme should produce good information regarding treatment.

Problems

Data collection

Various domains of data retrieval are easy whereas others are more difficult. There is good quality information from the screening process, slightly more patchy information regarding screening treatment and very few data at this stage regarding follow-up and results. Part of this depends on the surgeon's lack of time to give attention to such detail, but more importantly there is not enough resource built into the screening programme to pay for data collection of follow-up. An example of this situation from the Jarvis Centre, Guildford can be cited. Details of 191 screen-detected cancers from 1988 to 1993 were requested. Information was found in 171 of these and 158 were disease free. In 20 patients (10%) the hospital notes could not be found. Of 13 patients with further disease, five had died from breast cancer, three had died from other causes, and five had suffered relapse but not death. The time taken for a data manager to obtain this information was 105 hours, with a further 21 hours needed to enter data on computers. The task ahead for collection of data for follow-up purposes is enormous and needs more resource.

Interval cancers

For the screening project to be successful mammography must detect small cancers, but at the same time the number of cancers presenting in the first, second and third years after a normal screen must be low. True interval cancers are those which were definitely not present on review of previous screening mammograms. False negatives are those presenting between screens where review of the previous mammographic films shows that the cancer had been missed. Other cancers presenting between screens are not easily classifiable either because they are occult, have minimal signs, or because mammography was not carried out at the time of symptomatic presentation. Woodman in 1995, from the North Western Region, described 297 interval cancers from a screening population of 137 421 screened between 1988 and 1992. The results were compared against a cancer detection rate by screening of 59 per 10 000 and the assumption that the background overall cancer rate was 18.3 per 10 000. The results showed an interval cancer rate in the range 5–7.5 per 10 000 in the first year after screening, 9.3–10.5 per 10 000 in the second year, and 13.5–18.0 in the third year.[27] It was concluded that more interval cancers were being found than had originally been predicted, and although the levels were acceptable in the first 2 years, in the third year the level was very close to the expected background rate without screening. It was suggested that the screening interval of 3 years was too long.

The data from the North Western Region were similar to those from Nijmegen and Stockholm, but considerably higher than the interval rates from the Swedish two-county study. Figures from other screening units in the UK have confirmed that interval cancer rates are disconcerting. The results from the Avon screening service, for example, from 1989 to 1992 showed rates of 7 per 10 000 for year 1, 12.5 per 10 000 for year 2, and 14 per 10 000 for year 3 (J.R. Farndon, personal communication). Figures from South Thames West Region for the same time period (excluding DCIS) range from 3.3 to 4.7 per 10 000 for year 1, 6.7 to 12.9 per 10 000 for year 2, and 7.5 to 14.2 per 10 000 for year 3. The problem of interval breast cancers was highlighted at the beginning of 1995 and as a result of this, new national QA targets were set for interval cancers, these being up to 12 per 10 000 for years 1 and 2 combined, and less than 13 per 10 000 for the third year.[28]

The problem of interval cancers has been attacked in various ways, all of which aim to decrease the false negative rate. These measures include the introduction of two view mammography, the concept of films being double read independently by two trained radiologists, increases in the mean optical density of the films and improved and increased staff training, especially for the appreciation of subtle mammographic signs. The problem of interval cancers may be solved by the results of the randomised study comparing 1 versus 3 year mammography. If the excess interval cancer rate is purely a problem of the third year, then the reduction of the screening interval to 2 yearly cycles may radically streamline the whole screening project. This would have considerable cost implications and this then becomes a political decision regarding implementation. Epidemiologically it is important to establish whether cancers developing in the first, second and third year after screening have a different prognostic index profile to those detected either by screening or presenting in the background population.

Background cancer rate

Calculations regarding interval cancer rates and whether they approach the background cancer rate depend on knowing what the background cancer rate is. The Cancer Registry information may have underestimated the number of cancers in the population and the interval cancer data, therefore, may not be as worrying as they first seem. One of the primary targets of the breast screening project is a reduction in mortality by the year 2000, but it must be stressed that the background mortality from breast cancer is in a state of dynamic change even without screening and may be due to the introduction of more effective therapies. It has been pointed out that the breast cancer death rate in England and Wales stopped increasing in the late 1980s and has now started to fall. This means approximately 10% less cancer deaths in 1993 compared to 1985–9 in the age range 20–79 years.[29] This decline has occurred too soon to be influenced by the implementation of breast screening, but it is hoped that screening will accelerate the fall still further. A similar reduction in breast cancer mortality has been reported for Scotland.[30] This decrease in breast cancer death may be an indirect 'spin off' for the improved services delivered to women with breast disease that have come about due to the reorganisation of services mandated by the screening project as a whole.

The patient

For the majority of women who attend for breast screening the process is a positive experience. Questionnaire studies have shown a high level of satisfaction with many positive comments regarding its organisation, professionalism and communication. Nonetheless it is well recognised that it also induces considerable anxiety and for every 1000 women attending for screening 995 will not have cancer but may experience potentially negative experiences while waiting for results to be given. Indeed some 65 per 1000 will have been recalled for further assessment and some form of biopsy for what proves to be benign disease. Additional concerns have been voiced regarding the hidden dangers of screening mammography, particularly in younger women.[31] These include overdiagnosis of irrelevant lesions particularly DCIS (lag time bias), overdiagnosis of small invasive cancers resulting in treatment at a time when a woman is asymptomatic (lead time bias), and potential increased cancer formation due to repeat exposure to radiation, particularly in women carrying the ataxia-telangiectasia gene.

The health economics research group at Brunel University have conducted studies into the effects of screening on the psychological profile of women in the relevant age band. A total of 219 detailed healthcare questionnaires were carried out on women aged 40–44 years, and 231 in women aged 50–64 years. The assessments concentrate on aspects of the breast screening process such as a clear screen result, an assessment, a cancer and an interval cancer as well as aspects of treatment such as mastectomy, tamoxifen, and breast conservation with radiotherapy. Compared to a value of 1.0 for good health, a clear screening result description was valued at 0.92 and all other remaining descriptions were at values of 0.66. There was no difference between the younger and the more mature women except with regard to breast conservation. Of the women attending screening 20% said they felt more anxious than usual when they received their invitation for screening, 16% said they were more anxious while waiting for the appointment on the day, but only half of these said they felt very anxious. About 30% felt more anxious than usual while waiting to be seen for assessment and 42% were more anxious than usual while waiting for their results, half of these again being extremely anxious. The main finding of the study was that not only does screen-detected breast cancer have an adverse effect on the woman's quality of life, but so does that of a clear screen following assessment and the development of an interval cancer. The value obtained for a clear screening result was very close to the value for good health, suggesting that screening as a whole does not have any adverse quality of life effects.

Conclusions Trials have shown that screening mammography can reduce breast cancer mortality. In the UK a bold plan of screening for the whole nation has been adopted in an effort to help reduce the high mortality rates from this disease. National programmes exist in Australia, Holland and Iceland. In other countries relatively small proportions are covered such as only 6% in Italy and across five provinces in Canada. In some countries, such as Norway, the programmes are only just starting. Having implemented the screening process and defined targets and guidelines the programme is beginning to analyse its achievements. At this stage surrogate measures of survival are used rather than actual mortality rates.

There is no doubt that guidelines and targets can be met and can improve the services delivered for the diagnosis and treatment of breast cancer as a whole.[32,33]

Phenotypic drift

Although surrogate measures such as the Prognostic Index predict that lives will be saved by breast screening, it is useful to reflect on the later outcomes from some of the already published screening trials. Tabar found in the Swedish Two County trial that very small cancers of 10 mm or less were associated with a 12-year survival of 95% independent of nodal status or grade, and that for tumours less than 15 mm there was a 90% survival for node negative or grade 1 to 2 cancers. His conclusions were that screening arrests the disease[34] and that phenotypic drift occurs. Cancers need to be found as small as possible before phenotypic drift occurs and this means that it is not the number of interval cancers that is important, but their size and biological potential. Klemi believed that phenotypic drift occurs but if cancers can be found when they are biologically favourable it is important not to overtreat them.[35] The implication of phenotypic drift would be that the rescreening interval should be as short as possible. Hakama has put forward the alternative explanation that phenotypic drift does not occur since the DNA content of tumours did not change throughout the screening rounds.[36] If this is the case there is a need to detect aggressive cancers when they are as small as possible, and as it is unlikely that screening could be offered frequently enough to detect all of these, there needs to be improvement of the diagnostic services for minimally symptomatic women. Thomas has emphasised the need to improve services for diagnosing minimally symptomatic patients and this should take precedence over decreasing the screening interval if such a choice has to be made.[37]

Costs

When screening was set up there were many critics who felt that the whole process would not be worthwhile in human terms. The debate has moved forwards into the financial arena. Kattlore made a detailed analysis of the costs and benefits of screening and the treatment of early breast cancer.[38] The recommendation was that screening mammography had benefit only for women aged 50–69. This is an expensive luxury compared to the benefits of adjuvant therapy and the abandonment of routine follow-up. Baum, extracting data from this paper, commented that there may be a price tag of £1 000 000 for each woman who benefits from screening. Others put the cost of a life saved in the region of £100 000. Nonetheless as Baum comments, 'it is invidious to put a price on a woman's life'.[39]

The future

Sometime in the future a better test than mammography may be devised as a means to screen populations with a high and natural incidence of breast cancer. Until such time the UK screening programme gathers pace, is producing data and is filled with the right balance of enthusiasm and self-reflection. It is already known that two view mammography is better than one, the screening interval at 2 years is likely to be better than screening at 3 years and there may be a benefit for screening 40 year olds, although the cost–benefit ratio will be high. Further developments for the younger woman are now taking place, particularly in a context of a family history breast cancer clinic. The Nottingham group reported a cancer detection rate of eight per 1000 women screened, which is comparable to that in the routine screening process over the age of 50.[40]

The latest evidence for screening 40–49 year olds suggests that there will be a reduction in mortality by 25% provided a 15-month screening interval is used. Sweden employs a wide age range of screening from 40–79, but only half of their health councils enforce the recommendations. Undoubtedly screening prolongs life, but it now goes back into the political arena as to how scarce resources should be spent. The new Swedish guidelines are awaited with anticipation.[41]

References

1. Breast cancer screening report to the health ministers of England, Wales, Scotland and Northern Ireland by working group chaired by Professor Sir Patrick Forrest, 1986, London: Her Majesty's Stationery Office.
2. Kertilowske K, Grady D, Rubin S, et al. Efficacy of screening mammography, a meta-analysis. JAMA 1995; 273: 149–54.
3. Nystrom L, Lutquist RLE, Wall S, et al. Breast cancer screening with mammography overview of Swedish randomised trials. Lancet 1993; 341: 973–8.
4. Tabar L, Fagerberg G, Duffy S, et al. Update of the Swedish two county programme of mammographic screening trial. Radiol Clin North Am 1992; 20: 187–210.
5. Dillner L. Older woman ignorant of breast screening. Br Med J 1996; 312: 75–6.
6. Bird DL, Fox JN, Ashley S, et al. Results of the first year of breast cancer screening in a district hospital. Br J Surg 1992; 79: 922–4.
7. Wald N, Murphy P, Major P, et al. UKCCCR multi-centre randomised control trial of one and two view mammography in breast cancer screening. Br Med J 1995; 311: 1189–92.
8. Kissin MW, Cooke J, Kissin C, et al. Radial scars – a screen detected lesion that must be removed. Proceedings Nottingham, EORTC Joint Breast Cancer Meeting 1993; 1.
9. Holland PA, Walls J, Boggis CRM, et al. A comparison of axillary node status between cancers detected at the prevalence and first incidence breast screening rounds. Br J Cancer 1996; 74: (in press).
10. Nicholson S, Webb AJ, Coghlan D, et al. Will screening for breast cancer reduce mortality? Evidence from the first year of screening in Avon. Ann R Coll Surg Engl 1993; 75: 8–12.
11. Roberts JCH, Rainsbury RM. Tactile sensation: a new clinical sign during fine needle aspiration of breast lumps. Ann R Coll Surg Engl 1994; 76: 136–8.
12. Gui PH, Marygold-Curling O, Allum WH, et al. One-step diagnosis for symptomatic breast disease. Ann R Coll Surg Engl 1995; 77: 24–7.
13. Guidelines for cytology procedures and reporting in breast cancer screening. Cytology sub-group of the National Coordinating Committee for Breast Cancer Screening Pathology. NHSBSP Publication no 22; 1993, Sheffield.
14. Ciatto S, Cariggi P, Bulgraesi P, et al. Fine needle aspiration cytology of the breast. A review of 9533 consecutive cases. The Breast 1993; 2: 87–90.
15. Robinson IA, McLittle G, Nicholson A, et al. Prognostic value of cytological grading of fine-needle aspirates from breast carcinomas: Lancet 1994; 343: 947–9.
16. Yeoman LJ, Michell MJ, Humphreys S, et al. Radiographically guided fine needle aspiration cytology and core biopsy on the assessment of impalpable breast lesions. The Breast 1996; 5: 41–7.
17. Litherland JC, Evans AJ, Wilson ARM, et al. The impact of core-biopsy on pre-operative diagnosis rate of screen detected breast cancers. Clin Radiol 1996; 51: 562–5.
18. Chave MJB, Flowers CI, O'Brien CJ, et al. Image-guided core biopsy in patients with breast disease. Br J Surg 1996; 83: 1415–16.
19. Querci Della Rovere G, Benson JR, Morgan M, et al. Localisation of impalpable breast lesions – a surgical approach. Eur J Surg Oncol 1996; 22: 478–82.
20. Quality Assurance Guidelines for Surgeons in breast cancer screening. Prepared by the national coordination group for surgeons working in breast cancer screening. NHSBSP Publication no 20, Sheffield, 1996.
21. Dixon JM, Raviseker O, Cunningham M, et al. Factors affecting outcome of patients with impalpable breast cancer detected by breast screening. Br J Surg 1996; 83: 997–1001.
22. Chinyama CN, Davis JR, Rayter Z, et al. Factors affecting surgical margin clearance in screen-detected breast cancer and the effect of cavity biopsies on residual disease. Eur J Surg Oncol 1997, in press.
23. Dixon JM, Raviseker O, Walsh J, et al. Specimen-orientated radiography helps define excision margins of malignant lesions detected by breast screening. Br J Surg 1993; 80: 1001–2.
24. Armstrong JS, Weinzweig IP, Davies JD. Differential marking of excision planes in screened breast lesions by organically coloured gelatins. J Clin Pathol 1990; 43: 604–7.

25. Fisher ER. Pathologic findings from the National Surgical Adjuvant Breast Project (NSABP) protocol B-17. Intraductal carcinoma (ductal carcinoma in situ). Cancer 1995; 75: 1310–19.

26. Todd JH, Dowle C, Williams MR, *et al.* Confirmation of a prognostic index in primary breast cancer. Br J Cancer 1987; 56: 489–92.

27. Woodman CBJ, Threlfall AG, Boggis CRM, *et al.* Is the three year breast screening interval too long? Occurrence of interval cancers in NHS breast screening programmes North Western Region. Br Med J 1995; 310: 224–6.

28. Field N, Michelle NJ, Wallis MGW, *et al.* What should be done about interval breast cancers? Two view mammography and possibly a shorter screening interval. Br Med J 1996; 310: 203–4.

29. Beral V, Hermon C, Reeves G, *et al.* Sudden fall in breast cancer death rates in England and Wales. Lancet 1995; 345: 1642–3.

30. Brewster D, Everington V, Hakness E, *et al.* Incidence of and mortality from breast cancer since the introduction of screening. Br Med J 1996; 312: 639–40.

31. Jatoi I, Baum M. American and European recommendations for screening mammography in younger women: a cultural divide. Br Med J 1993; 307: 1481–3.

32. Winstanley JHR, Leinstern SJ, Wake TN, *et al.* The value of guidelines in a breast screening service. Eur J Surg Oncol 1995; 21: 140–2.

33. Birch D, Chia Y, Payne M, *et al.* Good prognosis tumours in breast cancer screening. Ann R Coll Surg Engl 1995; 77: 185–7.

34. Tabar L, Fagerberg G, Day ME, *et al.* Breast cancer treatment and natural history: new insights from results of screening. Lancet 1992; 339: 412–14.

35. Klemi PJ, Joensuu A, Toikkanen S, *et al.* Aggressiveness of breast cancers found with and without screening. Br Med J 1992; 304: 467–9.

36. Hakama M, Holli K, Isola J, *et al.* Aggressiveness of screen-detected breast cancers. Lancet 1995; 345: 221–4.

37. Thomas BT. Population breast cancer screening: theory, practise, and service implications. Lancet 1995; 345: 205–7.

38. Kattlore H, Liberati A, Keller E, *et al.* Benefits and costs of screening and treatment for early breast cancer. JAMA 1995; 273: 142–8.

39. Baum M. Screening for breast cancer, time to think – and stop? Lancet 1995; 346: 436–9.

40. Kollias J, Sibbering BM, Holland PAM, *et al.* Prevalent screen results from a family history breast cancer clinic. The Breast 1997, in press.

41. Awuonda M. New breast screening guidelines for Sweden. Lancet 1996; 347: 963.

9 Treatment of early stage breast cancer and breast reconstruction

Richard Sainsbury

Introduction

Breast cancer remains one of the commonest solid epithelial neoplasms with an annual incidence of about 20 000 new patients per year in the UK. The estimated world-wide incidence is of a million new patients per year. The prevalence is some five times higher so for a unit with 100 new cancers per year there will be approximately 500 women alive with the disease at any one time.

Breast cancer accounts for 50% of all cancers for women aged between 40 and 55 years and thus remains a major health problem. The modal age of presentation is 58 years. The incidence is rising[1-3] but the mortality rate in the UK appears to have fallen in the last three years. Comparisons with European data show a poorer outcome (5-year survival rate) for patients treated in the UK of the order of magnitude of 5–10%.[4] The reasons for this are unclear but may include greater use of adjuvant therapies on mainland Europe.

The organisation of cancer services in England and Wales is in the process of change. Following the report of the Expert Advisory Group on Cancer Services to the Chief Medical Officer (known as the Calman report)[5] a three-level cancer service is proposed with a primary health care led service referring to cancer units which will be district based and provide quality care locally for the common cancers. The cancer centres will provide tertiary services. After reports from the British Breast Group[6] and the British Association of Surgical Oncology (BASO),[7] a consensus on how breast cancer will be managed is emerging. It is envisaged that breast cancer will be managed locally provided a multidisciplinary breast team is functioning and that there are enough patients passing through the unit to make such a team viable. Two geographically close units might combine to provide such a service but this conflicts with the current theme of NHS reforms

Figure 9.1
Percentage of screen-detected cancers in 1992–95 for women aged 50–65 years.

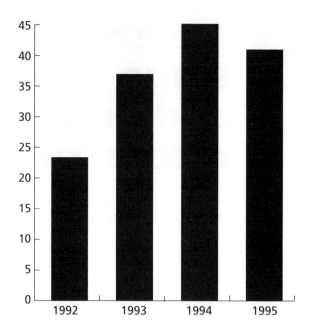

where competition is preferred to cooperation. There is evidence that patients under the care of clinicians with a special interest in the disease or those who treat larger numbers have improved outcomes.[8,9]

The breast care team will have dedicated surgical sessions for outpatient and operative activity. There will be identified radiologists and pathologists and breast care nurses in the team. Regular, documented meetings with clinical and or medical oncologists are essential although the necessary radiotherapy may well be provided off site. Dedicated inpatient beds and facilities for chemotherapy will be provided locally with suitable supervision. Protocols of care will be essential as will regular audit. A suitable computer program for such audit has recently been developed. Access to psychological services and reconstruction (if not provided locally) are essential.

The majority of patients with breast cancer still present with a lump as the dominant symptom. In the 50–65 age group (for whom screening is available) the percentage of screen-detected cancers rose through the first years of screening to about 45% but has declined as the prevalent tumours have been detected (Fig. 9.1). Other symptoms (in descending order of frequency) include lumpiness, distortion of the breast, nipple discharge and breast pain although the latter is uncommonly associated with malignancy. Fig. 9.2 shows patient numbers attending a breast clinic serving a population of 212 000. Guidelines on referral of patients with breast symptoms were issued in 1995 to all general practitioners by the Department of Health in an attempt to reduce the number of inappropriate referrals.[10] This has had the opposite effect and more patients are being referred. The ratio of malignant to benign disease was 10:1 but this has now risen to 15:1.

Figure 9.2
Relative proportion of referred symptoms to breast clinic (consultations about family history excluded).

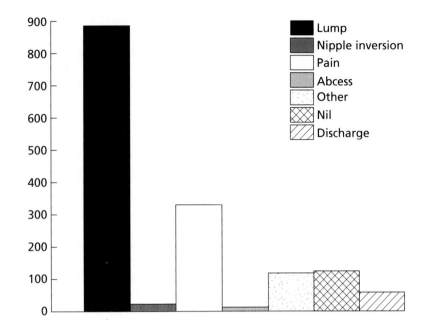

Aetiology and risk factors

The cause of breast cancer remains unknown. It is rare before the age of 25 but the incidence increases with age until the menopause when there is a slight levelling off (the menopausal hook of Clemmenson) before the incidence again rises although at a reduced rate compared to the premenopausal years. The incidence in increasing world-wide despite screening and is expected to involve about 1 000 000 women a year by 2000.

There is a marked geographical variation in the incidence and mortality from breast cancer. The level of fat consumption has been implicated. Immigrants from a country with a low incidence of breast cancer to one of higher incidence experience an increase in incidence to levels just below that of the adopted country within three generations. Breast cancer is commoner in women of higher than lower socioeconomic status.[11,12]

Women who have more menstrual cycles (i.e. an early menarche and late menopause) have an increased risk. Women whose menopause is before 45 have half the risk compared to those whose menopause occurs after 55. Those who have had an oophorectomy below 35 have a 40% reduction in the risk of breast cancer compared to those who have had a natural menopause.

Nulliparity and late age at first birth both increase the lifetime incidence of breast cancer. Women who have their first child after age 35 appear to have a risk higher than that associated with nulliparity. Breast feeding was thought to reduce the risk of breast cancer but this view has recently been challenged.

Family history is important. The extent of the risk depends on the number and relationship of relatives affected, the age of onset of the disease and relations with multiple sites of cancers. Fewer than 10% of all breast cancers are due to autosomal dominant susceptibility genes which may be transmitted through either maternal or paternal lines.[13,14] The main characteristics of an inherited susceptibility are:

- early age of onset
- bilateral disease
- multiple primaries in the same woman
- at least two different affected first degree relatives.

Referral to a genetics service may be appropriate to discuss risk and to see whether testing for BRCA1 or BRCA2 or p53 abnormalities is indicated.[15]

Other risk factors include obesity in the postmenopausal woman, previous radiation to the breast and a previous biopsy which has shown proliferative disease (especially if combined with a positive family history). There may be a small risk for prolonged use of hormone replacement therapy (HRT) but this may well be outweighed by its protective effect for osteoporosis and cardiovascular disease.

The above risk factors can be implicated in no more than 30% of breast cancers.[16]

Screening

Screening by regular mammography has been shown to reduce the risk of death from breast cancer for populations aged 50–65 by approximately 29%.[17] There is no evidence from randomised trials that screening the 40–50 age group is cost effective but screening those aged 65–70 detects significant numbers of cancers and may yet be introduced. In the UK eligible women are identified by general practitioners and are screened every three years using two views of each breast (from 1995). The films are usually read by a single radiologist although double reading detects an additional 5–10% of abnormalities. Based on studies in Scandinavia many feel that two years would be a more appropriate screening interval. This is being studied prospectively within the National Screening Programme.

Screen-detected cancers are likely to be of better histological grade or of special type and are less likely to be node positive than symptomatic cancers of the same size. Ductal carcinoma in situ (DCIS) is detected in about 30% of instances compared to less than 2% of symptomatic women.

Objectors to the programme point out the large costs involved in screening (about £27 million per year), the uncertainty of whether screen-detected disease would ever cause the patient harm and whether the anxiety generated by screening is worthwhile. It is, however, the only proven technique currently available of reducing mortality and is unlikely to be halted.

Prevention of breast cancer

Effective ways of reducing breast cancer incidence (although not preventing it totally) include prophylactic mastectomy or oophorectomy before age 35. Neither is generally acceptable. There is a trial of prevention using tamoxifen which has been shown to reduce the incidence of contralateral breast cancer when used as adjuvant treatment.[18] This trial aims to recruit 10 000 women world-wide who will be randomised to either 5 years tamoxifen or placebo. Concerns about the effects of tamoxifen on the uterus have slowed trial entry.[19]

Other possible preventative interventions include dietary manipulation with reduction of fat intake[20] or use of vitamin A analogues such as the retinoids.[21]

Diagnosis and investigations

Optimal treatment for patients with breast cancer is a multimodality activity requiring an input from surgeon, radiologist, pathologist, medical and clinical oncologist, general practitioner, breast care nurse and the woman herself. There is evidence that women treated by specialists seeing sufficient workloads to maintain such teams have better outcomes.[9] All primary care doctors in England and Wales have been circulated with guidelines on referral prepared on behalf of the Department of Health.[10]

The patient should be encouraged to participate in any decisions and psychological distress may be reduced by informed discussion before treatment.[22]

A preoperative diagnosis of breast cancer is essential and this is achieved through history, clinical examination and imaging with a cytohistological confirmation (the triple assessment).

History

This includes details of age of menorche, number of children and breast feeding, oral contraceptive use, family history, age of menopause, use of HRT and current medication.

Clinical examination

Both breasts and nodal drainage areas (axilla and supraclavicular fossa) should be carefully examined by palpation after a visual inspection. This should be performed with the patient placed in a good light. She should raise her arms above her head and return them to her side. This allows minor degrees of distortion or skin tethering to be seen as well as more obvious lumps.

Clinical examination is not completely reliable and over 55% of screen-detected cancers are impalpable. In younger women the sensitivity of clinical examination is lower with only 37% of cancers being detected.[23]

Detection of axillary nodes is difficult and, on examination, is accurate in only 50% of patients.[24] Ultrasonography, mammography and radioantibody scanning fare not much better and histological examination of resected tissue remains the only reliable method for determining axillary nodal status.

Imaging

Mammography remains the commonest imaging tool. The breast is compressed between two plates and usually two exposures of each breast are made in the oblique and craniocaudal (CC) positions although a true lateral view, axillary extended views and magnification views can be obtained. If an abnormality is detected further techniques such as paddle magnification views can be performed. These are often combined with stereotactic fine needle sampling for cytology. If a screen-detected lesion in impalpable it may be localised by mammography and a wire placed to mark the site of the lesion. The patient then has the area resected and a check radiograph will demonstrate complete removal. A mammogram is important even with a clinical diagnosis of breast cancer as it allows assessment of the contralateral breast as well as demonstrating multifocal disease. In women with DCIS mammography is better than clinical examination at determining the extent of the disease, but, even so, often underestimates the full extent of the disease.[25] Ultrasonography is good at distinguishing between solid lesions and cysts. It is useful for assessment of tumour size in most invasive breast cancers and may be more useful than mammography in demonstrating the margins in the younger woman with denser breasts.[26] It can be used to provide serial measurements of tumours being treated by induction chemotherapy or long-term endocrine therapy and is increasingly being used to localise impalpable disease prior to biopsy.

Not all breast cancers are detectable by mammography and ultrasonography. Persistence of a lump or other clinically suspicious area necessitates further investigation. The common pitfall is the lobular type of breast cancer which may present as diffuse lumpiness rather than a discrete lesion.

Biopsy techniques

Fine needle aspiration cytology (or biopsy) (FNAC) has been used for many years to confirm a diagnosis of palpable breast cancer.[27] In addition it may be used to confirm a clinically benign lump. The accuracy of FNAC is high when the operator is experienced and the cytologist is expert. It is reported on a C(cytology) 0–5 scale and a C5 report in conjunction with clinical and radiological evidence of a carcinoma is sufficient evidence to proceed to definitive surgery.[28] There are reported false positives but these tend to be where the cytology has given a discordant result from mammography and/or clinical findings. In such a case either an open or core biopsy should be taken. An acellular (C0) specimen may be appropriate if a random cytology of a fibrous area has been performed but should not be accepted if a discrete solid lesion is being aspirated. The biopsy must be repeated.

It is possible to obtain hormone receptor status on fine needle specimens. Core biopsies are now taken using a 14 gauge spring driven device. The skin is infiltrated with local anaesthesia and a scalpel used to nick the skin to allow passage of the core needle. Many women find it more comfortable than FNAC. A core of tissue is examined histologically thus allowing architectural detail to be shown. It can be used on impalpable disease using localisation techniques.[29] The cores should be X-rayed if microcalcifications were present on the original radiograph. Core biopsy should not be used instead of FNAC but is a valuable adjunct.

The use of FNAC and core biopsies should allow the majority of breast cancers to be diagnosed preoperatively thus allowing an informed discussion with the patient about treatment options and will allow definitive surgery to be performed. The combination of FNAC, mammography and clinical examination provide the highest diagnostic yield and the lowest risk of diagnostic error. The accuracy of the different investigations is shown in Table 9.1.

There is a tendency for all the above investigations to be provided at the time of the patient's first visit (the One Stop clinic) thus allowing repetition of FNAC should the result be inadequate. Whether the results are given to the patient the same day is a matter of local practice. A breast nurse should be present when the results are given as should a companion of the patient.

Open biopsy is occasionally needed if FNAC and core biopsy have failed to provide a diagnosis. This can be carried out as a day case procedure. A biopsy is not a definitive procedure and should not be confused with a treatment procedure such as a wide local excision (although sometimes, for a small lesion, the two may coincide). Frozen section is seldom used but may be helpful to confirm a suspicious

Table 9.1 *Accuracy of investigations*

	Clinical examination	US	Mammo-graphy	FNAC
Sensitivity	88	85	88	95
Specificity	91	88	90	95
Positive predictive value (PPV)	95	92	94	99.8

Sensitivity = % of cancers considered malignant.
Specificity = % of lesions diagnosed benign which are benign.
PPV = % of lesions diagnosed malignant which are cancer.

cytology result. The lesions which are difficult to diagnose on FNAC and core may also be difficult to diagnose histologically. In these instances the pathologist can provide better information with properly fixed tissue which has undergone routine processing than poorly fixed frozen sections.

Other preoperative investigations

For patients with early stage breast cancer (stages I and II) there has been a move away from staging investigations which have repeatedly been shown to give little useful information.[30] Currently a full blood count, liver function tests and a chest radiograph are all recommended along with investigation of specific complaints such as bone pain. For patients with larger cancers, where there is a higher chance of metastatic disease, bone and liver scans should be added. Tumour markers such as CEA or CA 15.3 may be helpful in monitoring response to treatment[31] but are generally non-specific and unreliable.

The above advice may change if the preliminary results of skeletal magnetic resonance imaging (MRI) are borne out. There is some evidence to show a correlation between MRI-detected bony lesions (in asymptomatic women) and early symptomatic relapse in bone. Patients with circulating tumour cells have earlier relapses and a greatly reduced chance of 5-year survival.

Pathology

Breast cancer arises in the terminal duct-lobular unit. The terminology used continues to change. The majority of cancers are of no special type (NST), also known as invasive ductal cancer or ductal NOS (not otherwise specified), and these account for about 70% of unselected tumours. Those with specific features which allow characterisation are associated with a better prognosis.

Carcinoma cells which have not yet broken through the basement membrane and are thus confined within the terminal ducto-lobular units are termed carcinoma in situ. These were historically broken down into ductal (DCIS) and lobular (LCIS) types. DCIS was described according to architectural features such as comedo or cribriform but this has given way to cytological features such as high grade and low grade which has improved prognostic significance.

Pathological examination of the resected specimen is used not just to provide a diagnosis but to confirm completeness of excision and to provide extra management information such as hormone receptor status.

If breast conservation has been performed the resected specimen should be orientated by clips or sutures and if the margins are involved a re-resection should be performed. Some try to avoid the need for this by performing cavity shavings and only return the patient to theatre is the shavings are involved.[32]

The pathology report should include the size of tumour, its type and grade (the Bloom and Richardson grading system is used for NST tumours), clearance of resection margins, presence and absence of tumour multifocality, the presence of DCIS in and around the tumour, lymphovascular invasion and axillary node positivity. This should be given as both number of nodes retrieved and number involved. In addition hormone receptor status (oestrogen (ER) and progesterone (PR)) can be performed with other biological markers such as epidermal growth factor receptor (EGFr), cell cycle kinetics or proliferative markers. Most of the latter have yet to be proven to give additional prognostic information.

Staging and prognostic factors

The TNM classification is still used for breast cancer although it is not well suited for this purpose. It was designed to be used clinically but the nodal status and size frequently change when the pathological measurements are given and there is thus little conformity as to which groups of patients are being compared. The UICC staging encompasses the TNM system and is still widely used. Of more importance is the full pathological description which allows patients to be compared in a meaningful manner.

Various pathological measurements influence prognosis, either individually or in combination. Nodal status is the single most important factor with an increasing loss of life expectancy with number of involved nodes. Grade, size, presence of lymphovascular invasion, S-phase fraction, Ki-67 staining, EGF receptor, ER and PgR all have prognostic significance. The combination of tumour size, grade and nodal status (the Nottingham Prognostic Index)[33] has been shown to have good discriminant function. Patients can thus be separated into a group whose survival mirrors the normal population, a group whose outcome is so poor that either no therapy or very aggressive therapy will be needed. The intermediate group may be the important one where the course of the disease might be influenced by means of chemotherapy or other adjuvant treatments.

Management options

Surgery

The aim of surgery is to achieve local control by eradication of the primary tumour. From screening studies it is clear that surgical intervention of early disease affects outcome although there are no randomised control studies of surgery against other treatment modalities. Because of its ability to influence local control, surgery remains the first treatment modality for early breast cancer.

Surgical treatment consists of breast conservation by wide local excision (WLE) or mastectomy, combined with axillary dissection. Wide local excision consists of removal of the tumour with about 1 cm of surrounding normal tissue (and skin if necessary). It is essential to achieve clear resection margins otherwise a high incidence of local recurrence is seen. This procedure is suitable for unifocal tumours generally smaller than 4 cm (although the overall breast size will modify this).[34] There is an increasing incidence of local recurrence with increasing tumour size. Patients with EIC (extensive intraductal component) are best treated with mastectomy as are patients where the cosmetic result is likely to be poor (such as large central tumours). Skin incision should be planned with both cosmesis and the need for postoperative radiotherapy in mind. If the scar is distant from the tumour bed the clinical oncologist must be informed as the scar is often used to plan any top-up boost of radiotherapy. Postoperative radiotherapy is part of conservation treatment and should be given unless restricted as part of a trial for specific groups of patients such as those with small, special types of tumours (The BASO II trial, British Association of Surgical Oncology). It is important to orientate the lumpectomy specimen for the pathologist and the AIM technique is recommended (one suture Anteriorly, two Inferiorly and three Medially).

Many randomised controlled trials have shown equal survival benefits after wide local excision combined with radiotherapy and mastectomy (when both have included axillary dissection).[35-37] The incidence of local recurrence in a conserved breast is of the order of 1% per year[38] compared to 0.5% per year after a mastectomy.[39] About 70% of mammographically detected cancers and 50% of symptomatic cancers are suitable for conservation therapy.[40]

Mastectomy is appropriate for those with multifocal disease, those with ill-defined margins, with the presence of EIC, where the tumour directly involves the nipple or central skin, or where the patient chooses such an operation. Mastectomy requires removal of all the breast tissue with conservation of the pectoral muscles and dissection of the axilla. Radiotherapy is not needed to the axilla after dissection but may be used to the mastectomy flaps if the tumour was large, of high grade or had extensive lymphovascular invasion.

It was once thought that conservation therapy reduced the risk of anxiety and depression postoperatively but it now seems that being offered a choice is more important than the procedure actually performed.[41] Many women who need a mastectomy can have reconstruction either as an immediate or delayed procedure (see below).

Timing of surgery for premenopausal women may be important. A report from Guy's Hospital, London and subsequent retrospective studies from other units have shown a survival benefit for patients operated on in the luteal phase (second half) of the menstrual cycle. Operating when unopposed oestrogens are present may allow dissemination and implantation of cells. Other centres have been unable to find such an effect and others an opposite effect with improved survival in the follicular phase. A prospective non-randomised study (the Intervention, Timing and Survival study) is currently examining this question.

Axillary dissection

Axillary dissection is either performed in continuity with a mastectomy or through a separate incision with a WLE. It allows assessment of the nodal status for prognostic purposes, eradication of metastatic disease within the nodes and assessment of nodal status to determine adjuvant treatment. There is as yet no reliable method of determining nodal status without surgical resection of nodes. Clinical examination of the axilla is unreliable. Sentinel node biopsy has been proposed as a more sensitive method of staging the axilla.

An axillary sample is an operation favoured by some who pick out the four largest nodes in the axilla but it neither allows full staging nor treats the axilla properly.[42]

Both the number of nodes retrieved and the number involved should be reported. The former may well be more a function of the pathologist rather than the surgeon. Surgery should not be combined with axillary radiotherapy as an unacceptable incidence of lymphoedema will occur.[43] As radiotherapy has been associated with brachial neuropathy and frozen shoulder many teams favour an axillary clearance. After an axillary clearance the axilla should be empty – the axillary vein should be clear and the nerve to serratus anterior and the thoracodorsal trunk should be preserved. The intercostobrachial nerve may have been divided although some try and preserve it – this defeats the object of an oncological clearance. The interpectoral nodes need attention as do the very lowest nodes which may be inadvertently left if too low an incision is made. This may occur if the axilla is being cleared as a separate procedure. Pectoralis minor usually needs division to allow access to the highest nodes.

Adjuvant treatment

Radiotherapy

Radiotherapy is an essential part of the treatment of breast cancer if conservation therapy has been performed and is used selectively after a mastectomy. Failure to give radiotherapy after WLE exposes the patient to an increased risk of local recurrence and the need for subsequent mastectomy.[44] The need for radiotherapy after small tumours of special type detected through screening is debated and the current BASO II trial addresses this problem. The need for a boost to the site of surgical resection is also debated. Radiotherapy after mastectomy used to be a standard treatment, but the results from several trials have shown that the routine addition of radiotherapy gave no additional benefit over a watch policy with radiotherapy used at the site of local recurrence.[45] In addition it was shown that single mastectomy and radiotherapy gave results equivalent to mastectomy and axillary dissection. Techniques for giving radiotherapy have changed since the early trials and the excess of cardiac deaths seen for left-sided tumours have subsequently disappeared.[46] As a result of these studies there was a move away from radiotherapy after mastectomy but it has become clear that there are patients at high risk of local recurrence. These patients have large tumours which were node positive and of high grade and with marked lymphovascular invasion.

Radiotherapy is associated with complications that occur either early (redness and soreness of skin which normally resolve within a few weeks) or late. Some are dose and fraction dependent and good skin care is an important part of the management of these patients. The excess of cardiac deaths is now no longer seen, but the rare complications of brachial plexopathy, second malignancy, lymphoedema and small degrees of pulmonary fibrosis still occur.[47] Radiotherapy is given by the clinical oncology team. It is usually based at cancer centres where the necessary technology is available.

Systemic adjuvant therapy

This includes hormonal treatments as well as cytotoxic chemotherapy and is normally started immediately after the surgical episode with the aim of reducing the micrometastatic burden and thus improve overall survival. It is now clear that adjuvant systemic therapy with multi-agent chemotherapy, tamoxifen[48] or ovarian oblation (in the under 50s)[49] will reduce the risk of recurrence and death for both node-positive and node-negative women. The effects of systemic adjuvant treatment are reviewed every five years where all trials utilising these agents are combined and subjected to meta-analysis.[48] This has shown a highly significant improvement for both recurrence free and overall survival (8.4% and 6.3%, respectively, at 10 years). These effects were twice as large for women under 50 and for those over 50. There is some evidence that anthracycline-based regimens are more effective than traditional cyclophosphamide, methotrexate and fluorouracil (CMF). Adjuvant chemotherapy has little effect on local control and should not, therefore, be substituted for radiotherapy where the risk of local regional recurrence is high.[50] Dose intensity is important[51,52] and reduction of doses may merely allow development of clones of resistant cells. The use of high-dose chemotherapy in the adjuvant setting is under investigation.[53] Currently patients at high risk (usually defined as having more than 10 nodes positive) are offered this treatment as part of a trial. The treatment is complicated and potentially hazardous. It involves extraction of peripheral stem cells in order to repopulate the marrow after high dose chemotherapy has had its effect. Chemotherapy has well-known side effects of nausea, vomiting, alopecia and tiredness.[54] The sickness can be reduced by the use of the HT3 antagonists such as ondansetron. Chemotherapy may induce amenorrhoea which may be temporary. Prolonged or high doses of anthracycline may be associated with congestive cardiac failure.

Tamoxifen

This drug was developed as a possible contraceptive but was not selective enough in its actions. It is now classed as one of the first selective oestrogen receptor modulators (SERM) and has both agonist and antagonist actions. Many individual trials as well as overview analyses[48] have shown the benefit for women who take tamoxifen postsurgery. The necessary duration of exposure is still unclear and trials continue to determine this but a minimum of two years dosing gives a reduction in odds of death of approximately 27% for post-menopausal women. Recent data from the CRC over 50s trial and other studies suggest that treatment with tamoxifen for 5 years gives prolonged survival. The effect appears to be greater in women whose tumours were oestrogen-receptor (ER) positive although an effect was also seen in 5–15% of ER-negative women.

The major side effect of tamoxifen which has emerged in recent years is the oestrogenic effect on the endometrium causing hyperplasia, and rarely, neoplasia. The beneficial effects of tamoxifen on reduction in deaths from breast cancer and reduction in the incidence of contralateral breast cancers[48] outweighs the risk from endometrial carcinoma.

Tamoxifen is currently undergoing investigation as a preventative agent in women at increased risk of breast cancer (as judged by family history). A placebo controlled trial is underway, with 10 000 women world-wide being recruited. The rationale for this is the finding of a 25% reduction in the incidence of contralateral breast cancers in women taking tamoxifen in the adjuvant setting.[55]

Newer selective oestrogen receptor modulators include a pure antioestrogen (ICI 182 117) which seems to have few side effects and drugs such as raloxifene, a compound originally developed for post menopausal osteoporosis prevention. Work continues on their efficacy and side effects.

Ovarian ablation

Reducing or stopping ovarian secretion in premenopausal women confers long-term benefit: a 25% reduction in mortality and 26% for recurrence – results similar to those achieved by polychemotherapy. There is debate over how much of the chemotherapy effect is achieved by ovarian suppression – over 50% of patients have a menopause induced by chemotherapy. There is less information about the combination of ovarian ablation with chemotherapy but this is being addressed by the current ABC trial.

Ovarian ablation can be achieved by radiotherapy (usually three fractions), open or laparoscopic surgery. In the short term an LH-RH analogue will achieve similar effects but these are expensive and currently have to be given by injection.

Trials currently available

The major national trials underway can be divided into those addressing issues of dosage (both intensity and density), combinations of treatments and duration of treatments. Quality of life measurements and economic evaluations are now essential parts of most studies. Some of the trials available in the UK are shown in Table 9.2.

An overview analysis of trials of chemotherapy, endocrine therapy and endocrine ablation is performed by the Oxford group every five years. Using the techniques of meta-analysis small, individual trials can be combined to allow firm conclusions to be drawn.[48] Clinical trials remain important in guiding the future management of patients with breast cancer. Even small differences in treatment arms may be significant because of the large number of women with the disease. Large numbers of patients are needed to provide such answers but

Table 9.2 *Trials available for patients with breast cancer (national studies)*

Trials for prevention of breast cancer
IBIS – tamoxifen vs. placebo for 5 years for women at increased risk.

Trials available at initial presentation
ITS – interval, timing and survival. To examine timing of surgery and menstrual cycle.
TOPIC – Infusional chemotherapy as neoadjuvant treatment.

Trials of surgical management and adjuvant treatments
UKCCCR DCIS – Role of R/T ± tamoxifen in management of DCIS.
BASO II – Role of R/T ± tamoxifen in management of small, special type node negative.
ABC – role of ovarian suppression and chemotherapy in addition to tamoxifen.
ATAC – place of anastrazole compared to tamoxifen in postmenopausal women.
DCIS – role of radiotherapy in management of DCIS.

Trials of dose intensity
Anglo-Celtic – Use of high dose vs. high dose and PBSC transplantation in high risk breast cancer.

Trials of duration of therapy
CRC over 50 – 2 years vs. 5 years tamoxifen.
ATTOM – length of duration of tamoxifen, UK study
ATLAS – length of duration of tamoxifen, international study

Trials involving screening
AGE – role of screening 40–50 year olds.
Frequency – optimum frequency of screening.

the randomisation rate remains very low with less than 10% of eligible patients entering studies in the UK. 'Excuses' for this include the time taken to talk to patients about studies and lack of support staff.

Breast reconstruction

The aim of breast reconstruction is to restore the normal shape and, to some extent, consistency of the breast after excisional or ablative surgery. It is commonly associated with mastectomy but the realisation that a quadrantectomy or a large wide local excision can lead to a significant cosmetic defect has also led to techniques for filling such defects.

Reconstruction after mastectomy is performed either at the time of initial surgery or as a delayed procedure. The advantages of the former include the patient having to undergo only one operation. Many patients do not wish to come back into hospital for further surgery 6–9 months after mastectomy when their lives are getting back to normal and do not take up the offer of a delayed reconstruction. There is evidence that the psychological benefit is greater after immediate reconstruction[56] and the techniques used do not prevent administration of adjuvant chemotherapy or hormone therapy. Disadvantages of immediate reconstruction include the time taken and the need for cooperation between breast and plastic surgeon in many cases (although more breast surgeons are being trained in such procedures).

The simplest form of reconstruction is an external prosthesis worn within the bra. This is, however, unsatisfactory for many as it feels unnatural and may move. Newer techniques include adhesive prostheses where a shaped plaster is stuck to the chest wall and a prosthesis attached to the plaster. Coloured prostheses are available for those whose skin is not white.

Tissue expansion allows stretching of the skin and muscle at a mastectomy site by means of placement of a temporary expander. This is an inflatable bag with a short connecting tube to an injection port which is usually placed under the pectoralis major muscle. Gradual inflation allows a pocket to be created into which a definitive (usually silastic) prosthesis can be placed. Care must be taken to site the expander and prosthesis correctly – it must not be allowed to sit too high or laterally towards the axilla. Dissection under the upper part of the rectus musculature may be necessary. Newer more expensive prostheses combine both functions and reduce the need to return the patient to theatre for a change of expander to prosthesis. A period of relative overexpansion of the expander is recommended as it allows some postoperative shrinking to occur without deforming the outline of the new breast. Complications include haematoma, infection, pain and capsular contracture. The incidence of capsular contracture has decreased since textured (rough) prostheses have been introduced. Late rupture can occur as can damage if fine needle cytology is inappropriately performed. Silastic prostheses were thought to be associated with new cancers or autoimmune diseases but subsequent research has shown no increased incidence of either condition and they are now judged to be safe.[57,58] A newer fill material is soya oil and these prostheses are marketed as a safe option if capsular rupture occurs.

Tissue expansion and silastic implants can provide an adequate breast mound, but the degree of ptosis of the normal breast may be difficult to mimic. The procedure is, however, relatively quick and does not require a large investment of time or trouble for the patient. Tissue expansion is often difficult after radiotherapy and tissue transfer is then to be preferred.

Flap reconstruction provides natural skin, fat and muscle to recreate the breast mound. The commonest flaps include the latissimus dorsi muscle and the transverse rectus abdominis myocutaneous flap (TRAM). The former is based on the thoracodorsal vessels and provides skin and muscle but little fat. It is useful to cover chest wall defects but often requires a supplemental silastic prosthesis to provide a realistic breast. It can be used to fill small defects associated with lumpectomy and quadrantectomy.

The TRAM flap can be swung on a pedicle based on the superior epigastric vessels or transferred as a free flap with a microvascular anastomosis between inferior epigastric and intercostal or axillary vessels. The blood reaches the skin and fat by means of perforator vessels which have to be carefully preserved during the operation. Large amounts of subcutaneous tissue can be moved with a TRAM flap thereby mimicking a normal breast whereas a latissimus flap often needs supplementing with a silastic prosthesis.

Complications are commoner with free flaps and include loss of part (uncommonly all) of the flap. Blockage of venous drainage rather than problems with arterial inflow result in impaired circulation within the flap. Fat necrosis may occur leaving hard areas of tissue which can be confused with local tumour recurrence. The donor site may cause problems; an unsightly, stretched scar can occur after transfer of part of latissimus whereas herniation through the rectus sheath can occur after a TRAM flap. The large abdominoplasty that occurs in the creation of a TRAM flap is often appreciated by the patient.

A TRAM flap is the current 'gold-standard' reconstruction but is time consuming and requires much commitment from patient and surgeon. Results are less good in those with an impaired micro-vasculature such as smokers, the obese and diabetics who may be excluded in some centres.

Nipple reconstruction is possible but the number of alternative techniques is testament to none having an outstanding claim to success. An artificial nipple may be created by taking a plaster cast of the opposite nipple and constructing a colour-matched silastic prosthesis.

Whether reconstructive surgery is the domain of the plastic surgeon or the breast surgeon is debated. Providing appropriate training in the techniques involved has occurred then the surgery may be performed by a breast surgeon.

References

1. Ewert Z, Duffy S. Incidence of female breast cancer in relation to prevalence of risk factors in Denmark. Int J Cancer 1994; 56: 783–7.
2. Holford TR, Roush GC, McKay LA. Trends in female breast cancer in Connecticut and the United States. J Clin Epidemiol 1991; 44: 29.
3. Persson I, Bergstrom R, Sparen P, *et al.* Trends in breast cancer incidence in Sweden 1958–1988 by time period and birth cohort. Br J Cancer 1993; 68: 1247–53.
4. Coleman MP, Esteve J, Damiecki P, *et al.* Trends in cancer incidence and mortality. IARC Scientific Publications 1993; 121: 411–32.
5. Expert Advisory Group on Cancer to the Chief Medical Officers of England and Wales. A policy framework for commissioning cancer services: a consultative document, 1994.
6. Report of a working party of the British Breast Group. Provision of breast services in the UK: The advantages of specialist units, 1994.
7. The Breast Surgeons Group of the British association of Surgical Oncology. Guidelines for surgeons in the management of symptomatic breast disease in the United Kingdom. Eur J Surg Oncol 1995; 21 (suppl A): 1–13.
8. Gillis CR, Hole DJ. Survival outcome of care by specialist surgeons in breast cancer: a study of 3786 patients in the West of Scotland. Br Med J 1996; 312: 145–8.
9. Sainsbury JRC, Haward R, Rider L, *et al.* Influence of clinician workload and patterns of treatment on survival from breast cancer. Lancet 1995; 345: 1265–70.
10. Austoker J, Mansel R, Baum M, *et al.* Guidelines for referral of patients with breast problems. NHS Breast Screening Programme, 1995.
11. Williams J, Clifford C, Hopper J, Giles G. Socioeconomic status and cancer mortality and incidence in Melbourne. Eur J Cancer 1991; 27: 917–21.
12. Fleming NT, Armstrong BK, Steiner HJ. The comparative epidemiology of breast lumps and breast cancer. Int J Cancer 1982; 30: 147–52.
13. Newman B, Austin MA, Lee M, King MC. Inheritance of human breast cancer: evidence for autosomal dominant transmission in high risk families. Proc Natl Acad Sci USA 1988; 85: 3044–8.
14. Iselius L, Slack J, Little M, Morton ME. Genetic epidemiology of breast cancer in Britain. Ann Hum Genet 1991; 55: 151–9.
15. Bishop DT. BRCA1, BRCA2, BRCA3 . . . a myriad of breast cancer genes. Eur J Cancer 1994; 30A: 1738–9.
16. Seidman H, Stellman SD, Mushinski MH. A different perspective on breast cancer risk factors: some implications of non attributable risk. Ca; Clin J Cancer 1982; 32; 301–13.
17. Nystrom L, Rutqvist LE, Wall S, *et al.* Breast cancer screening with mammography: overview of Swedish randomised trials. Lancet 1993; 341: 973–6.
18. Powles TJ. The case for clinical trials of tamoxifen for prevention of breast cancer. Lancet 1992; 340: 1145.
19. Fisher B, Constantino JP, Redmond CK, *et al.* Endometrial cancer in tamoxifen treated breast cancer patients: findings from the National Surgical Adjuvant Breast and Bowel Project (NSABP) B14. J Natl Cancer Inst 1994; 88: 527–34.
20. Hursting SD, Thornqvist M, Henderson MM. Types of dietary fat and the incidence of cancer at five sites. Prev Med 1990; 19: 242–8.
21. Willett WC, Hunter DJ. Vitamin A and cancers of the breast, large bowel and prostate: epidemiologic evidence. Nutr Rev 1994; 52: S53.
22. Fallowfield LJ, Hall A, Maguire GP, Baum M. Psychosocial outcome of different treatment policies in women with early breast cancer outside a clinical trial. Br Med J 1990; 301: 575–80.
23. Ashley S, Royle GT, Corder A, *et al.* Clinical, radiological and cytological diagnosis of breast cancer in young women. Br J Surg 1989; 76: 835–7.
24. Davies GC, Millis RR, Hayward JL. Assessment of axillary node status. Ann Surg 1980; 192: 148–51.
25. Holland R, Hendriks JHCL, Verbeek ALM, *et al.* Extent, distribution and mammographic/histological correlations of breast ductal carcinoma in situ. Lancet 1990; 335: 519–22.
26. Hirst C. Sonographic appearances of breast cancers 10 mm or less in diameter. In: Madjar H. *et al.* (eds) Breast ultrasound update. Basel: Karger, 1994, pp. 127–39.

27. Furnival CM, Hocking MA, Hughes LE. Aspiration cytology in breast cancer: its relevance to diagnosis. Lancet 1975; ii: 446–9.

28. Sterrett G, Harvey J, Parsons RW, et al. Breast cancer in Western Australia in 1989: III. Accuracy of FNA cytology in diagnosis. Aust NZ J Surg 1994; 64: 745–9.

29. Parker SH, Lovin JD, Jobe WE, et al. Non-palpable breast lesions: stereotactic, automated large core biopsies. J Radiol 1991; 180: 403–7.

30. del Turco R, Palli D, Carridi A. et al. Intensive diagnostic follow-up after treatment for primary breast cancer: a randomised controlled trial. JAMA 1994; 271: 1593–7.

31. Ward BG, Joy GJ, Ramm LE, et al. Comparative study of mammography and mammary serum antigen estimation for breast cancer screening. Med J Aust 1992; 157: 161–4.

32. MacMillan RD, Purushotham AD, Mallon E, Ramsay G, George WD. Breast conserving surgery and tumour bed positivity in patients with breast cancer. Br J Surg 1994; 81: 56–8.

33. Haybittle JL, Blamey RW, Elston CW, et al. A prognostic index in primary breast cancer. Br J Cancer 1982; 45: 361–6.

34. Calais G, Berger C, Descamps P, et al. Conservative treatment feasibility with induction chemotherapy, surgery and radiotherapy for patients with breast carcinoma larger than 3 cm. Cancer 1994; 74: 1283–8.

35. Blichert-Toft M. A Danish randomised trial comparing breast conservation with mastectomy in mammary carcinoma. Br J Cancer 1990; 62(S12): 15.

36. Veronisi U, Banfi A, Slavadori B, et al. Breast conservation is the treatment of choice in small breast cancer: longer term results of a randomised trial. Eur J Cancer 1990; 26: 668–70.

37. Fisher B, Redmond C, Poisson R, et al. Eight-year results of a randomised clinical trial comparing total mastectomy with or without radiation in the treatment of breast cancer. N Engl J Med 1989; 320: 822–8.

38. Fisher B, Anderson S, Fisher ER. Significance of ipsilateral breast tumour recurrence after lumpectomy. Lancet 1991; 338: 327–31.

39. Fisher B, Redmond C, Fisher ER. 10-year results of a randomised clinical trial comparing radical mastectomy and total mastectomy with or without irradiation. N Engl J Med 1985; 312: 674–81.

40. Collins J. The role of the surgeon. Cancer Forum 1994; 18: 92–5.

41. Fallowfield LJ, Baum M, Maguire GP. Effects of breast conservation on psychological morbidity associated with diagnosis and treatment of early breast cancer. Br Med J 1986; 293: 1331–4.

42. Kissin MW, Thompson EM, Price AB, et al. The inadequacy of axillary sampling in breast cancer. Lancet 1982; i: 1210–11.

43. Bundred NJ, Morgan DAL, Dixon JM. Management of regional nodes in breast cancer. Br Med J 1994; 309: 1222–5.

44. Gelber RD, Goldhirsch A. Radiotherapy to the conserved breast: is it avoidable if the cancer is small? J Natl Cancer Inst 1994; 8: 652–4.

45. Stewart HJ. Controlled trials in the treatment of 'early' breast cancer: a review of published results. World J Surg 1977; 1: 309–13.

46. Cuzick J, Stewart HJ, Peto R, et al. Overview of randomised trials of postoperative adjuvant radiotherapy in breast cancer. Recent Results Cancer Res 1988; 111: 108–29.

47. Pierquin B, Mazeron JJ, Glaubiger D. Conservative treatment of breast cancer in Europe: report of the Groupe Europeen de Curie-therapie. Radiother Oncol 1986; 6: 187–98.

48. Early Breast Cancer Trialists' Collaborative Group. Systemic treatment of early breast cancer by hormonal, cytotoxic or immune therapy. 133 randomised trials involving 31 000 recurrences and 24 000 deaths among 75 000 women. Lancet 1992; 339: 1–15, 71–85.

49. Early Breast Cancer Trialists' Collaborative Group. Ovarian ablation in early breast cancer: overview of the randomised trials. Lancet 1996; 348: 1189–96.

50. Fisher ER, Leeming R, Anderson S, et al. Conservative management of intraductal carcinoma (DCIS) of the breast. J Surg Oncol 1991; 47: 139–47.

51. Wood WC, Budman DR, Korzun AH, et al. Dose and dose intensity of adjuvant chemotherapy for stage II, node-positive breast cancer. N Engl J Med 1994; 330: 1253–9.

52. Bonadonna G, Valagussa P. Dose–response effect of adjuvant chemotherapy in breast cancer. N Engl J Med 1981; 304: 10–15.

53. Peters WP, Ross M, Vredenburgh JJ, et al. High-dose chemotherapy and autologous

bone marrow support as consolidation after standard-dose adjuvant therapy for high-risk primary breast cancer. J Clin Oncol 1993; 11: 1132–43.

54. Coates AS, Abraham S, Kaye SB, *et al*. On the receiving end – patient perception of the side effects of cancer chemotherapy. Eur J Cancer Clin Oncol 1983; 19: 203–8.

55. Fisher B, Constantino J, Redmond C, *et al*. A randomized clinical trial evaluating tamoxifen in the treatment of patients with node-negative breast cancer who have estrogen receptor-positive tumors. N Engl J Med 1989; 310: 479–84.

56. Dean C, Chetty U, Forrest APM. Effect of immediate breast reconstruction on psychosocial morbidity after mastectomy. Lancet 1983; i: 459–61.

57. Brooks PM. Silicone breast implantation: doubts about the fears. Med J Aust 1995; 162: 432–4.

58. Fisher J. The silicone controversy: when will science prevail? N Engl J Med 1992; 326: 1696.

10 Treatment of advanced breast cancer

Richard Sainsbury

Patients with breast cancer may present with advanced disease or may acquire this as part of the natural history of disease progression. A working definition of advanced stage breast cancer is 'that which is no longer curable by local treatments'. As such, this stage requires systemic therapy although surgery may still have an important role.

The standardised mortality rate for breast cancer remains approximately 50% with a median survival of 8 years. Most patients go through one or more recurrences before death and these episodes may span many months – as such the management of this phase is important. Even after dissemination the median survival is 14–20 months.[1] Breast cancer can recur at the site of previous surgery (local recurrence), in the area of the chest wall and lymph nodes (locoregional recurrence), or as disseminated disease. Each of these types of recurrence may present in isolation or combination.

It is common to stage or restage a patient when they present with recurrent disease as this may provide information which will affect management. Staging at the time of initial treatment has been shown to be unhelpful and costly, at least for T_1 and T_2 tumours.[2] Normally a chest radiograph, bone scan, liver function tests and a full blood count will suffice although tests specific to any local complaint may also be necessary such as a liver scan or radiographs of a painful bony area.[3] The role of tumour markers to assess disease recurrence is still unclear although they may be useful in monitoring progression or response to therapy.[4]

The diagnosis of recurrent disease may cause the patient more distress than that experienced at the time of the original diagnosis due to the realisation that the disease has not been cured and is likely to prove terminal. Appropriate support to the patient and her family is vital as patients frequently express a view that whereas the initial diagnosis and management was good the delivery of the news of recurrence and its subsequent management was less so. Although multidisciplinary working is increasingly seen it is still common for the onset of recurrence to mark a change in the personnel caring for the patient as the surgeon hands over to clinical or medical oncologist. This can be a difficult time for physician and patient. The diagnosis of recurrence may be difficult. It is more common for the patient to re-present with new symptoms than for those signs to be detected at routine follow-up. The role of large follow-up clinics run by junior staff is increasingly questioned.

Presentation with advanced stage breast cancer

There is a group of patients who present with large, locally inoperable cancers in whom radical local surgery (Halstead radical mastectomy) or chest wall resection would once have been the only option. Long-term survivors from such treatments confirm the non-metastatic nature of this form of disease in some patients. The majority, however, quickly suffered from extensive local recurrence.

Some of these patients have harboured tumours for a long time and have concealed them. In these, estimation of oestrogen receptor status (ER) by fine needle or core biopsy and treatment with tamoxifen may well be worthwhile. If ER positive greater than 60% response rates can be expected.

Younger patients, those with ER-negative tumours and those in whom the disease is progressing rapidly are now treated with neo-adjuvant (up front or primary) chemotherapy. After diagnosis and staging induction chemotherapy (usually four cycles of cyclophosphamide, adriamycin and 5-fluorouracil) is given. Response is then assessed and patients who fail to respond have radiotherapy and second-line chemotherapy.[5] The outlook for this group is generally poorer. Those who respond either go on to mastectomy, then radiotherapy and further chemotherapy or radiation therapy and chemotherapy alone. Although clinical response rates are high there may be viable tumour cells in the mastectomy specimen and many feel it prudent to include excision of the original tumour site in the treatment package.

Inflammatory cancers are a special subgroup of the above and present as an indurated, reddened breast with peau d'orange from lymphatic blockage. Once universally fatal within a short time they are now treated with chemotherapy and radiotherapy with surgery being used to resect any residual disease. Response rates over 70% are now seen with 5-year survival rates of 10–55% reported.[6] Further increases in response rates may be expected with the use of high-dose chemotherapy and stem cell transplantation although it is not yet clear if this translates into long-term survival.

Aims of treatment

Advanced stage breast cancer is, by definition, incurable but worthwhile symptom control and extension of survival are achievable. Such concepts should be discussed with the patient and her family especially if toxic treatments are being proposed. If cure is no longer possible quality of life becomes of paramount importance and should be formally assessed both before and during treatment. There are validated formal measures of quality of life but one simple method is to ask patients if they felt better at the end of treatment, if they thought the treatment was worthwhile and whether they would undergo it again.

Local recurrence

After conservation therapy

The ideal management of local recurrence after conservation treatment is prevention! This means selection of patients for whom this treatment is appropriate and the use of radiotherapy as part of the treatment. The choice of conservation treatment does not, by itself, influence survival. It is important to recognise that some patients are unsuitable for conservation treatment and should be advised to have a mastectomy. This applies to both invasive and non-invasive cancers as there is now recognition of subtypes of duct carcinoma in situ (DCIS) with a higher predilection of local relapse. Although this is reduced by radiotherapy there is still a high enough incidence to warrant primary treatment by mastectomy (with the addition of immediate reconstruction should the patient wish). Resection margins must be clear of disease (by 1 cm) and the axilla should be surgically treated to provide staging information and to prevent the need for radiotherapy to the axilla. High grade, node-positive tumours with extensive lymphovascular invasion are likely to be associated with recurrence. Appropriate chemotherapy is also necessary although it is not clear to what extent this affects local recurrence rates.

Radiotherapy is indicated as part of conservation treatment for invasive cancers and reduced local recurrence. The evidence whether it influences long-term survival is less strong. A recent randomised trial found no beneficial effect[7] whereas others report an improved long-term survival for those treated with radiotherapy especially in the node-positive subgroup.[8]

Whether radiotherapy is needed for all types of cancers is debated. The BASO II (British Association of Surgical Oncology) trial is examining this. Patients with small, well-differentiated node-negative tumours are randomised to radiotherapy or none and/or tamoxifen or none. This is an important area as the number of patients with such lesions has increased greatly as the NHS Breast Screening Programme has been introduced.

Detection of recurrence in the conserved breast is not always easy. Mammography has a lower sensitivity and specificity, cytology may produce abnormal looking cells and clinical examination may be difficult if the postradiotherapy changes have led to fibrosis. Magnetic resonance imaging (MRI) appears to be useful but needs a special breast coil and is not readily available.[9] Newer techniques using gadolinium contrast and short acquisition times appear to give improved results. The current recommendation for post-conservation treatment monitoring is for mammography every 18–24 months.

If an isolated local recurrence is detected the options may include further local excision or completion mastectomy. If radiotherapy has already been given it is not repeated and chemotherapy or a change in hormone therapy is not usually indicated. As some recurrence at the original tumour site may be due to inappropriate or inadequate initial therapy it would seem better to correct these measures than to have to salvage the situation later.

After mastectomy

Large aggressive tumours predispose to local recurrence which is more often of the locoregional type. It is, unfortunately, still possible to see a true local recurrence after mastectomy if the operation has left large amounts of breast tissue behind. A mastectomy may not be an easy operation in a woman with a large breast especially if unequal skin flaps are needed. Attention to detail over axillary surgery and radiotherapy to the flaps, when recurrence is likely, are important.

A spot recurrence in the flaps in the absence of disseminated disease is best treated by a local resection. Although further skin nodules are to be expected there is a group of (often elderly) women who can be dealt with by repeated local excisions. A change in hormone therapy is often tried and may slow down the appearance of more nodules. Multiple spot recurrences can be dealt with by a wide excision and either primary closure under tension or by means of a skin graft or rotation flap.

Radiotherapy to the area should be employed if it has not already been used. Occasionally a second treatment may be used if the original adjuvant radiotherapy occurred some time previously using a different technique such as electrons. Skin changes such as telangiectasia are then to be expected. Newer treatments include photodynamic therapy in which laser light is used to destroy cancer cells which have been sensitised with the oral administration of certain compounds. This technique appears to be successful for small isolated recurrences.[10]

The role of systemic chemotherapy in the management of local recurrence is not clearly defined. In the absence of proven systemic spread many would reserve it for later use and try a change of hormone treatment initially. The range of hormonal manipulations has increased lately and the use of the new generation of oral aromatase inhibitors has allowed extra options.

Chemotherapeutic agents have been tried topically but do not seem particularly active although this is an area that may well change in the near future. Regional chemotherapy with infusion of agents into the feeding vessels to the chest wall has been used with some success. It requires cannulation of the internal mammary and lateral thoracic arteries or infusion into the subclavian artery depending on the extent of the infusion required.[11] This was initially performed as an open operation but is now carried out via the femoral route by interventional radiologists.

High doses of drug are delivered locally and good responses are seen if the vascular supply is intact. Unfortunately, however, the blood supply has all too often been compromised by previous surgery and radiotherapy and so little drug reaches the affected area. In addition previous adjuvant chemotherapy may have bred out a clone of resistant cells. If untreated, such patients can go on to develop cancer-en-cuirasse – a particularly distressing form of the disease. The cancer creeps round in the subcutaneous plane and often does not metastasise elsewhere. The benefits of regional chemotherapy are best when previously untreated disease is being treated in which case clinical response rates of 80% are common.

Continual infusion of 5-fluorouracil via a Hickman or peripherally inserted central catheter line appears to be effective in local recurrence. This can be given alone[12] or in combination with boluses of cisplatin and an anthracycline as in the ECF regimen.

Locoregional recurrence

Disease recurring in the ipsilateral axillary nodes can be treated by axillary clearance if this has not previously been performed although the risks of lymphoedema are high. If the nodal disease is fixed or growth has occurred into the surrounding fat then local radiotherapy or chemotherapy may be more appropriate.

Supraclavicular fossa nodal recurrence represents systemic spread as does recurrence in the jugular chain. Occasionally a node may need to be biopsied to confirm the nature of the recurrence but radiotherapy and not surgery is the main therapeutic manoeuvre. Patients whose primary tumours were heavily node positive often receive a supraclavicular field as part of the primary radiotherapy to try and prevent recurrence here.

Systemic recurrence – dissemination

This marks the onset of disease which is incurable but still very treatable. There are distinct types of recurrence with different outcomes. Recurrence in bone and soft tissue is associated with a longer survival and is more responsive to treatment than disease in liver, lung or brain. The length of time to dissemination after original presentation is important as patients who have a longer disease-free interval tend to respond better to subsequent therapy.

Restaging with bone and liver scan, chest radiograph, full blood count, liver function tests, bone biochemistry as well as tumour markers in addition to investigation of any specific patient signs is indicated.[3] A treatment plan needs to be agreed between the patient and treating doctors with involvement of relevant specialists as part of the multidisciplinary team. Support from breast nurse specialists/counsellors is essential.

Various treatment strategies can be used depending on site and speed of relapse. An isolated painful bony metastasis can, for instance, be treated by a single fraction of radiotherapy with or without a change in endocrine therapy whereas rapidly progressive disease in the liver requires chemotherapy.

An indication of how patients may respond to treatment can be obtained from the disease free interval – those who relapse quickly after primary treatment are less likely to respond to hormone therapy and should probably start on chemotherapy.

Endocrine treatment

Oophorectomy was the first hormonal manipulation attempted and was performed in 1896 by Beatson whose first two (of six) patients with advanced disease responded to this treatment.[13] This response rate of 30% is typical of endocrine treatments in unselected patients. Surgical oophorectomy is still used if histology is needed or if scanning has shown any evidence of ovarian abnormality, otherwise a radiation menopause using three fractions of radiotherapy can be performed. The other surgical operations for advanced disease, adrenalectomy and hypophysectomy, are no longer performed as endocrine manipulations have advanced. The endocrine agents currently available are shown in Table 10.1. Tamoxifen remains the mainstay of treatment for adjuvant treatment but is being used less for advanced disease as patients have already been exposed to it. Rechallenge with tamoxifen is possible after time off treatment. The majority of oestrogens in the postmenopausal women are made in peripheral fat and muscle by aromatisation of steroid precursors.

Table 10.1 *Current endocrine therapies*

Specific oestrogen receptor modulators (SERMS)	Tamoxifen
	Raloxifene
	Toremifine
	ICI 181 117 (a pure antioestrogen undergoing trials)
Aromatase inhibitors	
Injectable	4-Hydroxyandrostenedione
Oral	Anastrozole
	Vorozole
	Letrazole
LHRH agonists	Leuprorelin
	Goserelin
Others	Medroxyprogresterone acetate (MPA)
	Megestrol

Table 10.2 *Endocrine options for patients with advanced breast cancer*

Premenopausal	Oophorectomy
	  Surgical
	  Radiotherapy
	LH RH antagonist

Postmenopausal	Tamoxifen unless previously received otherwise Oral aromatase inhibitor MPA Megestrol

A similar effect also occurs in the tumour itself. Aminoglutethimide was the first aromatase inhibitor but had the side effect of adrenal suppression requiring patients to take supplemental hydrocortisone. It also caused a rash, nausea and depression and is now no longer used. The second generation aromatase inhibitors required injections but the third generation compounds such as vorozole, letrazole and anastrozole are orally available and their use is increasing and is likely to displace megaprogesterone acetate and megestrol. There are recent reports that there may be a survival advantage for patients taking aromatase inhibitors compared to other second line agents.

Endocrine treatments are more likely to be effective in patients whose tumours were ER positive (approximately 60%) although there is a 5–15% response rate in those with ER negative tumours. If response to one endocrine agent is seen then a second agent should be tried as long as the disease is not progressing rapidly since a second endocrine response is likely. Table 10.2 shows the options for the various endocrine treatments.

Chemotherapy

Combination chemotherapy is given in a similar manner to adjuvant therapy though different regimes may be used. There is no evidence that treating patients with asymptomatic metastases improves overall survival and chemotherapy should be reserved for those patients with symptoms which can not be controlled by other means.

Aggressive disease or recurrence in sites likely to progress (liver and lung) is treated aggressively with anthracycline-based drugs. Patients who have relapsed on or after such drugs may be treated with the taxoids.[14] These newer agents work by inhibiting formation of the tubules needed for cell division and were originally derived from the Pacific Yew tree needles. They have different side effects but seem effective in anthracycline-resistant disease. High-dose chemotherapy with bone marrow rescue or support has attracted much

Table 10.3 *Current chemotherapy regimens*

Single agent	Mitoxantrone
	Epirubicin
	Adriamycin
	Taxoids (Taxotere and Taxatol)
Combination regimens	CMF – cyclophosphamide, methotrexate, 5FU
	MMM – mitoxantrone, methotrexate and mitomycin-C
	FEC – 5FU, epirubicin, cyclophosphamide
	ECF – epirubicin, cisplatin and infusional 5FU

attention. Bone marrow can be harvested prior to a dose of chemotherapy, which would otherwise kill the patient, and it can be reinfused for rescue. A more modern alternative is to mobilise the marrow stem cells into the peripheral circulation where they can be extracted and reinfuse them after treatment. The early mortality (circa 10%) has dropped and this technique gives higher response rates. Whether this translates into long-term survival is unclear and trials are under way to determine this.[15]

A summary of chemotherapy regimens is given in Table 10.3. Given that these drugs are being given for palliation it is important that side effects are minimised and full use of supportive measures to reduce nausea and vomiting is essential. Quality of life must be assessed. Response rates to chemotherapy for patients with advanced disease is of the order of 40–60% with a median time to relapse of 8–14 months. Further courses achieve lower response rates (around 25%) and third courses lower still. Trials of palliative chemotherapy against best supportive care are under way to see which provides better quality of life.

Specific sites of metastatic disease

Brain

Between 15 and 25% of patients with breast cancer develop nervous system metastases as detected at postmortem. They are commoner in young women with ER-negative tumours. Headache occurs in half the patients, with focal weakness and fits occurring in another 20%. MRI is the diagnostic test of choice although computed tomographic (CT) scanning is more commonly employed in the UK. About 50% of brain metastases are single and some, very selected, patients may be helped by metastasectomy.[16] Radiation is the treatment used most often although 20% of patients fail to complete the course and less than 10% are alive 1 year after completion of treatment. Radiosurgery with stereotactically delivered high dose focused radiotherapy may be useful for isolated metastases.

Steroids are used to control the symptoms and neurological signs but their use is short-lived and their side effects are high. Anticonvulsants should also be used if the patient has had a fit.[17]

Cord compression

This is caused by metastasis to the epidural space. Their recognition and early treatment are essential to avoid the complication of paraplegia. Over 90% of patients have symptoms for over a week before diagnosis and most have concurrent bony metastases elsewhere. Pain is the commonest first symptom but by diagnosis weakness, autonomic dysfunction and sensory loss all occur. Plain radiograph, bone scanning, CT and MRI are all used in diagnosis. Corticosteroids are used to reduce oedema. Laminectomy with or without radiotherapy should be used early although there is debate as to which order these should be performed.[18] This condition is a true emergency and patients with breast cancer who complain of back pain must be investigated appropriately.

Bone metastases

About 80% of patients with secondary breast cancer develop bony metastases which are most prevalent in the marrow rich skeleton, i.e. the long bones, pelvis and axial vertebral skeleton. Bony secondaries lead to pain, fractures and hypercalcaemia each of which may need treatment.[19] Investigation is by bone scan, plain radiograph and, occasionally, MRI. Localised bony metastases may be dealt with by a single fraction of radiotherapy. Specific sites may require orthopaedic surgery to prevent (or treat) fractures. Specific therapies directed against the skeleton include strontium-89 which is effective in 90% of patients with generalised bone pain.[20] Unfortunately its expense prevents wiser use in the UK. The bisphosphonates stabilise bone mineral and are effective treatments for malignant hypercalcaemia and allow healing of some lytic metastases.[21] They are poorly absorbed orally and are given as i.v. infusions. The patient with hypercalcaemia is often dehydrated and rehydration remains an important part of treatment.

Bone pain can be distressing and effective treatment with nonsteroidal anti-inflammatory agents with or without opioids should be used. Care should be taken over side effects such as constipation.

Pleural effusions

Up to 50% of patients will develop a pleural effusion, the majority of which need no treatment. After a small sample has been removed to confirm the diagnosis symptomatic tube drainage rather than simple aspiration is indicated as the latter leads to rapid reaccumulation. Pleurodesis with talc, tetracycline or bleomycin after drainage reduces reaccumulation.[22] Better still is formal drainage by thoracoscopy and instillation of a talc–mitoxantrone mixture under direct vision.

Bone marrow metastases

Marrow involvement leads to a leuko-erythroblastic picture with anaemia being common.[23] Chemotherapy and/or endocrine therapy are necessary although the dose of chemotherapy may need to be reduced.

Isolated liver and thoracic nodules

Metastasectomy may be indicated for true solitary isolated metastases. Unfortunately, on investigation most patients have multiple sites of disease and surgery is not possible. Liver metastases from breast cancer respond better to hepatic artery chemotherapy than colorectal metastases as they have a better blood supply allowing drug to reach the tumour deposits.

Pain and symptom control

The help of a pain control or palliative specialist is an important contribution to the team. Many patients have pain as part of their illness.[24] This pain may occur in more than one site and may be caused by different mechanisms. The patient's perception of the pain will depend on their emotional state and a thorough assessment is necessary. The concept of a ladder of pain control is a good one and patients can move up and down this ladder as the disease progresses or is treated. Simple measures such as paracetamol may suffice but opioids should not be withheld if needed. Concomitant administration of drugs with no analgesic component may help – antidepressants and anxiolytics used judiciously may allow reduction in the need for analgesics. Attention to fluid intake and the avoidance of known side effects is also important.

Other symptoms such as nausea, anorexia, headache, breathlessness and constipation all need addressing. The help of specialist teams such as Macmillan and Marie Curie nurses and the hospice movement can make the difference between a death with dignity and a painful, peaceless end.

The future

Newer cytotoxic drugs are being introduced but their impact is likely to be small. More exciting are some of the biological agents such as inhibitors of angiogenesis and metastatic-related proteins. The monoclonal antibodies against cellular epitopes have, so far, proved disappointing although they may yet be combined with labels to allow detection of metastatic foci. Newer concepts to be explored include that of tumour-stasis rather than further development of drugs aimed at cell killing. Trials of therapies continue to be required which need patient involvement.

References

1. Leonard RCF. Oncology in practice. Palliative chemotherapy for advanced breast cancer. J Cancer Care 1995; 4: 127–30.
2. del Turco, R, Palli D, Carridi A, *et al.* Intensive diagnostic follow-up after treatment for primary breast cancer: a randomised controlled trial. JAMA 1994; 271: 1593–7.
3. Glynne-Jones R, Young T, Ahmed A, *et al.* How far investigations for occult metastases in breast cancer aid the clinician. Clin Oncol 1991; 3: 65–72.
4. Hayes DF, Kaplan W. Evaluation of patients after primary therapy. In: Harris JR *et al.* (eds) Diseases of the breast. Philadelphia: Lippincott–Raven, 1996, pp. 630–42.
5. Scholl SM, Fourquet A, Asselain B. *et al.* Neoadjuvant versus adjuvant chemotherapy in premenopausal patients with tumours considered too large for breast conserving surgery: preliminary results of a randomized trial. Ann Oncol 1991; 30A: 645.
6. Hortobagyi GN, Buzdar AU. Locally advanced breast cancer: a review including the MD Anderson experience. In: Ragaz J, Ariel IM (eds). High risk breast cancer. Berlin: Springer-Verlag, 1991, pp. 382–403.
7. Forrest AP, Stewart HJ, Everington D, *et al.* Randomised controlled trial of conservation therapy for breast cancer: 6-year analysis of the Scottish trial. Lancet 1996; 348: 708–13.
8. Arriagada R, Rutqvist LE, Mattsson A, *et al.* Adequate locoregional treatment for early breast cancer may prevent secondary dissemination. J Clin Oncol 1995; 13: 2869–78.
9. Dao Th, Rahmouni A, Campana F, *et al.* Tumor recurrence versus fibrosis in the irradiated breast: differentiation with dynamic gadolinium-enhanced MR imaging. Radiology 1993; 187: 751–9.
10. Khan SA, Dougherty TJ, Mang TS. An evaluation of photodynamic therapy in the management of cutaneous metastases of breast cancer. Eur J Cancer 1993; 29A: 1686–91.
11. Lewis W, Walker V, Ali HH, Sainsbury JRC. Intraarterial chemotherapy for patients with breast cancer – a feasibility study. Br J Cancer 1995; 71: 605–9.
12. Ng JSY, Cameron DA, Lee L, *et al.* Infusional 5-fluorouracil given as a single agent in relapsed breast cancer: its activity and toxicity.

The Breast 1994; 2: 87–90.
13. Beatson GT. On the treatment of inoperable cases of carcinoma of the mamma: suggestions for a new method of treatment, with illustrative cases. Lancet 1896; ii: 104–7.
14. Gollins SW, Barrett-Lee PJ. Response and side effects of Taxotere in advanced breast cancer. Breast cancer treatment today – focus on Taxotere (docetaxel), Meeting at the Royal College of Physicians, London, 1996, p. 12.
15. Myers SE, Williams SF. Role of high-dose chemotherapy and autologous stem cell support in the treatment of breast cancer. Hematol Oncol Clin North Am 1993; 7: 631–56.
16. Hendrickson FR. The optimum schedule for palliative radiotherapy for metastatic brain cancer. Int J Radiat Oncol Biol Phys 1977; 2: 165–8.
17. Galicich JH, French LA, Melby J. Use of dexamethasone in treatment of cerebral oedema associated with brain tumours. Lancet 1961; i: 46–8.
18. Gorter K. Results of laminectomy in spinal cord compression due to tumours. Acta Neurochir 1978; 42: 177–95.
19. Hortobagyi GN, Libshitz HI, Seabold JE. Osseous metastases of breast cancer: clinical, biochemical, radiographic and scintigraphic evaluation of response to therapy. Cancer 1987; 53: 577–82.
20. Robinson RG, Blake GM, Preston DF, *et al.* Strontium-89: treatment results and kinetics in patients with painful metastatic prostate and breast cancer in bone. Radiographics 1989; 9: 271–8.
21. Theriault RL. Hypercalcaemia of malignancy: pathophysiology and implications for treatment. Oncology 1993; 7: 47–51.
22. Fentiman IS, Rubens RD, Hayward JL. Control of pleural effusions in patients with breast cancer: a randomized trial. Cancer 1983; 52: 737–82.
23. Webster DJT, Preece PR, Bolton PM *et al.* Leukoerythroblastosis in breast cancer. Clin Oncol 1975; 1: 315–17.
24. Portenoy RK, Foley KM. Management of cancer pain. In: Holland JC, Rowland JH (eds). Handbook of psychooncology: psychological care of the patient with cancer. New York: Oxford University, 1989, pp. 369–83.

11 Hormones and chemotherapy

J. Michael Dixon
Robert C. F. Leonard

Introduction

Patients who present with breast cancer can be classified into three groups, those with:

1. operable breast cancer (T_{0-3}, N_{0-1}, M_0);
2. locally advanced breast cancer (T_4, N_{0-2}, M_0); or
3. metastatic disease (M_1).

Up to 50% of patients with operable breast cancer and over 80% of those with locally advanced disease will ultimately die of metastatic disease even though many of these patients never develop local recurrence. These observations indicate that even in those patients with apparently localised disease, the majority have systemic metastases present at the time of diagnosis. A possible way of improving the survival of these patients and those with overt metastatic disease is to give some form of systemic therapy to eradicate or slow down the growth of these metastases. There are two major forms of systemic therapy in common usage, hormonal therapy and chemotherapy.

Hormonal therapy

Introduction

Oestrogen and progesterone regulate the growth and differentiation of normal breast tissue. Evidence for this includes a reduced breast cancer risk in women who have an early menopause[1] and an increased risk of breast cancer in women treated with oestrogen replacement therapy.[2] Oestrogens probably play an important role in the progression of breast cancer which, like progestogens, exert their effects on cells through binding to specific nuclear receptors.[3] Oestrogen receptors (ER) and to a lesser extent, progesterone receptors, determine the responsiveness to endocrine therapy, given either as treatment for locally advanced or metastatic breast cancer or given as an adjuvant after locoregional therapy.[4,5] Patients with oestrogen receptor positive tumours have a 50–70% chance of responding to hormonal therapy and this increases to over 70% in patients whose tumours have both

Figure 11.1
Enzymes involved in oestrogen biosynthesis. (17ß-HSD, 17ß hydroxysteroid dehydrogenase)

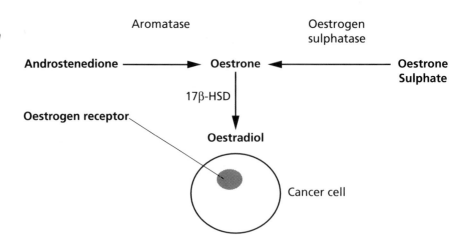

oestrogen and progesterone receptors.[5] There appears to be a direct correlation between the quantity of oestrogen receptors and the probability and extent of response, at least for the biochemical assay for oestrogen receptors.[6] Tumours with high ER levels are more likely to respond and have a greater quantitative response than tumours with lower ER levels.[6] Absence of ER predicts for early recurrence and poor short-term survival of patients with breast cancer.[7] Oestrogen and progesterone receptor-positive tumours are also more likely to be well differentiated, to be diploid and to have a lower cellular proliferation rate than hormone receptor negative tumours.[8]

Sources of oestrogens

The major source of oestrogens in premenopausal women is the ovary. Levels of oestrogen in postmenopausal women are much lower and oestrogens are synthesised peripherally, principally in fat (including breast fat), skin, muscle and liver from androstenedione which is produced in the adrenal gland. The production of oestrogens requires the presence of the hormone aromatase (Fig. 11.1).

Historical background

Hormonal therapy or perhaps more correctly anti-hormonal therapy for breast cancer dates back to 1896 when Beatson treated premenopausal women with metastatic breast cancer by oophorectomy and documented regression of skin nodules.[9] Subsequently, DeCourmelles used ovarian irradiation in patients with breast cancer in 1905.[10] More recent studies have confirmed the benefit of oophorectomy as a treatment for metastatic breast cancer[11,12] or as adjuvant therapy following surgery and/or radiotherapy.[13]

Oophorectomy is not effective in postmenopausal women[10] and adrenalectomy was formerly used in these patients as a means of interrupting hormone synthesis.[14] Hypophysectomy has also been used to produce total endocrine blockade.[15] Of the surgical methods only oophorectomy continues to be used currently, although with the introduction of luteinising hormone-releasing hormone agonists (LHRH) there is a decreasing need for surgical oophorectomy.[14]

A number of other hormonal agents have been used over the years. These include oestrogen preparations such as diethylstilboestrol, ethinyloestradiol and conjugated oestrogen.[11] Exactly how they work is unclear but they produced a 20–40% response rate. Toxicity with high-dose oestrogens was a problem and for this reason they are no longer used. Progestogens have been and continue to be used, although their mechanism of action is unknown.[11,14] Androgens were formerly used in premenopausal women with advanced breast cancer with an average reported response rate of about 20%.[11]

Current hormonal therapies and agents

Oophorectomy

This procedure can now be performed laparoscopically. It increases survival from breast cancer in the adjuvant setting but is now rarely used in advanced disease where it has been superceded by LHRH agonists.[13,14]

Luteinising hormone releasing hormone (LHRH) agonists

LHRH agonists suppress ovarian production by de-sensitising pituitary LHRH receptors.[14] Administration of these agents stimulates gonadotrophin production initially but thereafter blocks release of FSH and LH with a net decrease in production of both oestrogen and progesterone from the ovary, resulting in endocrine blockade with cessation of menstruation. These drugs only have activity in premenopausal women.[16] LHRH receptors have been demonstrated on the surface of human breast cancer cell lines and in human breast tumours suggesting that this drug may also have a direct action on breast cancer cells.[17] This does not translate into a benefit for postmenopausal women.

Goserelin is the best known LHRH agonist. It is given as a monthly depot injection subcutaneously in a dose of 3.6 mg. Efforts are underway to produce a three-monthly depot injection. Response rates with LHRH are identical to those of oophorectomy.[18]

Tamoxifen

Tamoxifen is a synthetic partial oestrogen agonist which acts primarily by binding to the oestrogen receptor. It is the most widely used hormonal treatment for breast cancer. It has a half-life of seven days and it takes approximately four weeks for the drug to reach a steady state in the plasma.[19] The standard dose is 20 mg once a day, although at this dose there are wide variations in plasma concentrations of the drug between individual patients; there does not appear to be a direct correlation between the level of the drug in plasma and response.[20]

Between 0 and 10% of patients with oestrogen receptor-negative tumours apparently have a response to this drug.[21] Technical problems associated with ER assays and lack of quality control may account for some of the variations in reported response rates. Other non-receptor mechanisms of action for tamoxifen have been proposed to explain the claimed occasional effectiveness of tamoxifen in oestrogen-negative tumours.[10]

Response rates to tamoxifen are similar to those of other endocrine agents, but some tumours develop resistance to tamoxifen. Tumours which have become resistant to tamoxifen do not appear to lose oestrogen receptor and overgrowth of oestrogen receptor negative clones cannot explain the development of tamoxifen resistance.[22]

Although tamoxifen appears to be antagonistic in its action on breast cancer cells, it has oestrogen agonist activity at other sites which account for both the benefits and side effects of the treatment. Benefits include preservation of bone density,[23,24] decrease in plasma cholesterol levels[25] with an associated reduction in cardiovascular morbidity[26] (both agonist effects) and a 35–40% decrease in second primary breast cancers (antagonistic effect).[13] Only 3% of patients given tamoxifen stop taking the drug because of side effects. Hot flushes are among the most common complaints of treatment.[27] Clonidine is occasionally effective in reducing flushing. Evening primrose oil has not been shown to be of any benefit, but megestrol acetate (20 mg twice a day) appears to be effective at reducing this troublesome symptom.[28,29] In premenopausal women, tamoxifen can decrease vaginal secretions and produce atrophy and vaginal dryness. This should be treated initially with a non-hormonal cream (such as Replens®) but if this is not effective and symptoms are severe, pessaries containing oestrogen should be prescribed.[29] Systemic absorption of oestrogen is a potential concern but appears minimal with Vagifem®. Tamoxifen has oestrogenic effects on the uterus which accounts for the approximately fourfold increase in the risk of uterine cancer in women on this drug.[30] The number of endometrial cancers developing on tamoxifen is less than the number of contralateral breast cancers that tamoxifen prevents. In the United States, women have endometrial screening prior to starting tamoxifen but this is not common practice in the United Kingdom and Europe. Whether patients on tamoxifen should have periodic endometrial screening is not clear. Retinal problems have occasionally been reported but are rare.[30] Although placebo-controlled trials have not shown an excessive weight gain in women on tamoxifen, this is the most common complaint of women on long-term treatment.[30]

Dose
The recommended dose of tamoxifen is 20 mg a day and there is no indication for giving tamoxifen at a greater dose.[10] The optimal dura-

tion of treatment is being addressed by current trials; available data suggest the optimal duration is 5 years.[13]

Role in premenopausal women

Tamoxifen has been used both as an adjuvant and as therapy for metastatic breast cancer in premenopausal women.[30] Tamoxifen does not appear to have a major effect on follicle stimulating hormone activity and luteinising hormone levels but oestradiol and oestrone levels are increased.[31] Many premenopausal women taking tamoxifen still have regular menses and it is important to advise that pregnancy can occur.

In the treatment of metastatic disease tamoxifen produces equivalent rates of response to oophorectomy[32,33] and in the adjuvant setting it improves survival of premenopausal women who have hormone receptor-positive tumours with little or no apparent benefit in oestrogen receptor-negative tumours.[13]

Other anti-oestrogens

Other synthetic antioestrogens have been developed and some such as toremifene are in clinical use and others are in clinical trials.[10,34] Toremifene has little effect on the uterus but has similar efficacy to tamoxifen on breast cancers. Other non-steroidal antioestrogens include draloxifene, raloxifene and idoxifene. Some of the newer agents retain agonist effects on bone but have little effect on the uterus. Pure antioestrogens have been developed such as ICI 182 70 but problems with formulation of this compound remain, although in clinical trials it appears to be very effective.[34]

Aromatase inhibitors

The production of oestrogen requires the presence and activity of the aromatase enzyme (Fig. 11.1). Oestrogen production in postmenopausal women is by peripheral aromatisation of androgens produced from the adrenal.[35] A number of aromatase inhibitors have been used in the treatment of breast cancer and a number are under development.[36,37]

Aminoglutethimide

Aminoglutethimide is not a pure aromatase inhibitor as it also blocks production of cortisol.[14] This drug was developed as an alternative to adrenalectomy and in randomised clinical trials produced similar response rates to the surgical procedure. Initially it was given in a dose of 1 g a day combined with hydrocortisone 40 mg a day. Later it was used in doses of 125–500 mg per day without hydrocortisone. Toxicity includes lethargy in 36% of patients, rash in 22%, nausea and vomiting in 14%, dizziness in 16% and ataxia in 9%. The rash which can be dramatic and worrisome usually remits spontaneously. Other side effects usually lessen within 2–3 weeks.[38]

4-Hydroxyandrostenedione (Formestane)

This is 30–60 times more potent than aminoglutethimide at inhibiting aromatase and studies indicate that this drug inhibits circulating oestradiol levels by 60% in postmenopausal women, but it has little effect on an oestradiol suppression in premenopausal women. The problem with 4-hydroxyandrostenedione is that it has to be given by intramuscular injection at a dose of 250 mg twice per week.[39] Local pain and/or hypersensitivity reactions at the injection site can be a problem with this agent.

Newer aromatase inhibitors

The new-generation aromatase inhibitors are non-steroidal inhibitors with an imidazole or triazole structure.[36] These agents have a far better specificity for the aromatase enzyme and are much less toxic than aminoglutethimide. The first of these agents, fadrozole, inhibits aromatase *in vivo* by more than 90% whereas the newer agents anastrozole and letrozole produce 96.7–98.1% and 98.4–98.9% aromatase inhibition, respectively.[36] Vorozole appears to be at least as effective as an aromatase inhibitor letrozole. The agents which currently have product licences are anastrozole which is given in a dose of 1 mg per day and letrozole in a dose of 2.5 mg per day. Letrozole produces higher response rates that megestrol acetate in the second line setting. In another second line study, patients with anastrozole had a significantly longer survival than patients treated with megestrol acetate. Toxicity with these new drugs is much less of a problem and side effects which are uncommon include nausea and lethargy.[36] A new steroidal aromatase inhibitor, exemestane, is currently in clinical trials.

Progestogens

These agents are used in the treatment of metastatic breast cancer.[11,14] Medroxyprogesterone acetate (MPA) and megestrol acetate are the best-known agents. MPA has been most commonly used as an intramuscular injection. Doses of 500–1000 mg per day intramuscularly per day for 30 days have been used followed by a maintenance dose given weekly. Response rates are similar to that of tamoxifen when used as a second-line agent. Between 10 and 15% of patients on MPA develop cushingoid features and oedema, uterine bleeding, hot flushes and thromboembolic phenomena have all been observed.[40] In the UK and United States, megestrol acetate is the most commonly used progestogen in patients with breast cancer. As with MPA the main problem is weight gain. The mechanisms of action of progestogens are unknown but they may interfere with the binding of oestrogen to the oestrogen receptor, they may accelerate oestrogen catabolism or they may interfere with aromatisation of androgens to oestrogens. The reason these agents are reserved for second or third line treatment is the frequency with which they cause side effects. The standard dose is 160 mg once a day and the response rates to megestrol acetate are the same as those seen with MPA.[10]

Antiprogestogens

Synthetic antiprogestogens are in clinical trials at the present time.[10]

Use of hormonal agents

Hormonal agents have classically been used alone or in combination with chemotherapy. Some studies have assessed the combination of different endocrine agents. The optimal sequencing of hormonal agents is not clear.[10] In postmenopausal women the endocrine agent of choice is tamoxifen but with the advent of the new aromatase inhibitors, this may change. In premenopausal women LHRH agonists, oophorectomy and tamoxifen are all used for adjuvant therapy and treatment of metastatic breast cancer.[40] Although some studies suggest that combining hormonal agents given either simultaneously or in sequence, may initially produce a higher response rate, combination therapy appears to offer no survival advantage over sequential single agent therapy.[10]

Chemotherapy

Many active agents are available for the treatment of breast cancer and numerous combination chemotherapy regimens have been reported. Certain drugs form the cornerstone of treatment and these include the following.

Anthracyclines

Doxorubicin

Anthracyclines have long been considered to be the most active agents in the treatment of breast cancer. The antitumour antibiotic, doxorubicin (adriamycin) is the most widely used of these agents. When used as a single agent (50–60 mg 3 weekly) in untreated patients with metastatic breast cancer the response rate ranges from 40 to 50%.[41,42] When combined with other agents the response rates are much higher. Although it is usually given as a bolus once every three weeks, weekly administration allows some intensification of dosage and possibly reduces cardiac toxicity. Other side effects include myelosuppression and mucositis. Doxorubicin produces alopecia in most patients.[10]

Epirubicin

This is a semisynthetic doxorubicin stereoisomer. Its single agent response rate is comparable to that of doxorubicin, ranging from 25% in previously treated patients to 62% in untreated patients.[43] It is associated with less cardiac toxicity,[44] the risk of clinical cardiac impairment rising rapidly at doses of 1000 mg m^{-2} or above, compared with a cumulative toxic dose of 550 mg m^{-2} for doxorubicin. It is used most frequently in combination regimens such as ECF (epirubicin, cisplatin, 5-fluorouracil (5-FU)).

Mitoxantrone

Because the cumulative dose and dose rate of doxorubicin are limited by cardiac toxicity, other anthracycline analogues have been developed to circumvent this problem. Although mitoxantrone is reported to produce less cardiac toxicity than doxorubicin, clinical trials have demonstrated cardiac effects with increasing cumulative doses.[45] Response rates when used as a single agent vary from 17 to 35%.[43] Side effects are similar but less severe than those with doxorubicin. In particular, severe alopecia is avoided. It is most commonly used in a combined regimen.

Cyclophosphamide

Cyclophosphamide is inert until activated by microsomal enzymes in the liver which then produce the potent alkylating cytotoxic metabolite phosphoramide mustard.[46] Although cyclophosphamide is an active single agent, it is usually used in combination regimens such as CMF (cyclophosphamide, 5-fluorouracil and methotrexate). Response rates in advanced breast cancer with CMF vary between 29 and 68% and this regimen is the commonest used in the adjuvant setting.[46] Specific side effects include mucositis and occasionally a chemical cystitis.[10]

5-Fluorouracil

This is a pyrimidine analogue which has been used in cancer chemotherapy for more than 30 years. The drug first has to be metabolised and then binds to the enzyme thymidylate synthase thus inhibiting DNA synthesis.[47] Activity of 5-FU depends on peak concentrations and duration of exposure. In early trials, 5-FU was administered as a bolus but more recently it has been used as an infusional therapy, initially over 24 hours, then over 5 days and now continuously for many months.[47,48] Specific problems with continuous 5-FU include the 'hand foot' syndrome where the patients develop erythema and eventually blistering of the epithelium over the hands and feet and mucositis. These problems rapidly disappear if the infusion is discontinued for a few days.

Methotrexate

Methotrexate is an analogue of folic acid and works by blocking indirectly thymidylate synthesis. In breast cancer it is primarily used in the CMF regimen. Debate continues as to whether substitution of doxorubicin or epirubicin for methotrexate increases the efficacy of this combination therapy.[10]

Platinum compounds

Platinum compounds were first used in the treatment of germ cell tumours. These compounds work by forming adducts with DNA which inhibit replication.[49] Cisplatin is the most widely used agent.

Toxicity is, however, a problem with the platinum compounds and includes peripheral neuropathy, renal toxicity and ototoxicity.[10] Carboplatin has a similar efficacy to cisplatin but fewer toxic effects. Cisplatin is most frequently used in combination with epirubicin and infusional 5-fluorouracil in the ECF regimen. Response rates over 90% have been reported with this regimen in patients with large operable or locally advanced breast cancers.

Mitomycin

Mitomycin is an antitumour antibiotic that forms covalent cross-links with DNA and inhibits DNA, RNA and protein synthesis.[50] Mitomycin-C causes cumulative myelotoxicity. In the UK it is used in combination with mitoxantrone and methotrexate (MMM combination) and although it is a well-tolerated treatment for breast cancer,[51] neutropenia, thrombocytopenia and treatment delays can be a problem.

Taxoids

Paclitaxel is a novel chemotherapeutic agent derived from the Western Pacific yew tree. Paclitaxel has been the most widely used taxane. It has a unique mechanism of action and stabilises microtubular assembly.[52] This prevents cell division. Another semisynthetic taxoid, docetaxel has been derived from the European yew tree. Dose-limiting toxicity seems to be myelosuppression. These agents are very active against breast cancer although to date the interest in their activity has been based on observations in anthracycline resistant or refractory patients.[53] Continued trials will define their role and the correct dosing schedule in primary and adjuvant combination therapy.[10]

General side effects of chemotherapy

Although hair loss is the most common concern of patients before starting chemotherapy, 80% report fatigue and lethargy as the most troublesome side effect. The occurrence of alopecia with some chemotherapy regimens may be reduced by scalp cooling. Patients should be measured for a wig before losing hair and should be reassured that hair regrows after treatment. Nausea and vomiting are unpleasant side effects but can be controlled in most patients by appropriate anti-emetic drugs. Younger patients seem more at risk of nausea and vomiting and are more likely to suffer from extrapyramidal side effects from standard anti-emetics such as metoclopramide. It is thus appropriate to give serotonin-3 (5-HT$_3$)[35] antagonists to women aged under 45 as first-line treatment even for moderately emetogenic chemotherapy, the main argument against their universal use being that of cost. Occasional patients, however, can develop severe constipation as a side effect.

White count nadirs occur 10–14 days from the start of treatment. Using more intensive chemotherapy specific infective complications can develop including neutropenia (increasing in likelihood with white cell counts below 1000 mm^{-3}) and Gram-negative septicaemia, requiring immediate investigation and treatment by broad spectrum antibiotics before the results of culture are known.[54–56]

Extravasation of cytotoxics with necrosis and ulceration of the skin and subcutaneous tissues is a rare complication and is the single most powerful argument for employing trained and experienced teams of doctors and nurses to deliver cytotoxic chemotherapy.[54]

Complications of adjuvant chemotherapy may occur many months and years after completion of treatment. The major potential toxicities are cardiac dysfunction, premature menopause and the development of second cancers. Cardiomyopathy due to doxorubicin may occur during treatment, shortly after its completion or many months later. However, by screening women for pre-existing heart conditions (a single radionucleotide injection fraction measurement) cardiac problems are rare. Menopausal symptoms and cessation of periods are quite common and affect approximately 70% of premenopausal women after treatment. Very often menstrual function returns in the weeks following completion of chemotherapy. Sometimes the menopause is permanent and the severity and completeness of the menopause varies in relation to the patient's age and the intensity of the chemotherapy.[56] Even if menstruation returns, the eventual natural menopause may be advanced by several years. There is some evidence that after chemotherapy there is an increased risk of second cancers, particularly leukaemias.[56] As with Hodgkin's disease, the risk is probably drug and dose related, being more common with alkylating agents.

Operable breast cancer

In those with operable breast cancer systemic treatment can be given following local surgery and/or radiotherapy – **adjuvant treatment**. In large operable breast cancers systemic therapy can be given initially (**primary systemic therapy or neoadjuvant therapy**) prior to loco-regional therapy. Whereas the effectiveness of adjuvant treatment has been demonstrated in clinical trials, the benefits of primary systemic therapy is still under evaluation.

Primary systemic therapy

One potential problem with primary systemic treatment is that, if the diagnosis of cancer is made by fine needle aspiration cytology alone, *in situ* disease could be overtreated by chemotherapy (cytology cannot differentiate invasive and *in situ* disease).[55,56] A biopsy to obtain a histological diagnosis of invasive cancer should therefore be obtained before embarking on primary medical treatment. A major concern with this approach is that axillary nodal status is not known prior to the selection of systemic therapy and this information is the most useful prognostic factor for long-term survival.[56] This may become particularly important if the current generation of dose-intensive adjuvant trials demonstrates benefits in multiple node-positive patients. There is no evidence that leaving a primary tumour in the breast during primary systemic treatment increases a patient's anxiety.

Primary systemic therapy was introduced initially as treatment for inoperable and locally advanced disease to achieve tumour reduction and to make locally advanced tumours operable.[56] Its use has now been extended to patients with large operable breast cancers in an attempt to avoid mastectomy. Response rates ranging from 62% in tumours larger than 5 cm to 93% in tumours of 3–4 cm have been reported.[57] The response rates approach 80% and there appears to be no difference between different chemotherapy regimens. After chemotherapy, breast conserving surgery (quadrantectomy) was possible in 91% of patients in one series with just over 73% of the patients with tumours over 5 cm becoming candidates for breast conservation. At 18 months 1 of 201 patients treated by primary systemic therapy, quadrantectomy and postoperative radiotherapy suffered a local recurrence. Preliminary results have been published from two randomised trials. A French study of 272 women with tumours larger than 3 cm were randomised to primary chemotherapy followed by appropriate local treatment or mastectomy followed by the same chemotherapy to patients who were node positive or ER negative.[58] Of the patients receiving primary chemotherapy 63% were treated by breast conservation. More than 1300 patients have been randomised in an NSABP study comparing surgery followed by four cycles of AC or four cycles of AC followed by surgery.[59] The initial response rate to chemotherapy was 80% including 37% with a complete clinical response. More than 65% of patients in the primary chemotherapy group underwent breast conservation, compared with 57% in the adjuvant chemotherapy group. At surgery 59% of those receiving primary chemotherapy were node negative compared with 42% in the immediate surgery group. The first report of this study has shown no survival differences between the two treatment groups.

Although the majority of studies have treated patients prior to surgery with chemotherapy, there is an increasing interest in treating patients with hormone-sensitive disease with initial hormonal therapy.

The use of primary medical (neoadjuvant) treatment for operable breast cancer has increased over the past decade.[55] A theoretical advantage is the ability to assess response *in vivo*, clinically according to the criteria of the International Union Against Cancer (UICC) or by using mammography or ultrasonography.[60] Ultrasonography is the most accurate of these three methods.[61] Both the primary tumour and lymph node metastases can be shown to respond (Fig. 11.2), and invasive cancer seems to be more sensitive to chemotherapy than *in situ* disease. Early detection of resistance to treatment allows the oncologist to discontinue ineffective therapy, which avoids unnecessary toxicity and

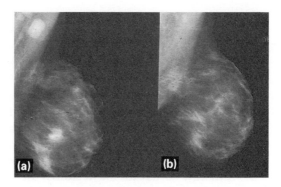

Figure 11.2 *Mammograms showing primary cancer involving axillary node before (a) and after (b) primary chemotherapy. At subsequent surgery, the patient was found to have no residual carcinoma in the breast or axilla – a complete pathological response. From Dixon JM ABC of breast diseases, BMJ Publishing Group, 1995.*

may facilitate a change to a potentially more effective regimen. Primary systemic therapy also has the theoretical advantage that by treating disease earlier, it is less likely that resistant tumour clones will have emerged spontaneously.[60] The advantages and disadvantages of primary systemic therapy are summarised in Table 11.1.

Chemotherapy

Regimens used for primary chemotherapy have generally been the same as those used for adjuvant treatment and about 70% of patients show a partial response, 20–30% a complete clinical response and a small number (about 10–15%) achieve a complete pathological response.[55,60] There is preliminary evidence that continuous infusional chemotherapy with agents such as fluorouracil combined with intermittent agents such as epirubicin and cisplatin achieve even higher response rates (over 90%) when compared with standard regimens of bolus chemotherapy.[62]

Table 11.1 *Advantages and disadvantages of adjuvant and primary systemic treatment*

Systemic treatment	Advantages	Disadvantages
Adjuvant	Proved efficacy Prognostic information available after surgery	Uncertainty whether treatment is effective in individual patients
Primary	Allows direct assessment of effectiveness Tumour shrinkage may allow breast conservation Early treatment of micrometastases	Loss of prognostic information May treat *in situ* disease (if diagnosis made by fine needle aspiration cytology alone)

Figure 11.3
Patient with large inflammatory cancer of right breast before (a) and after (b) infusional chemotherapy showing a complete clinical response.

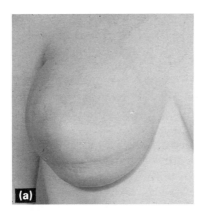

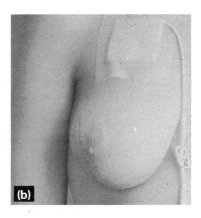

Primary hormonal therapy

Tamoxifen (20 mg a day by mouth) produces a partial response in 60% of elderly patients with hormone responsive (oestrogen receptor positive) tumours (Fig. 11.3) and a complete clinical response in 15%.[63]

The use of gonadotrophin releasing hormone analogues (goserelin 3.6 mg monthly given subcutaneously or leuprorelin 3.75 mg monthly given subcutaneously or intramuscularly) as primary medical treatment for premenopausal women with oestrogen receptor positive tumours is under evaluation.[63] Few patients show a complete pathological response after hormonal treatment but the side effects are generally much less than with chemotherapy.[63]

Tumours treated with primary systemic therapy are generally treated for up to three months with primary medical treatment.[55,63] During this period, patients should be monitored carefully using clinical and ultrasonographic assessment of tumour volume at monthly intervals. Overall, between 50 and 70% of patients with large operable tumours will have sufficient tumour regression to avoid mastectomy. All patients require some other form of local treatment (surgery or radiotherapy) after primary systemic treatment. It is not yet clear whether primary medical treatment prolongs survival. It is acceptable treatment for patients with large operable breast cancers but the use of primary systemic therapy for other groups of patients cannot be recommended except in clinical trials.[55]

Adjuvant therapy for operable breast cancer

The effectiveness of adjuvant therapy has been shown in clinical trials, but its effectiveness in individuals cannot be assessed as there is no overt disease to monitor.[55] Because small randomised trials can produce misleading results, data from all trials have been analysed in an overview or meta-analysis.[13] Large numbers of patients included in such an analysis provide great statistical power and enables these analyses reliably to detect modest advantages of one treatment over another.

Adjuvant endocrine therapy and chemotherapy in women with operable breast cancer each reduce the annual risk of death by about 30% for at least 10 years. Benefits of adjuvant therapy add up to about 10 extra women alive at 10 years for every 100 women with stage II disease and five extra women alive at 10 years for every 100 women with stage I disease.

The relative reductions in mortality are the same in axillary node negative and positive women. This suggests that adjuvant therapy is equally active in both low and high risk groups. Absolute reduction in death rate depends on the chances of a woman dying from the disease. A 30% reduction in the relative risk of the odds of dying reduces a 10% mortality at 10 years by 3% and 60% mortality at 10 years by 20%. The shape of the disease free and overall survival curves over time indicates that for most patients the benefit is that of a delay in the onset of recurrence rather than long-term cure.

Hormonal therapy

Premenopausal patients

Results from the Early Breast Cancer Trialists' Overview demonstrate that in women under 50 years of age ovarian suppression as the sole adjuvant therapy is associated with a 30% reduction in the annual risk of death and this effect lasts for at least 15 years.[13] The overview

Table 11.2 *Direct estimates of reduction in the annual odds of recurrence and death among women aged less than 50 in trials of adjuvant therapy*

Adjuvant therapy	No. aged <50 years randomised	Reductions % (SD) in annual odds of	
		Recurrence or prior death	Death from any cause
Trials of single modality therapy with untreated controls			
Polychemotherapy vs nil	2976	37 (5)	27 (6)
Ovarian suppression vs nil	878	30 (9)	28 (9)
Tamoxifen (mean 2.6 years) vs nil	2216	27 (7)	17 (10)
All tamoxifen trials, including those in which both arms also received chemotherapy			
Tamoxifen 1 year	2478	5 (7)	4 (8)
2 years	4794	10 (5)	4 (6)
>2 years	1311	43 (11)	27 (17)

From reference 13.

Table 11.3 *Overview of adjuvant tamoxifen trials*

Patient group	No. randomised	Reduction (SD) in annual odds	
		Recurrence (%)	Death (%)
All patients	30 081	25 (2)	16 (2)
<50 years	8586	12 (4)	6 (5)
⩾50 years	21 505	29 (2)	20 (2)
<50 years, premenopausal	7905	12 (4)	6 (5)
50–59 years, premenopausal	1583	33 (7)	23 (9)
<50 years, postmenopausal	681	12 (15)	*
50–59 years, postmenopausal	7804	28 (3)	19 (4)
60–69 years, all	9452	29 (3)	17 (4)
70+ years	2656	28 (5)	21 (6)

*To few patients. Adapted from Early Breast Cancer Trialists' Collaborative Group.[13]

suggests that prolonged tamoxifen appears to produce benefits in premenopausal women as well as postmenopausal women (Table 11.2). Benefits of oophorectomy appear greatest in oestrogen receptor-positive patients. The evidence that is available on duration of tamoxifen in premenopausal patients suggests that they should be treated for five years (Table 11.2).

Postmenopausal patients
Compared to a 6% reduction in the annual risks of deaths in women below the age of 50, tamoxifen produces a 20% reduction in the annual odds of death in women aged 50 or older (Table 11.3). The optimum duration of tamoxifen is not yet clear. The meta-analysis included five studies which compared three to five years of tamoxifen treatment with one to two years and although the analysis showed a reduction in recurrence ($22\% \pm 8\%$) which was significant, and there was an apparent reduction in mortality ($7\% \pm 11\%$), this reduction in mortality did not reach statistical significance (Table 11.4). With the concerns about the long-term effects of tamoxifen on the uterus, the current recommendation is that patients should take adjuvant tamoxifen for a maximum of five years. There appears to be significant interaction between the oestrogen receptor status of the tumour and the benefit obtained from tamoxifen in postmenopausal patients, although patients with oestrogen receptor-poor tumours may obtain a small benefit (Table 11.5).

Table 11.4 *Indirect comparison of the optimal duration of tamoxifen*

	Reduction (SD) in annual odds	
Patient group	Recurrence	Death
Tamoxifen for 2 years	28 (2%)	19 (3%)
<50 years	10 (5%)	4 (6%)
≥50 years	33 (3%)	23 (3%)
Tamoxifen for >2 years	39 (4%)	25 (6%)
<50 years	43 (11%)[a]	27 (17%)[a]
≥50 years	38 (5%)	23 (6%)

[a] Statistically unreliable; too few patients.
Adapted from Early Breast Cancer Trialists' Collaborative Group.[13]

Table 11.5 *Effects of tamoxifen by oestrogen receptor*

	Reduction (SD) in annual odds	
Patient group	Recurrence	Death
ER-poor (<10 fmol/mg)	13 (4%)	11 (5%)
ER+ (19–100 fmol/mg)	29 (3%)	19 (4%)
ER+ (>100 fmol/mg)	43 (5%)	29 (7%)

Adapted from Early Breast Cancer Trialists' Collaborative Group.[13]

Chemotherapy

The Overview concluded that when using chemotherapy, a combination of drugs produced better results than a single drug alone and that six courses produced similar benefits to more prolonged treatment schedules.[13]

Chemotherapy given at the time of or just after surgery has theoretical advantages. Drugs given at the time of surgery would theoretically kill any circulating tumour cells dislodged by surgery. Cumulative data suggest, however, that there is little added benefit from administering perioperative chemotherapy.

Premenopausal patients

Adjuvant chemotherapy appears to produce similar reductions in odds of death to oophorectomy (Table 11.3). Data from a Scottish trial suggest that the greatest benefit from chemotherapy is in patients with oestrogen receptor negative tumours.[64] Adjuvant chemotherapy given for at least two months produces a highly significant 36% reduction in annual odds of recurrence in women aged under 50 and 24%

Table 11.6 *Overview of adjuvant chemotherapy trials: recurrence and mortality with prolonged polychemotherapy*

Patient group	No. randomised	Reduction (SD) in annual odds	
		Recurrence (%)	Death (%)
All patients	11450	28 (3)	17 (3)
<50 years	3363	36 (5)	24 (5)
≥50 years	8087	24 (3)	13 (4)
<50 years, premenopausal	3138	36 (5)	25 (6)
50–59 years, premenopausal	911	25 (9)	23 (9)
<50 years, postmenopausal	225	37 (19)	*
50–59 years, postmenopausal	3128	29 (5)	13 (7)
60–69 years, all	3774	20 (5)	10 (6)
70+ years	277	*	*

*To few patients. Adapted from Early Breast Cancer Trialists' Collaborative Group.[13]

reduction in the annual odds of death (Table 11.6).[13] Chemotherapy appears to be most effective in younger patients. One third or more of recurrences and one quarter of the deaths in premenopausal women appear to be avoided or delayed at 10 years by adjuvant chemotherapy. Adjuvant chemotherapy appears, therefore, to produce highly significant benefits for premenopausal patients with breast cancer (Table 11.6).

Postmenopausal patients
Ten-year survival data do show a statistically significant reduction in recurrence and improved survival in postmenopausal patients given adjuvant chemotherapy. Overall, a 13% reduction in the odds of dying was observed in women of 50 years of age or older (Table 11.6). This reduction is about half that seen in younger patients. The benefits appear to be less pronounced in women aged 60–69 years when compared with younger, postmenopausal women. Too few women aged over 70 years of age were included in the Overview to provide a valid estimate of the effects of adjuvant chemotherapy in these patients. Some of these differences have been attributed to the added endocrine effects of chemotherapy in premenopausal patients. Since publication of the Overview, recent trials have raised doubts about the lack of effectiveness of chemotherapy in older patients.[56]

Optimal regimen for adjuvant chemotherapy
The most commonly used treatment is six cycles of CMF over 6 months. Studies have demonstrated that four cycles of AC (given over

approximately 3 months), appear to be as effective as six cycles of CMF.[65] Interestingly, in this direct comparison the days of nausea were fewer with the CMF regimen; cardiac toxicity was not a major problem although alopecia was worse with the AC regimen.

In a randomised trial from Milan of patients with four or more positive nodes comparing the sequence of doxorubicin for four cycles followed by intravenous CMF for eight courses with CMF for two cycles followed by doxorubicin for one cycle repeated to a total of 12 courses of chemotherapy, there was a highly significant improvement in disease free and overall survival in the patients treated with adriamycin and then CMF.[65] The survival curve of patients having the sequential regimen flattens out a few years after the start of treatment suggesting this regimen may be 'curing' some patients. No CMF arm alone was included in this trial but comparison with earlier results with CMF suggests that a sequence of four cycles of adriamycin and eight of CMF is a potent regimen for high-risk node-positive patients.

Although many physicians routinely use a doxorubicin regimen such as CAF or AC especially for node-positive patients, definitive proof of their superiority over CMF is lacking.[56] Results of ongoing trials should provide a definitive answer to this question.

Dose intensive adjuvant chemotherapy

The issue of dose intensity first received attention in 1981 when the Milan group reported that only those patients who received at least 85% of the planned CMF dose benefited significantly, whereas those receiving less than 65% of the planned dose had the same disease free and overall survival as the control group treated by surgery alone.[66] Later, in a retrospective analysis of published randomised trials, Hryniuk and Levine[67] showed a direct correlation between survival and dose intensity. One prospective study compared three doses of CAF and after a median follow-up of 3.4 years, the higher and moderate dose intensity regimens yielded superior disease free and overall survivals compared with the low dose.[68] The 'low-dose' chemotherapy was well below the intensity most oncologists would accept. There may be a threshold rather than a dose–response effect, i.e. a minimum dose below which cytotoxics are not effective. In a second study where the dose of cyclophosphamide in the AC regimen was intensified there was no difference in outcome in the three groups given different doses of cyclophosphamide.[69]

Studies of dose intensity using extremely high dose chemotherapy and autologous bone marrow transplant or peripheral stem cell rescue are being evaluated. A non-randomised study from Duke University estimated a 72% three-year disease-free survival with high dose chemotherapy and marrow rescue.[70] This was clearly superior to the survival of local historical controls and of 'matched' cohort from the CALGB database. High dose therapy with bone marrow or peripheral stem cell rescue as adjuvant therapy remains unproven and should be restricted to patients entering randomised clinical trials.

Table 11.7 *Definitions of risk groups and associated risk of relapse*

Risk group	Definition	Survival without relapse after 5 years
Node-negative patients		
Low risk	Tumour ≤1 cm in diameter >90%	
Intermediate risk	Tumour >1 cm, grade I or II	75–80%
High risk	Tumour >1 cm, grade III	50–60%
Node positive patients		
Low and intermediate risk	1–3 axillary nodes involved	40–50%
High risk	4–9 axillary nodes involved	20–30%
Very high risk	≥10 axillary nodes involved	10–15%

Table 11.8 *Adjuvant treatment for patients with breast cancer*

Risk group	Premenopausal patients	Postmenopausal patients
Node-negative patients		
Low risk	Tamoxifen or no treatment	Tamoxifen or no treatment
Intermediate risk	Tamoxifen	Tamoxifen
High risk	Consider chemotherapy[a] (with or without tamoxifen) or Ovarian ablation (with or without tamoxifen) if tumour is oestrogen receptor positive	Tamoxifen (with or without chemotherapy)
Node positive patients		
Low and intermediate risk	Chemotherapy[a] (with or without tamoxifen) or Ovarian ablation (with or without tamoxifen) if tumour is oestrogen receptor positive or Chemotherapy[a] and ovarian ablation (with or without tamoxifen)	Tamoxifen with or without chemotherapy
High and very high risk	Consider more intensive chemotherapy[b] (with or without tamoxifen)	Tamoxifen and chemotherapy if fit

[a] For example, cyclophosphamide, methotrexate and fluorouracil

[b] For example, regimen containing anthracycline. Some units are investigating use of intensive chemotherapy supported by rescue using autologous bone marrow or peripheral stem cells for patients at very high risk.

Current view on adjuvant therapy

The benefit of adjuvant therapy, possible treatment side effects, long-term toxicities and their impact on quality of life need to be taken into consideration when selecting adjuvant therapy for individual patients. Absolute improvements in survival appear greatest in those patients at high risk of recurrence and death. Patients in these categories may therefore be prepared to accept higher degrees of toxicity and side effects. The current philosophy in adjuvant therapy is to stratify patients in relation to their risk of recurrence and death and to tailor the adjuvant treatment to that risk. Patients can be stratified on the basis of number of involved nodes (Table 11.7) using tumour size and grade to stratify the node negative group.[55] Alternatively, patients can be stratified on the basis of a single index such as the Nottingham Prognostic Index which combines tumour size, histological tumour grade and node status.[71] Having identified the different risk group, the plan is then to tailor the adjuvant treatment to that risk. An outline of the current recommendations for adjuvant treatment for patients with operable breast cancer is given in Table 11.8.

Combinations of hormonal and chemotherapy

The overview predicted that in postmenopausal women there were additional survival gains from addition of chemotherapy to tamoxifen.[13] These gains, although not statistically significant in terms of survival, did make major differences in terms of recurrence and these are expected eventually to translate into improvements in survival. Trials are currently underway to investigate combinations of hormonal therapy and chemotherapy in pre- and postmenopausal women.

Adjuvant immunotherapy

More than 20 randomised trials of adjuvant immunotherapy have been completed and currently no evidence exists to support the use of this modality.[56]

Locally advanced breast cancer

Definition

Locally advanced disease is characterised clinically by features suggesting infiltration of the skin or chest wall by tumour or matted involved axillary nodes (Table 11.9).[72] Large operable cancers and tumours fixed to muscle should not be considered locally advanced. Depending on referral patterns and clinical definitions between 1 in 12 and 1 in 4 patients present with locally advanced disease.[72] Differences in definition and the different forms of breast cancer explain why the reported five-year survival rates for locally advanced disease vary between 1 and 30%. Overall median survival is about 2 to 2.5 years which is not very different from the survival described for breast cancer in the late 19th and early 20th centuries.

Table 11.9 *Clinical features of locally advanced breast cancer*

Skin
Ulceration
Dermal infiltration
Erythema over tumour
Satellite nodules
Peau d'orange

Chest wall
Tumour fixation to
Ribs
Serratus anterior
Intercostal muscles

Axillary nodes
Nodes fixed to one another or to other structures

Locally advanced breast cancer may arise because of it position in the breast (for example if the lesion is peripheral), because of neglect, or because the cancer is biologically aggressive (inflammatory cancers and the majority of those with peau d'orange). Inflammatory cancers are uncommon and are characterised by brawny, oedematous, indurated and erythematous skin changes; these cancers have the worst prognosis of all locally advanced breast cancers.

Treatment

Current treatments have had some impact on local control but have had little overall impact on survival.[73] Patients with hormone-sensitive disease have a much longer survival than those with hormone-insensitive disease. Local and regional relapse is a major problem in locally advanced disease and affects approximately half of all patients.

Surgery

Mastectomy is generally not indicated in the presence of features of locally advanced disease, but following treatment with a combination of cytotoxic drugs or initial hormonal treatment, surgery may become feasible some weeks or months later.[74] It may be possible to perform a wide excision although mastectomy is the most commonly performed procedure. Some cancers, principally, those with direct skin involvement because of position or neglect are suitable for primary surgical treatment.

The role of systemic and local treatments

The mainstay of local treatments has been radiotherapy because surgery is associated with high rates of local recurrence.[74–76] Radiotherapy can produce high rates of local remission in both the

Table 11.10 *Factors affecting choice of systemic treatment for locally advanced breast cancer*

Hormonal treatment
  Slow growing or indolent disease
  Oestrogen receptor positive cancer
  Elderly or unfit patients

Chemotherapy
  Inflammatory cancer
  Oestrogen receptor negative cancer
  Rapidly progressive cancer

breast and axilla but when radiotherapy is used alone, only 30% of patients remain free of locoregional disease at death. By combining appropriate systemic therapy and radiotherapy, response rates of over 80% have been reported and over two thirds of patients retain locoregional control at death. Radiotherapy should be given to patients managed initially by surgery or to those who have operations after a course of systemic therapy.

Choice of systemic treatment

Systemic therapy should be administered as part of a planned programme of combined systemic and local therapies.[73] Factors affecting the choice of systemic therapy for locally advanced breast cancer are outlined in Table 11.10. Standard chemotherapy such as CMF increases rates of local control, but has little impact on survival. There are some data to suggest that infusional therapies based on 5-FU combined with doxorubicin (AF) sometimes with the addition of cyclophosphamide (ACF) or 5-fluorouracil combined with epirubicin and cisplatin (ECF) do produce higher local response rates than the intermittent regimens used for adjuvant chemotherapy (Fig. 11.3). Work is currently underway to determine whether intensifying drug dosage is worthwhile in this group of women and is associated with

Table 11.11 *Choice of treatment for patients with locally advanced breast disease*

Hormonal treatment
  Premenopausal women – ovarian ablation (surgery, radiation, or
    gonadotrophin releasing hormone antagonists)
  Postmenopausal women – tamoxifen

Chemotherapy
  Intravenous – infusion of fluorouracil combined with an anthracycline
    (e.g. doxorubicin, cyclophosphamide and fluorouracil;
    or epirubicin, cisplatin and fluorouracil)
  Intra-arterial

Figure 11.4
Locally advanced breast cancer before (a) and after (b) treatment with six months of tamoxifen. The mass in the supraclavicular region is a lipoma.

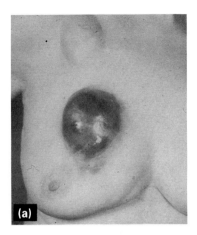
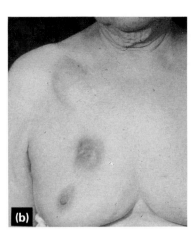

an improvement in operability rates, local control and survival.[77]

Primary hormonal therapy can be given to patients with locally advanced breast cancer providing that their cancers are oestrogen-receptor positive and appear to be relatively slow growing or indolent (Fig. 11.4). The choice of treatments in these patients is outlined in Table 11.11.

Despite the best efforts with combined treatments a substantial proportion of patients who present with locally advanced disease do develop uncontrolled disease of the chest wall. Impressive local control rates with low toxicity have been reported by giving chemotherapy intra-arterially via the internal mammary or lateral thoracic artery.[78] The drugs are administered following radiological placement of a catheter into the vessel which provides the major blood supply to the tumour. Drugs and doses used are similar to those given intravenously.

Metastatic breast cancer

The pattern of survival of patients with metastatic disease is variable. Some patients with hormone-sensitive disease survive many years after sequential hormone manipulation. Patients with disease which is not hormone sensitive have much shorter survivals.[29] The clinical pattern of relapse predicts future behaviour. Patients with a long disease-free interval (> 2 years following primary diagnosis) and favourable sites of recurrence (such as local lymph nodes and chest wall) survive much longer than patients who have either a short disease-free interval or recurrence at other sites.[79,80] Patients with lung, liver and brain disease have the poorest outlook (Fig. 11.5).

The aim of treatment is to produce effective control of symptoms and at the same time prolong survival. The primary aim, however, is to improve quality of life. At the present time, there is no evidence that treating asymptomatic metastases improves survival and it is not appropriate to perform regular routine screening investigations looking for systemic disease during follow-up.[10]

Figure 11.5
Median time of survival associated with sites of metastasis in patients with breast cancer.

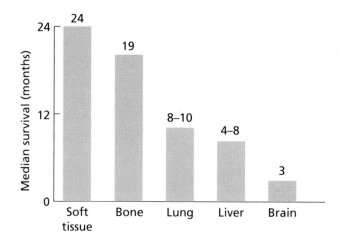

Figure 11.6
Choices of treatment for metastatic or recurrent breast cancer.

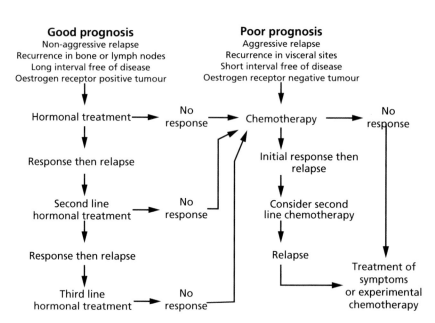

The choice of whether patients should have hormonal treatment or chemotherapy depends on the biology of the disease. Good prognosis disease is best treated by hormonal treatment, whereas poor prognosis usually requires chemotherapy (Fig. 11.6).[10,29]

Hormonal treatment

Although generally regarded as causing few side effects, all hormonal therapies can cause distressing symptoms. Objective responses to hormonal agents are seen in 30% of all patients and in 50–60% of patients with oestrogen receptor-positive tumours, although when symptomatic response rates are included the final clinical response rate (those who

Table 11.12   *Hormonal treatment of metastatic breast cancer*

	Premenopausal patients	Postmenopausal patients
First line treatment	LHRH agonists if not previously used If patients had previous oophorectomy, LHRH agonists and tamoxifen	Tamoxifen if not previously used or an aromatase inhibitor such as anastrozole or letrozole
Second line treatment		Following tamoxifen, anastrozole or letrozole Following anastrozole, or letrozole progestogens
Third line treatment		Following anastrozole, or letrozole, progestogens

gain a benefit from the drug) is usually much higher.[10] Response rates of 25% are seen with second line hormonal treatments, although less than 15% of patients who get no response to first line hormonal treatment, will respond to second line treatment.[29] Approximately 10 – 15% of patients respond to third line treatment. In premenopausal women second line treatment following tamoxifen would be LHRH agonists whereas in patients who have relapsed on LHRH agonists or following oophorectomy, then tamoxifen can be added.[29] In postmenopausal women, if tamoxifen has not already been used then this would at present be the first line agent.[10] If tamoxifen has already been used, one of the newer aromatase inhibitors such as anastrozole or letrozole is the hormonal treatment of choice. The next agents to be used are the progestogens, such as megestrol acetate or medroxyprogesterone acetate (Table 11.12).[29]

Chemotherapy

With chemotherapy a balance has to be achieved between obtaining a high rate of response and limiting side effects. The best palliation and subsequent quality of life is obtained with regimens which produce the highest response rates. Studies which have compared different intensities of chemotherapy show that quality of life is better on more intensive regimens with their associated side effects, rather than with less intensive regimens which have lower response rates and fewer side effects.[81,82] Overall rates of response to chemotherapy are about 40–60% with a median time to relapse of 6–10 months.[29] Subsequent courses of chemotherapy have low rates of response of less than 25%.[10,29] The agents used for treating metastatic disease are similar to those used in the adjuvant or primary systemic therapy settings.

Short-term results from high dose chemotherapy with bone marrow or stem cell rescue for metastatic breast cancer appear promising, with 15–20% of patients being disease free after 3–10 years.[83] One randomised study has shown a significant survival benefit for patients having stem cell rescue, but this study has been criticised, because the survival of patients given standard doses of chemotherapy was less than would have been expected and long-term tamoxifen was given only to the chemotherapy responders in a population of women that included a substantial number with ER+ cancers. Larger, long-term controlled studies are currently underway.[84]

Specific problems

Soft tissue or local chest wall disease

Although local disease can be isolated, up to half of patients have associated systemic relapse. Local recurrence after mastectomy can be classified as single spot relapse, multiple spot relapse or field change.[85] Treatment and prognosis differ for these three categories (Fig. 11.7, Table 11.13). If the recurrence is focal and occurs many years after the original, surgery alone can provide long-term control.[86] If the recurrence is multiple spot, but still localised, the options are radiotherapy or more radical excision.[29] In widespread recurrence, standard treatments are often disappointing, although intra-arterial chemotherapy and infusional 5-FU is sometimes effective for chest wall and soft tissue disease (Fig. 11.8).[87] The topical agent miltefosine is active for small volume multiple skin nodules, but it does not yet have a product licence in the UK. Failure to halt the progress of local

Figure 11.7
Survival of patients with local recurrence separated into three groups; single spot, multiple spot and field change compared with patients without local recurrence. Modified from reference 85.

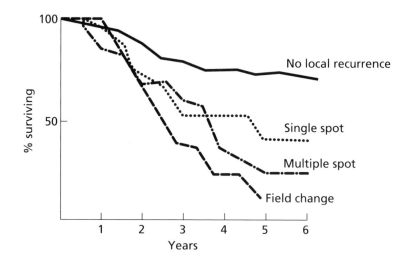

Table 11.13 *Treatment of local recurrence in chest wall*

Type of recurrence	Treatment
Single spot	Excise and consider radiotherapy
Multiple spot	Radiotherapy unless already given or more radical excision (possibly with coverage with myocutaneous flap)
Widespread	Consider radiotherapy unless already given or disease too widespread Appropriate systemic treatment (local application of chemotherapy such as miltefosine applied daily)

Figure 11.8
Patient with symptomatic skin and soft tissue disease in left supraclavicular fossa before (a) and after (b) a 12-week course of single agent continuous 5-fluorouracil.

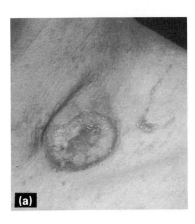
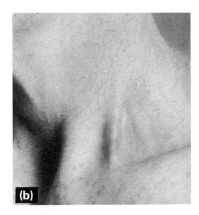

disease can lead to carcinoma en cuirasse where the chest wall is encircled by tumour – a most unpleasant situation for the patient.[86] The control of ulceration and focal malodorous infected tissue is a considerable problem for carers and patients. Excision of dead tissue and the use of topical and oral antibiotics with antianaerobic activity combined with charcoal dressings help to control the malodour.[29]

Recurrent axillary disease
If initial axillary therapy has been suboptimal, axillary disease can represent residual untreated disease rather than recurrence. Isolated mobile recurrences should be excised and combined with a level III dissection if this has not already been performed.[88,89] Patients with isolated, inoperable recurrence may be given radiotherapy (if not previously given) or systemic therapy, or both; these are sometimes effective at palliation but rarely produce long-lasting control of the disease.[86] When as is often the case, axillary recurrence occurs in association with metastases at other sites, then appropriate systemic therapy with or without local treatments are required.[90,91]

Figure 11.9
Radiograph showing metastatic lesions in humerus before (a) and after (b) course of hormonal treatment with consequent reduction in bone pain and increase in bone density.

From Dixon JM
ABC of Breast Diseases,
BMJ Publishing Group,
1995.

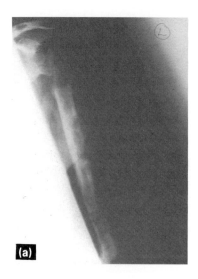
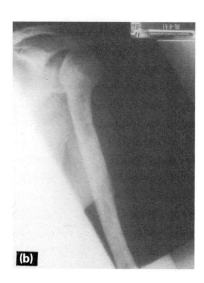

(a)   (b)

Bony disease

Bone is the most common site of secondary breast cancer with three quarters of patients having bone metastases. Widespread bone disease alone often responds well to hormonal treatment (Fig. 11.9) but when associated with visceral disease or it occurs in young patients, chemotherapy is usually required.[56] Assessing response to treatment is difficult and studies suggest that serological tumour markers may be of more use than repeated radiographs or bone scans.[92] Most clinicians use control of symptoms to determine response to therapy.

Localised bone pain can be treated by a single fraction of radiotherapy.[93] Widespread bone pain can be treated with radioactive strontium with few systemic side effects, with sequential upper and lower body hemibody radiotherapy being an alternative.[93,94] This latter treatment is associated with more toxicity. Bisphosphonates are useful for diffuse bone pain although their true role remains to be determined.[95]

When bone lysis threatens fracture, internal fixation followed by radiotherapy (low doses in a few fractions) will improve quality of life and maintain mobility (Fig. 11.10). Such treatment is often associated with a reasonable survival. If a pathological fracture does occur a combination of internal fixation and radiotherapy should be used although the functional result is usually inferior to that of prophylactic treatment.[93]

Detection of bone metastases can be a problem. Some patients have infiltration of marrow causing the pain rather than bony destruction. Such disease is often best detected by MRI or CT scanning rather than by bone scanning or plain radiographs.[29]

Widespread marrow infiltration can cause a leucoerythroblastic blood picture (immature cells in the peripheral blood). In such patients

Figure 11.10
Radiograph showing lytic lesion in the neck of the right femur before (a) and after (b) prophylactic replacement. Patient was alive and well three years later.

From Dixon JM
ABC of Breast Diseases,
BMJ Publishing Group,
1995.

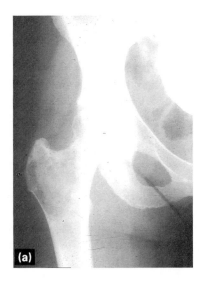
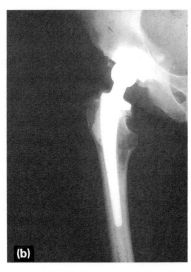

chemotherapy is generally required although it has to be given initially at reduced doses with careful monitoring and adequate supportive care.[96]

Malignant hypercalcaemia

The onset of confusion, thirst and polyuria can be insidious; in particular in patients with bone disease non-specific illness should always arouse the clinician to the possibility of malignant hyper-calcaemia. After diagnosis, patients should be treated with hydration with saline (about 3 litres are given over 24 h) and then intravenous bisphosphonates. Effective anticancer treatment reduces the risk of recurrence but patients who exhibit continuing hypercalcaemia can be treated with repeated intravenous bisphosphonates. Oral bisphosphonates (gastrointestinal absorption is poor and variable) are available and their role in recurrent hypercalcaemia is currently being investigated.[97]

Malignant pleural effusion

Up to half of patients with metastatic breast cancer will develop a malignant pleural effusion and only some of these require specific treatment. When examining the fluid aspirated only 85% of patients have malignant cells in the effusion.[98] Although aspiration is effective at establishing a diagnosis, it is not an effective treatment. Tube drainage followed by new or changed systemic therapy controls effusions in just over a third of patients.[29] For the other two thirds who get recurrent disease, installation of bleomycin, tetracycline or occasionally talc inserted under general anaesthesia is required to control recurrence.[99–101] The effusion should be aspirated to complete dryness and then a small amount of local anaesthetic placed before adding the active agent. This reduces the pain associated with the procedure. Patients often develop transient pyrexia following this procedure.

Neurological complications

Although non-metastatic syndromes of the central nervous system can occur with breast cancer any focal neurological symptom must be investigated. Computerised tomography or magnetic resonance imaging can detect even small volumes of disease in the brain or spinal cord.[102-105] Initial treatment of brain metastases is to reduce oedema with high dose corticosteroids (12–16 mg daily of dexamethasone) pending local treatment with fractionated radiotherapy.[29] Radiotherapy produces most benefit in patients whose neurological symptoms improve after taking steroids. Radiotherapy is delivered in five daily fractions.[106] The long-term results of treating CNS disease are disappointing with most patients dying within three or four months. Long-term survival has been reported in patients with isolated brain metastases following excision of metastasis and postoperative radiotherapy.[107]

Cord compression is not usually amenable to surgery and is seen most often in patients with thoracic spinal metastases.[100] Treatment is with steroids and fractionated radiotherapy. Treatment needs to be started as soon as possible and before any neurological deficits are severe. Occasionally patients do have isolated metastases causing cord compression and in these laminectomy can be effective.[29,108]

References

1. Vessey MP. The involvement of oestrogen in the development and progression of breast disease: epidemiological evidence. Proc R Soc Edinb 1989; 95B: 35.
2. Du Pont WD, Page DL. Menopausal oestrogen replacement therapy and breast cancer. Arch Intern Med 1991; 51: 67–72.
3. Fuqua SAW. Estrogen and progestogen receptors in breast cancer. In: Harris JR, Lippman ME, Morrow M, Hellman S (eds) Diseases of the breast. Philadelphia: Lippincott–Raven, 1996, pp. 261–71.
4. Bezwoda WR, Esser JD, Dansey R, et al. The value of estrogen and progesterone receptor determination in advanced breast cancer. Cancer 1991; 68: 867–72.
5. Osborne CK, Yochmowitz MG, Knight WA, et al. The value of estrogen and progesterone receptors in the treatment of breast cancer. Cancer 1980; 46: 2884.
6. Hawkins RA, Tesdale AL, Sangster K, et al. The quantitative importance of oestrogen receptor (ER) assays in elderly patients with breast cancer treated with tamoxifen. Br J Surg 1996; 83(Suppl 1): 11.
7. Hawkins RA, White, G, Bundred NJ, et al. Prognostic significance of oestrogen and progestogen receptor activities in breast cancer. Br J Surg 1987; 74: 1009–13.
8. Wenger CR, Beardslee S, Owens MA, et al. DNA ploidy, S-phase and steroid receptors in more than 127,000 breast cancer patients. Breast Cancer Res Treat 1993; 28: 9–20.
9. Beatson GT. On the treatment of inoperable cases of carcinoma of the mamma. Suggestions for a new method of treatment with illustrative cases. Lancet 1896; ii: 104–7 and 162–5.
10. Honig SF. Hormonal therapy and chemotherapy. In: Harris JR, Lippman ME, Morrow M, Hellman S (eds) Diseases of the breast. Philadelphia: Lippincott–Raven, 1996, pp. 669–734.
11. Muss HB. Endocrine therapy for advanced breast cancer: a review. Breast Cancer Res Treat 1992; 21: 15–26.

12. Hoogstraten B, Fletcher WAS, Gad-el-Mawla N, et al. Tamoxifen and oophorectomy in the treatment of recurrent breast cancer. Cancer Res 1982; 42: 4788.

13. Early Breast Cancer Trialists' Collaborative Group. Systemic treatment of early breast cancer by hormonal, cytotoxic or immune therapy. 113 randomised trials involving 31,000 recurrences and 24,000 deaths amongst 75,000 women. Lancet 1992; 339: 1–15 and 71–85.

14. Santen RJ, Manni A, Harvey H, et al. Endocrine treatment of breast cancer in women. Endocr Rev 1990; 11: 221–65.

15. Harvey HA, Santen RJ, Osterman J, et al. A comparative trial of transphenoidal hypophysectomy and estrogen suppression with aminoglutethimide in advanced breast cancer. Cancer 1979; 43: 2207.

16. Harris AL, Carmichael J, Cantwell BMJ, et al. Zoladex: endocrine and therapeutic effects in post-menopausal breast cancer. Br J Cancer 1989; 59: 97.

17. Miller WR, Scott WN, Morris R, et al. Growth of human breast cancer cells inhibited by a leutinizing hormone-releasing hormone agonist. Nature 1985; 313: 231.

18. Nicholson RJ, Walker KJ, Davies P. Hormone agonists and antagonists in the treatment of hormone sensitive breast and prostate cancer. Cancer Surv 1986; 5: 463.

19. Furr JA, Jordan VC. The pharmacology and clinical uses of tamoxifen. Pharmacol Ther 1984; 25: 127.

20. Langan-Fahey SM, Tormey DC, Jordan VC. Tamoxifen metabolites in patients with long-term adjuvant therapy for breast cancer. Eur J Cancer 1990; 26: 883–8.

21. Wittliff JL. Steroid-hormone receptors in breast cancer. Cancer 1984; 53: 630.

22. Osborne CK, Coronado E, Allred DC, et al. Acquired tamoxifen resistance: correlation with reduced breast tumour levels of tamoxifen and isomerization of trans-4-hydroxytamoxifen. J Natl Cancer Inst 1991; 83: 1477–82.

23. Turken S, Siris E, Seldin D, et al. Effects of tamoxifen on spinal bone density in women with breast cancer. J Natl Cancer Inst 1989; 81: 1086.

24. Love RR, Mazess RB, Barden HS, et al. Effects of tamoxifen on bone mineral density in postmenopausal women with breast cancer. N Engl J Med 1992; 326: 852–6.

25. Schapira DV, Kumar NB, Lyman GH. Serum cholesterol reduction with tamoxifen. Breast Cancer Res Treat 1990; 17: 3–7.

26. McDonald CC, Stewart HJ. Fatal myocardial infarction in the Scottish adjuvant tamoxifen trial. Br Med J 1991; 303: 435–7.

27. Fisher B, Costantino J, Redmond C, et al. A randomised clinical trial evaluating tamoxifen in the treatment of patients with node-negative breast cancer who had estrogen-receptor-positive tumors. N Engl J Med 1989; 320: 479.

28. Loprinzi CL, Michalak JC, Quella SK. Megestrol acetate for the prevention of hot flashes. N Engl J Med 1994; 331: 347–52.

29. Leonard RCF, Rodger A, Dixon JM. Metastatic Breast Cancer. In: Dixon JM (ed.) ABC of breast diseases. London: BMJ Publishing Group, 1995; pp. 45–8.

30. Jaiyesimi IA, Buzdar AU, Decker DA, Hortobagyi GN. Use of tamoxifen for breast cancer: 28 years later. J Clin Oncol 1995; 13: 513–29.

31. Jordan VC, Fritz NF, Langan-Fahey S, et al. Alteration of endocrine parameters in premenopausal women with breast cancer during long-term adjuvant therapy with tamoxifen as the single agent. J Natl Cancer Inst 1991; 83: 1488–91.

32. Ingle JN, Krook JE, Green SJ, et al. Randomized trial of bilateral oophorectomy versus tamoxifen in premenopausal women with metastatic breast cancer. J Clin Oncol 1986; 4: 178.

33. Buchanan RB, Blamey RW, Durrant KR, et al. A randomized comparison of tamoxifen with surgical oophorectomy in premenopausal patients with advanced breast cancer. J Clin Oncol 1986; 4: 1326.

34. Howell A, DeFriend DJ, Robertson JFR, et al. Clinical studies with the specific 'pure' antioestrogen ICI 182780. The Breast 1996; 5: 192–195.

35. Dowsett M. Biological background to aromatase inhibition. The Breast 1996; 5: 196–201.

36. Lønning PE. Pharmacology of new aromatase inhibitors. The Breast 1996; 5: 202–8.

37. Jonat W. Results of phase II and phase III trials with new aromatase inhibitors. The Breast 1996; 5: 209–15.

38. Stuart-Harris RC, Smith IE. Aminoglutethimide in the treatment of advanced breast cancer. Cancer Res Treat 1984; 11: 189.

39. Wiseman LR, McTavish D. Formestane: a review of its pharmacodynamic and pharmokinetic properties and therapeutic potential in the management of breast cancer and prostatic cancer. Drugs 1993; 45: 66–84.

40. Mattson W. Current status of high dose progestin treatment in advanced breast cancer. Breast Cancer Res Treat 1983; 3: 231.

41. Ahmann DL, Bisel HF, Eagan RT, et al. Controlled evaluation of adriamycin (NSC-123127) in patients with disseminated breast cancer. Cancer Chemother Rep 1974; 58: 877.

42. Hoogstraten B, George SL, Samal B, et al. Combination chemotherapy and adriamycin in patients with advanced breast cancer. Cancer 1976; 83: 13.

43. Robert J. Epirubicin: clinical pharmacology and dose-effect relationship. Drugs 1993; 45: 20–30.

44. Brambilla C, Rossi A, Bonfante V. et al. Phase II study of doxorubicin versus epirubicin in advanced breast cancer. Cancer Treat Rep 1986; 70: 261.

45. Myers CE, Chabner BA. Anthracyclines: In: Chabner B, Collins JM (eds) Cancer chemotherapy: principles and practice. Philadelphia: JB Lippincott, 1990, p. 356.

46. Engelsman E, Klijn JCM, Rubens RD, et al. 'Classical' CMF versus 3-weekly intravenous CMF schedule in postmenopausal patients with advanced breast cancer. Eur J Cancer 1991; 27: 966–70.

47. Diasio RB, Harris BE. Clinical pharmacology of 5-fluorouracil. Clin Pharmacokinet 1989; 16: 215.

48. Chang AYC, Most C, Pandya KJ. Continuous intravenous infusion of 5-fluorouracil in the treatment of refractory breast cancer. Am J Clin Oncol 1989; 12: 453.

49. Reed E, Kohn KW. Platinum analogues. In: Chabner B, Collins JM (eds) Cancer chemotherapy: principles and practice. Philadelphia: JB Lippincott, 1990, p. 465.

50. Verweij J, Den Hartigh J, Pinedo HM. Antitumour antibiotics. In: Chabner B, Collins JM (eds) Cancer chemotherapy: principles and practice. Philadelphia: JB Lippincott, 1990, p. 382.

51. Jodrell DI, Smith IE, Mansi JL, et al. A randomised comparative trial of mitozantrone/ methotrexate/mitomycin C (MMM) and cyclophosphamide/methotrexate/5 FU (CMF) in the treatment of advanced breast cancer. Br J Cancer 1991; 63: 794–8.

52. Rowinsky EK, Cazenave LA, Donehower RC. Taxol: a novel investigational antimicrobule agent. J Natl Cancer Inst 1990; 82: 1247–59.

53. Buzdar AU, Hortobagyi GN, Frye D, et al. Second-line chemotherapy for metastatic breast cancer including quality of life issues. The Breast 1996; 5: 312–317.

54. Yarnold J. Breast cancer. In: Price P, Sikora K (eds) Treatment of breast cancer. London: Chapman and Hall, 1995, pp. 413–36.

55. Richards MA, Smith IE. Role of systemic treatment for primary operable breast cancer. In: Dixon JM (ed.) ABC of breast diseases. London: BMJ Publishing Group, 1995, pp. 38–41.

56. Osborne CK, Clarke GM, Ravdin PM. Adjuvant systemic therapy of primary breast cancer. In: Harris JR, Lippman ME, Morrow M, Hellman S (eds) Diseases of the breast. Philadelphia: JB Lippincott–Raven, 1996, pp. 548–78.

57. Bonadonna G, Valgussa P, Brambilla C et al. Adjuvant and neoadjuvant treatment of breast cancer with chemotherapy and/or endocrine therapy. Semin Oncol 1991; 15: 515–24.

58. Mauriac L, Durand M, Avril A, et al. Effects of primary chemotherapy in conservative treatment of breast cancer patients with operable tumours larger than 3 cm: results of a randomised trial in a single center. Ann Oncol 1991; 2: 347–54.

59. Fisher B, Rockette H, Ribidoux A, et al. Effect of preoperative therapy for breast cancer (BC) on local-regional disease: first report of NSABP B-18. Proc ASCO 1994; 13: 64.

60. Smith IE. Primary (neoadjuvant) medical therapy: introduction. In: Powles T, Smith IE (eds) Medical Management of breast cancer. London: Martin-Dunitz, 1991, pp. 259–65.

61. Forouhi P, Walsh JS, Anderson TJ, Chetty U. Ultrasonography as a method of measuring breast tumour size and monitoring response to primary systemic treatment. Br J Surg 1994; 81: 223–5.

62. Smith IE, Walsh G, Jones A, *et al.* High complete remission rates with primary neoadjuvant infusional chemotherapy for large early breast cancer. J Clin Oncol 1995; 13: 424–9.

63. Anderson EDC, Forrest APM, Levack PA, *et al.* Response to endocrine manipulation and oestrogen receptor concentration in large, operable breast cancer. Br J Cancer 1989; 60: 223–226.

64. Scottish Cancer Trials Breast Group and ICRF Breast Unit, Guy's Hospital. Adjuvant ablation versus CMF chemotherapy in premenopausal women with pathological stage II breast carcinoma: the Scottish trial. Lancet 1993; 341: 1293–8.

65. Fisher B, Brown AM, Dimitrov NV, *et al.* Two months of doxorubicin–cyclophosphamide with and without interval reinduction therapy compared with 6 months of cyclophosphamide, methotrexate and fluorouracil in positive-node breast cancer patients with tamoxifen-nonresponsive tumours: results from the National Surgical Adjuvant Breast and Bowel Project B-15. Clin Oncol 1990; 8: 1483–96.

66. Bonadonna G, Valaguss P. Dose–response effect of adjuvant chemotherapy in breast cancer. N Engl J Med 1981; 304: 10.

67. Hryniuk W, Levine MN. Analysis of dose intensity for adjuvant chemotherapy trials in stage II breast cancer. J Clin Oncol 1986; 4: 1162.

68. Wood WC, Budman DR, Korzun AH *et al.* Dose and dose intensity of adjuvant chemotherapy for stage II, node-positive breast carcinoma. N Engl J Med 1994; 330: 1253–9.

69. Dimitrov N, Anderson S, Fisher B, *et al.* Dose intensification and increased total dose of adjuvant chemotherapy for breast cancer (BC): findings from NSABP B22. Proc ASCO 1994; 13: 64.

70. Peters WP, Ross M, Vrendenburgh JJ, *et al.* High-dose chemotherapy and autologous bone marrow support as consolidation after standard-dose adjuvant therapy for high-risk primary breast cancer. J Clin Oncol 1993; 11: 1132–43.

71. Galea MH, Blamey RW, Elston CE, Ellis IO. The Nottingham prognostic index in primary breast cancer. Breast Cancer Res Treat 1992; 22: 207–19.

72. Rodger A, Leonard RCF, Dixon JM. Locally advanced breast cancer. Dixon JM (ed.) ABC of breast diseases, London: BMJ Publishing Group, 1995, pp. 42–4.

73. Hortobagyi GN, Singletary SE, McNeese MD. Treatment of locally advanced and inflammatory breast cancer. In: Harris JR, Lippman ME, Morrow M, Hellman S (eds) Diseases of the breast. Philadelphia: Lippincott–Raven 1996, pp. 585–99.

74. Haagensen CD, Stout AP. Carcinoma of the breast: criteria of inoperability. Ann Surg 1943; 118: 859.

75. Zucali R, Islenghi C, Kenda R, *et al.* Natural history and survival of inoperable breast cancer treated with radiotherapy and radiotherapy followed by radical mastectomy. Cancer 1976; 37: 1422.

76. Harris JR, Sawicka J, Gleman R, *et al.* Management of locally advanced carcinoma of the breast by primary radiation therapy. Int J Radiat Oncol Biol Phys 1983; 9: 345.

77. Antman KH. Dose-intensive therapy in breast cancer. In: Armitage JO, Antman KH (eds) High-dose cancer therapy. Baltimore: Williams and Wilkins, 1992, p. 701.

78. de Dycker RP, Timmerman J, Neumann RLA. Regional induction chemotherapy in locally advanced breast cancer. The Breast 1992; 1: 82–6.

79. Valagussa P, Bonadonna G, Veronesi U. Patterns of relapse and survival following radical mastectomy. Cancer 1978; 41: 1170.

80. Perez JE, Machiavelli M, Leone BA, *et al.* Bone-only versus visceral-only metastatic pattern in breast cancer: analysis of 150 patients. Am J Clin Oncol 1990; 13: 294–8.

81. Carmo-Pereira J, Oliveira Costa F, Henriques E, *et al.* A comparison of two doses of adriamycin in the primary chemotherapy of disseminated breast carcinoma. Br J Cancer 1987; 56: 471.

82. Tannock IF, Boyd NF, DeBoer G, *et al.* A randomized trial of two dose levels of cyclophosphamide, methetrexate and fluorouracil chemotherapy for patients with metastatic breast cancer. J Clin Oncol 1988; 6: 137.

83. Myers SE, Williams SF. Role of high-dose chemotherapy and autologous stem cell support in treatment of breast cancer. Hematol Oncol Clin North Am 1993; 7: 631–45.

84. Bezwoda WR, Seymour L, Dansey RD. High-dose chemotherapy with hematopoietic rescue as primary treatment for metastatic breast cancer: a randomized trial. J Clin Oncol 1995; 13: 2483–9.

85. Blacklay PF, Campbell FS, Hinton SP, et al. Patterns of flap recurrence following mastectomy. Br J Surg 1995; 72: 719–20.

86. Recht A, Hayes DF, Eberlein TJ, Sadowsky NL. Local-regional recurrence after mastectomy or breast-conserving therapy. In: Harris JR, Lippman ME, Morrow M, Hellman S (eds) Diseases of the breast. Philadelphia: Lippincott–Raven 1996, pp. 649–67.

87. Ng JSY, Cameron DA, Lee L, et al. Infusional 5-fluorouracil given as a single agent in relapsed breast cancer: its activity and toxicity. The Breast 1994; 3: 87–9.

88. Halverson KJ, Perez CA, Kuske RR, et al. Isolated local-regional recurrence of breast cancer following mastectomy: radiotherapeutic management. Int J Radiat Oncol Biol Phys 1990; 19: 851–8.

89. Bundred NJ, Morgan DAL, Dixon JM. Management of regional nodes in breast cancer. In: Dixon JM (ed.) ABC of breast diseases. London: BMJ Publishing Group, 1995, pp. 30–3.

90. Recht A, Pierce SM, Abner A, et al. Regional nodal failure after conservative surgery and radiotherapy for early-stage breast carcinoma. J Clin Oncol 1991; 9: 988–96.

91. Gateley CA, Mansel RE, Owen A, et al. Treatment of the axilla in operable breast cancer (abstract). Br J Surg 1991; 78: 750.

92. Coleman RE. Evaluation of bone disease in breast cancer. The Breast 1994; 2: 73–8.

93. Aaron AD, Jennings LC, Springfield DS. Local treatment of bone metastases. In: Harris JR, Lippman ME, Morrow M, Hellman S (eds) Diseases of the breast. Philadelphia: Lippincott–Raven, 1996, pp. 811–19.

94. Robinson RG, Blake GM, Preston DF, et al. Strontium-89: treatment results and kinetics in patients with painful metastatic prostate and breast cancer in bone. Radiography 1989; 9: 271.

95. Theriault RL. Medical treatment of bone metastases. In: Harris JR, Lippman ME, Morrow M, Hellman S (eds) Diseases of the breast. Philadelphia; Lippincott–Raven, 1996, pp. 819–26.

96. Come SE, Schnipper LE. Bone marrow metastases. In: Harris JR, Lippman ME, Morrow M, Hellman S (eds) Diseases of the breast. Philadelphia: Lippincott–Raven, 1996, pp. 847–53.

97. Warrell RP Jr. Hypercalcemia. In: Harris JR, Lippman ME, Morrow M, Hellman S (eds) Diseases of the breast. Philadelphia: Lippincott–Raven, 1996, pp. 840–7.

98. Prakash UBS, Reiman HM. Comparison of needle biopsy with cytologic analysis for the evaluation of pleural effusion: analysis of 414 cases. Mayo Clin Proc 1985; 60: 158.

99. Hausheer FH, Yarbro JW. Diagnosis and treatment of malignant pleural effusion. Semin Oncol 1985; 12: 54.

100. Pearson FG, Macgregor DC. Talc poudrage for malignant pleural effusion. J Thorac Cardiovasc Surg 1966; 51: 732.

101. Ruckdeschel JC, Moores D, Lee JY, et al. Intrapleural therapy for malignant pleural effusions: a randomized comparison of bleomycin and tetracycline. Chest 1991; 100: 1528–35.

102. Shi M-L, Wallace S, Libshitz HI, et al. Cranial computer tomography of breast carcinoma. J Comput Assist Tomogr 1982; 6: 77.

103. Hayman LA, Evans RA, Henck VC. Delayed high iodine dose contrast computed tomography. Radiology 1980; 136: 677.

104. Shalen PR, Hayman LA, Wallace S, et al. Protocol for delayed contrast enhancement in computed tomography of cerebral neoplasia. Radiology 1981; 139: 397.

105. Kent DL, Larson FB. Magnetic resonance imaging of the brain and spine. Ann Intern Med 1988; 108: 402.

106. Borgelt B, Gelber R, Kramer S, et al. The palliation of brain metastases: final results of the first of two studies by the Radiation Therapy Oncology Group. Int J Radiat Oncol Biol Phys 1980; 6: 1.

107. Posner JB. Surgery for metastases to the brain. (Editorial). N Engl J Med 1990; 322: 544–5.

108. Freilich RJ, Foley KM. Epidural metastasis. In: Harris JR, Lippman ME, Morrow M, Hellman S (eds) Diseases of the breast. Philadelphia: Lippincott–Raven, 1996, pp. 779–89.

12 Palliative care in breast cancer

Janet Hardy

As metastatic breast cancer is an incurable malignancy the ability to palliate advanced disease is of major importance, particularly as around 15 000 women in the UK die of the disease each year. Palliative care is important not just in the terminal phase of disease but throughout the patient's illness. Chemotherapy, hormone therapy and radiotherapy (see Chapter 11) are probably the most effective means of palliation in breast cancer but it is not always possible or appropriate to deliver these treatment modalities. The common symptoms of breast cancer relate to the pattern of metastatic disease spread and any treatment should always be delivered in conjunction with symptom control measures.

Pain Pain is the most common and certainly the most feared symptom in patients with cancer. Chronic pain can be controlled, however, in 80–90% of patients by adhering to the WHO analgesic guidelines.[1] This is based on a 3-step ladder approach whereby increasing severity of pain is matched by increasing strengths of analgesia (Fig. 12.1). Analgesia at each step can be supplemented by the use of additive drugs or co-analgesics (see below). Drugs at each step of the ladder should be used up to the maximum dose and frequency prior to progression to the next step. The system is based on regular oral drug dosing rather than 'as required' medication. It is illogical to use an alternate drug of the same strength if the previous drug on the same step has failed to control pain. Recommended drugs at each step are shown in Fig. 12.2. At step 1, paracetamol is used in preference to aspirin because of its relative lack of gastrointestinal toxicity. A common mistake at step 2 is to use combination analgesics that comprise low doses of opioid which are in fact sub-therapeutic, e.g. co-codaprin and co-codamol 8/500 which both contain only 8 mg codeine in combination with aspirin and paracetamol. In contrast both coproxamol and co-codamol 30/500 (Tylex®) comprise adequate doses of paracetamol with dextropropoxyphene and codeine, respectively.

Figure 12.1 *WHO analgesic ladder.*

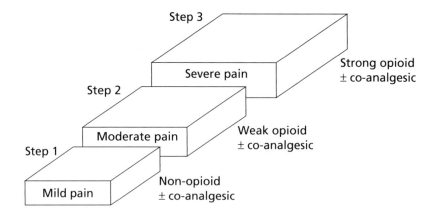

Figure 12.2 *Recommended analgesics at each step of the WHO analgesic ladder.*

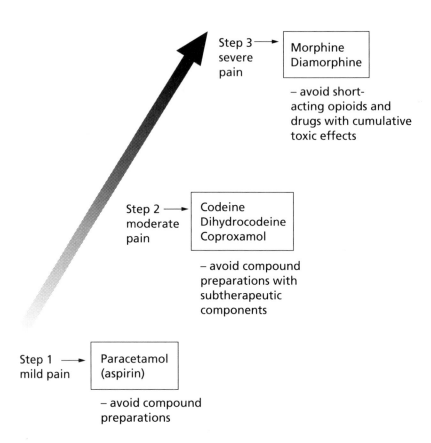

Table 12.1 *Morphine formulations commercially available for routine use*

Immediate release oral preparations
Duration of action 4 h

Morphine sulphate oral solution e.g. Oramorph®	10 mg/5 ml + taste mask, suitable for dose titration
Concentrated oral morphine sulphate solution	100 mg/5 ml (no taste mask)
Morphine sulphate unit dose vials	10 mg/5 ml, 30 mg/5 ml, 100 mg/5 ml
Morphine tablets (Sevredol®)	10 mg, 20 mg and 50 mg tablets suitable for those patients who prefer tablets
Morphine suppositories	10, 15, 20, 30, 50, 100 mg, similar bioavailability to oral morphine

Delayed release oral preparations -
Duration of action 12 h

Morphine sulphate controlled release tablets, e.g. MST – Continus® Oramorph® SR	Available in 5, 10, 30, 60, 100 and 200 mg strength Suitable for patients with good pain control on a stable dose of morphine
Morphine sulphate slow release suspension	Sachet of granules to mix with water: 20, 30, 60, 100, 200 mg

Duration of action 24 h

Morphine sulphate controlled release tablets e.g. MXL capsules®	Available in 30, 60, 90, 120, 150, 200 mg capsules
Morphine sulphate injection	Diamorphine is usually used in preference because of its greater solubility

Dihydrocodeine is a semi-synthetic analogue of codeine and has the advantage of being available in a delayed release preparation that can be given twice daily rather than 4-hourly as with coproxamol.

Although there are now a large number of alternate strong opioids available on the market morphine remains the opioid of choice at step 3.[2] There are a large number of preparations and strengths of morphine available as shown in Table 12.1.

When starting morphine, patients should ideally be prescribed one of the immediate release preparations, e.g. Sevredol® or Oramorph®, that are given every four hours at a dose of 5–10 mg. The dose can then be increased every 24 hours or so until pain control is achieved. The total daily dose can then be give as a delayed release preparation, either once or twice a day, e.g. 4-hourly 10 mg immediate release morphine can be given as MST Continuus® 30 mg bd or as MXL-capsules® 60 mg once a day. A 'breakthrough dose', which is

Table 12.2 *Guidelines for the prescription of morphine*

1. Start with a low dose of immediate release morphine
2. Prescribe a regular 4-hourly dose (with a double dose at night to avoid the middle-of-the-night dose).
3. The same 4-hourly dose should be given 'prn' for 'breakthrough pain'.
4. Review after 24–36 h and if pain is not controlled, increase 4-hourly dose by one-third e.g. 10 → 15 → 20 → 30 → 40 mg.
5. Once the pain is controlled, convert to once or twice daily slow-release morphine preparations.
6. Continue to supply appropriate 'breakthrough' doses equivalent to the 4-hourly dose in an immediate release preparation.
7. If pain control is lost, recalculate total daily dose required according to 'breakthrough' requirements.
8. *Always* prescribe a laxative to be taken concurrently.
9. Ensure that outpatients have a supply of antiemetics in case of opioid induced nausea.
10. Reassure that most of the initial side effects e.g. drowsiness, light-headedness and nausea, will pass.
11. Ensure appropriate patient review.

equivalent to the 4-hourly dose (or one-sixth the total 24 hours dose) can be given at any time in between planned doses for uncontrolled or 'breakthrough' pain. A patient should never be expected to wait the standard 4 hours for the next dose of morphine if they are in pain. The necessity for many breakthrough doses would suggest, however, that the baseline dose should be increased. It is unusual for patients to have to take delayed release morphine more often than recommended. Very rarely, a patient may have to take MST Continuus® 8-hourly rather than 12-hourly, for example, but this usually indicates that the baseline 12-hourly dose needs to be increased. There is no ceiling dose of morphine; the correct dose for any patient is the dose that controls the pain. Most patients can be controlled on ≤ 30 mg 4-hourly but the dose range is huge (5–> 500 mg 4-hourly). Guidelines for the prescription of morphine are shown in Table 12.2. Patients are advised to take morphine regularly rather than 'as required' as morphine is a relatively poor analgesic when given orally in single doses. Morphine-6-glucuronide (M6G), an active morphine metabolite, is a potent analgesic but is produced in very small quantities after single doses of morphine. It is thought that repeated dosing is necessary to allow accumulation of M6G to sufficient levels to provide analgesia and specifically to cross into the cerebral spinal fluid to reach central opioid receptors.[3]

Patients should always be prescribed laxatives along with morphine as constipation is an inevitable side effect of the drug. Other side effects include nausea and vomiting and drowsiness which usually resolve after a couple of days. Respiratory depression can be used to advantage to palliate breathlessness in a patient without pain, but in patients with pain this is not usually a problem. Pain does appear to provide physiological antagonism to the respiratory depressant effects of opioid analgesia.[4] Dry mouth is unfortunately a common side effect that does not tend to resolve. Itch and hallucinations are rarer side effects which are generally a contraindication to the continued use of the drug.

Morphine toxicity is reflected by increasing drowsiness, miosis, myoclonic jerks and respiratory depression. This often reflects deteriorating renal function as morphine-6-glucuronide accumulates in renal failure. This situation can usually be managed by stopping the drug for a while and re-starting at a lower dose but in severe toxicity the morphine effect may be reversed with naloxone, a synthetic opioid agonist that competitively antagonises the effects of opioids.

Unfortunately, many patients equate morphine with the 'end of the road' and feel that if they agree to take morphine they are somehow 'giving up'. It is crucial, therefore, to explain that this is not the case and that morphine may in fact allow people to live longer by allowing them greater activity and relieving stress. Another common concern is a fear of addiction. Although patients can develop a physical dependence to morphine (as detected by a withdrawal syndrome when the drug is stopped suddenly), addiction encompasses psychological and behavioural factors which do not apply when morphine is taken for pain. There is no reason why a woman on morphine cannot continue to undertake normal daily activities (including driving) assuming her pain is under control.[5]

When the oral route is not available, diamorphine is the agent of choice to be used parenterally at step 3 (see below). Fentanyl is a synthetic opioid that is available in a transdermal delivery system. Skin patches are applied every 72 h and a 'fentanyl depot' concentrates in the upper skin layers from which drug diffuses to the systemic circulation. The full clinical effects are not noted for 8–16 hours following application of the patch and persist for about 17 hours after patch removal. Fentanyl patches are therefore not suitable for patients with acute or changing pain as dose titration is difficult. It offers an alternate non-invasive parenteral approach for patients with chronic stable pain however.[6]

Some of the alternative opioids available and their respective advantages and disadvantages are listed in Table 12.3. There has been recent interest in the concept of opioid rotation whereby improved pain relief with fewer side effects can sometimes be achieved by changing a patient from one strong opioid to another. The exact underlying mechanism is not clear but it may be that changing to a new drug allows toxic metabolites of the previous drug to dispel and is subsequently better tolerated.[7]

Co-analgesics are drugs which often have little intrinsic analgesic effect but, when taken with standard analgesia, can confer an addi-

Table 12.3 *'Alternate' strong opioids*

Drug	Indication	Comments
Diamorphine	Nil by mouth Inability to take oral medications	Greater solubility than morphine allows injection of smaller volumes Drug of choice for subcutaneous strong opioid infusion
Phenazocine	Intolerance to morphine	Often better tolerated in the elderly, can be given sublingually; dose-limited by number of tablets (5 mg tablets only available)
Fentanyl transdermal patch	When oral route not available Gut absorption poor	Patch changed every 3 days ? less constipating than morphine Not suitable for dose titration in unstable pain
Methadone	Opioid rotation	Long half-life Should not be given more often than twice daily, toxic metabolites can accumulate with prolonged use.
Oxycodone	Headache secondary to raised intracranial pressure	Analogue of morphine available in both oral and PR formulations
Hydromorphone	Opioid rotation	Analogue of morphine with similar pharmaco-kinetic properties Widely used in the USA
Tramadol	WHO Step 2 to 3 analgesic (moderate to severe pain)	Opioid and non-opioid analgesia by enhancement of serotoninergic and adrenergic pathways; therefore fewer opioid side effects, but has ceiling dose
Pethidine	*Not* indicated in chronic pain because of short half-life	Less intense action at smooth muscle compared with morphine plus additional anticholinergic effects, toxic metabolites accumulate with prolonged use
Dextromoramide	Incident pain Painful procedures, e.g. wound dressings	Short half-life, duration of action 1–2 h, unsuitable for regular analgesia in chronic pain

tive benefit with respect to pain control at any step of the WHO ladder. Examples include the use of non-steroidal anti-inflammatory drugs (NSAIDs) in bone pain or anticonvulsants for neuropathic pain (Table 12.4.) (see below). Corticosteroids are valuable co-analgesics in several pain situations. As well as their non-specific benefit in mood elevation and general well-being they can often provide added analgesia for bone pain, neuropathic pain and inflammatory tumours. Side

Table 12.4 *Co-analgesics*

Indication	Appropriate agents	Comments
Bone pain	NSAIDs	Anti-inflammatory action via inhibition of prostaglandin synthesis
	Bisphosphonates	Potent inhibitors of osteoclast-mediated bone resorption
	Corticosteroids	
Neuropathic pain	Antidepressants e.g. amitriptyline dothiepin	Analgesic effect via increased levels of serotonin in spinal cord Indicated for dysaesthetic, aching neuropathic pain
	Anticonvulsants, e.g. sodium valproate carbamazepine	Analgesic effect via stabilisation of neuronal membrane Indicated for shooting, lancinating pain
	Antiarrhythmics e.g. flecainide, mexiletine	Membrane stabilisers, usually used '3rd line', caution in patients with cardiac history
	Corticosteroids	Reduce perineuronal oedema
Soft tissue inflammation	NSAIDs Corticosteroids Antibiotics	Useful for inflammatory breast tumours
Muscle spasm	Benzodiazepines Baclofen	Added anxiolytic effect Can be sedative

effects following long-term use are significant, however, and include proximal myopathy, Cushingoid habitus, oral candida, glucose intolerance, sleep disturbance and even psychosis. Patients on steroids should always be monitored so that the drug can be discontinued if the desired symptomatic benefit is not achieved. If effective, maintenance doses should be kept as low as possible.[8] One must also consider non-pharmacological means of pain control. Acupuncture, transcutaneous electrical nerve stimulator (TENS), relaxation therapy, massage and distraction therapy for example, can all be of great benefit to some patients. Similarly, anaesthetic techniques for pain control, e.g. spinal opioid administration and neurolytic blocks, are sometimes indicated for the control of particularly difficult pain or where standard analgesia cannot be tolerated because of unacceptable side effects.

Factors that predict for difficult or poor pain control are: neuropathic pain, incident pain (pain only on movement), high previous narcotic exposure, major psychological distress, high tolerance (necessitating rapid increase in dose) and a past history of alcoholism or drug addiction.

Special pain circumstances that are particularly common in metastatic breast cancer are as follows.

Bone pain secondary to metastatic bone metastases (Fig. 12.3)

Radiotherapy remains the treatment of choice for the palliation of bone disease. Single fractions have been shown to be as effective as multiple fractions in the achievement of pain control[9] and this is obviously more acceptable to patients, especially those with a poor performance status. NSAIDs are specifically indicated in this situation but should always be used as an adjunct to the basic analgesia as described above. There are a large number of these agents available and none is clearly superior to any other. They all share the most common toxicity which is gastrointestinal irritation. Many are now available in slow release preparations (which are valuable for patients who are on a large number of medications) as well as suppository and elixir form (see Table 12.5). It is important to remember that the prescription of an NSAID 'per rectum' does not protect from gastrointestinal toxicity as this is a systemic effect.[10] Other side effects include fluid retention and a reversible inhibition of platelet aggregation and they should not be used in patients with low platelet counts. All NSAIDs should be used with caution in the elderly and in those with cardiac or renal impairment.

Biphosponates are potent inhibitors of osteoclast-mediated bone resorption. There is now quite extensive experience with their use not only for the prevention of complications of bone disease, but also for

Figure 12.3
Bone scan showing widespread metastases from breast carcinoma.

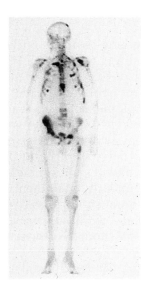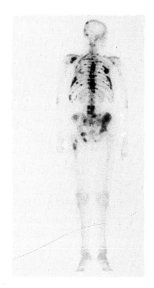

Table 12.5 *Non-steroidal anti-inflammatory agents*

Drug	Usual oral dose	Comments
Naproxen (S, E)	500 mg bd	Available as enteric coated preparation
Diclofenac (S, E)	50 mg tds	75 mg and 100 mg slow-release preparations available
Ibuprofen (E)	400 mg tds – 600 mg qds	Fewer side effects than other NSAIDs but weaker anti-inflammatory properties
Ketoprofen (S)	100–200 mg daily	Available as once daily slow-release preparation
Sulindac	200 mg bd	Least harmful in renal failure
Indomethacin (S, E)	50 mg tds	? greater gastrointestinal toxicity
Ketorolac	40 mg/day	? higher analgesic/anti-inflammatory ratio, can be given subcutaneously

S Available as suppository.

E Available as elixir/dispersible tablet.

Figure 12.4
Pathological fracture of a humerus that may have been prevented by prophylactic pinning

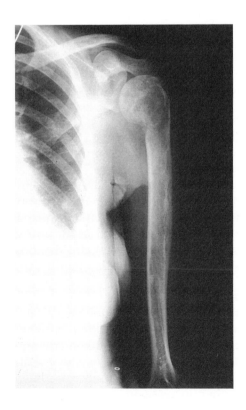

the palliation of bone pain.[11] The ideal route and scheduling of these agents remains unclear.

Orthopaedic procedures, e.g. pinning of a femur or a total hip joint replacement should be undertaken prophylactically where there is loss of integrity of bone cortex or as a palliative procedure following pathological fracture (Fig. 12.4).

Neuropathic pain

Neuropathic pain results from damage or compression to a peripheral nerve. The most common example of this in breast cancer is brachial plexopathy following treatment of the axilla or recurrent disease in the axilla. Neuropathic pain is classically resistant to standard analgesia and in this situation it is often necessary to use co-analgesics at an early stage. Agents that are widely used in this situation include antidepressants, anticonvulsants and some antiarrhythmics as shown in Table 12.4. The antiarrhythmics and anticonvulsants are thought to work via their membrane-stabilising activity and are possibly more effective for shooting, lancinating type pain, whereas antidepressants have a central and peripheral action on serotonin and noradrenaline-mediated neurotransmission and are indicated for burning or dysaesthetic type neuropathic pain. Each of these drugs has its own inherent side effects (sedation being the most common) and should be used with care. The doses required to achieve an analgesic effect are often well below the doses required to achieve the usual effect, e.g. the analgesic effect of amitriptyline is seen well below its antidepressant effect. Neurolytic blocks, for example intercostal or brachial plexus blocks, should be considered for neuropathic pain that does not respond to the measures described above.

Liver capsular pain

Right upper quadrant pain is frequent in patients with liver metastases. This follows not only swelling of the liver capsule but may also be particularly severe following a bleed into a liver metastasis.

Non-steroidal anti-inflammatory drugs may provide an excellent additive analgesic effect in this situation. Similarly corticosteroids can reduce swelling, inflammation and pain in an enlarged liver. Dexamethasone can be started at an oral dose of about 8 mg a day and then reduced to the lowest effective dose to avoid side effects. A maintenance dose of 2–4 mg is often necessary to maintain control.

Headache

In the scenario of metastatic breast cancer, especially if associated with vomiting, headache is often a sign of cerebral metastases. It is frequently taught that codeine and strong opioids should be avoided in this situation because of the possibility of respiratory depression associated with hypercapnoea leading to reflex cerebral vasodilation, a further increase in intracranial pressure and increased headache. Although this does not appear to be a common practical problem, especially if these agents are used in conjunction with dexamethasone, oxycodone, a strong opioid available in both oral and rectal preparations, can be particularly valuable in this situation.

Spiritual pain

Pain is multifactorial and is often exacerbated by added burdens such as fear, anxiety, anger, depression, sleep disturbance, uncertainty and other uncontrolled symptoms. These factors are often overlooked with the main focus of pain control being on the physical aspects. It is crucially important, therefore, to make every attempt to relieve these factors if 'complete pain control' is to be achieved. Simple measures such as explanation, reassurance, understanding and empathy can have profound pain-relieving effects. Anxiety and depression should be carefully assessed before deciding on a course of action but may require specific treatment with either anxiolytics (e.g. diazepam, lorazepam) or antidepressants (e.g. fluoxetine).

Dyspnoea It is not always the malignancy that causes shortness of breath in a patient with metastatic breast cancer. It is therefore important to look for and treat any underlying treatable cause, for example infection, pulmonary embolism or anaemia. Specific causes of breathlessness include malignant pleural effusions, lymphangitis carcinomatosis, intrapulmonary metastases, pericardal effusion and constricting chest wall disease.

Aspiration of a pleural effusion will often result in significant improvement of a patient's dyspnoea. Pleurodesis with bleomycin or tetracycline can be effective but only if the chest is drained to complete dryness. Talc pleurodesis via thoracoscopy is a most effective way of preventing reaccumulation of the fluid.[12] A pleuroperitoneal shunt should be considered in a fit patient whose major problem is of recurrent effusions. Lymphangitis carcinomatosis is an exceptionally common complication of metastatic disease. The patient presents with gradually progressive shortness of breath and dry cough. Auscultation of the chest is often non-contributory but a chest radiograph will show fine septal lines reflecting interstitial oedema. It is best palliated with corticosteroids at the lowest possible dose that controls symptoms. Corticosteroids can also help dyspnoea associated with intrapulmonary disease almost certainly be reducing inflammation around a tumour.

The respiratory depressive effect of opioids can often be used to great advantage in patients who are dyspnoeic, especially those without pain. A small dose of regular morphine is used in conjunction with anxiolytics such as diazepam to calm both the patient and the respiratory drive. Morphine can also suppress the production of respiratory secretions. Any reversible airways component can be well palliated with bronchodilators such as ventolin either orally or by a nebuliser. Morphine is also an effective cough suppressant. Small doses of methadone at night can successfully control troublesome nocturnal cough without leading to unbearable drowsiness. Lignocaine or bupivacaine nebulisers are rarely required. A short course of palliative radiotherapy to an obstructed bronchus, especially if this is associated with haemoptysis, is often worthwhile.

Nausea and vomiting

The commonest causes of this symptom in metastatic breast disease are therapy, specifically chemotherapy and radiotherapy. Other common causes are hypercalcaemia, liver metastases and constipation.

Nausea and vomiting is often multifactorial in origin, however, and a specific treatable cause may not be identified. There are a large number of antiemetics available, which act at different sites or via different mechanisms. The appropriateness of each in specific situa-

Table 12.6 *Antiemetics*

Drug	Specific indication	Comments
Metoclopramide[a]	Treatment related nausea and vomiting Gastric stasis	Dopamine antagonist ($5HT_3$ antagonist at high dose) Gastrokinetic may induce acute dystonic reaction
Domperidone	Speeds gastric emptying and gut transit time	Available in suppository form Gastrokinetic
Haloperidol[a]	Drug of choice for opioid-induced nausea and vomiting	Sedative at dose > 3 mg/24 h Long half-life; can be given once or twice daily
Cyclizine[a]	Nausea and vomiting associated with bowel obstruction	Antihistamine; can cause dry mouth Will not exacerbate bowel colic
Methotrimeprazine[a]	If sedation is desirable	Powerful, broad-spectrum antiemetic with activity at several different receptors
Prochlorperazine	Motion sickness	Phenothazine derivative
Ondansetron Granisetron	Chemo- and radiotherapy-induced vomiting; also post-operative	Potent $5HT_3$-receptor antagonists
Corticosteroids[a]	Vomiting, secondary to raised ICP or liver metastases	Broad spectrum antiemetic

[a] Can be given subcutaneously.

tions is shown in Table 12.6. Haloperidol and methotrimeprazine are probably the most appropriate 'broad spectrum' antiemetics when no obvious cause is identifiable. There is little evidence to support the use of the 5-HT$_3$-receptor blockers other than for chemo- or radiotherapy-induced vomiting. Corticosteroids can often give control when all other antiemetics have failed, especially in the case of metastatic liver disease. A cycle of protracted vomiting can sometimes be broken by giving antiemetics via a continuous subcutaneous infusion. Those drugs suitable for delivery by this route are shown in Table 12.6.

Anorexia and weight loss

This is not as common in breast cancer as it is in many other advanced malignancies, for example carcinoma of the pancreas or lung. Corticosteroids will improve appetite and general well-being but there is little evidence that they result in actual non-fluid weight gain.[13] Progestogens are commonly used as third-line hormonal therapy in breast cancer. Increased appetite and weight gain is a well documented side effect of these agents that can be used to advantage in metastatic disease.[14]

Sore mouth

One of the commonest causes of sore mouth is oral candida. This usually follows therapy (especially with corticosteroids) but can develop because of general debility. If a therapeutic dose of nystatin (5 ml qds) does not eradicate this, a 5-day course of fluconazole is indicated, care being taken in those patients with renal impairment. Most patients find amphotericin lozenges unpalatable as they are large and sticky.

A dry mouth is a side effect of opioid analgesia and can follow radiotherapy to the head and neck. Fluoride may stimulate saliva in some patients and fluoride mouth washes and toothpaste are recommended. Artificial saliva is available but distasteful. Tinned pineapple contains a proteolytic enzyme, ananase, that will stimulate saliva and cleanse the mouth. Regular tooth brushing and mouth care, including the regular use of a mouth wash (e.g. chlorhexidine gluconate 0.2%) should be encouraged to avoid infection.

The effervescent action of one-quarter of a vitamin C tablet will improve a coated tongue, and sucralfate suspension tends to coat and heal mouth ulcers.

Abdominal distension

The commonest cause of abdominal distension in metastatic breast cancer is ascites, usually associated with liver metastases or intraperitoneal disease. Abdominal paracentesis can lead to considerable relief and should be relatively painless when performed with a narrow bore tube, e.g. a suprapubic catheter. Leaving a tube 'in situ' provides a route of infection and therefore, the procedure should be repeated on an 'as required' basis. The use of diuretics in this situation serves only to dehydrate the patient and rarely results in satisfactory control of ascites.

Lymphoedema

Lymphoedema of the upper limb develops following recurrence in the axilla and as a complication of treatment (surgery and radiotherapy). It is associated with pain and often loss of mobility and function of the arm.

Diuretics may help but meticulous skin care, massage, elevation of the limb, bandaging and use of support sleeves to prevent recurrence are other practical measures. Oedematous limbs are prone to infection and antibiotics should be prescribed at the earliest suggestion of cellulitis.

Ankle swelling will often cause the patient great alarm even in the face of widespread metastatic disease. Hypoalbuminaemia, immobility and concurrent medications as well as mechanical blockage by tumour can all exacerbate this condition. Diuretics and support hose remain the mainstay of treatment. Intravenous albumin supplementation is of short-lasting benefit and not generally recommended.

Wounds

Many women live with extensive locally recurrent malignancy for many months before they die. Chest wall disease can be most distressing, particularly because of its detrimental effect on body image. Poor nutritional state, infection and oedema will all have an adverse effect on a malignant wound. There are a large number of dressings available with different properties appropriate for different types of wound (Table 12.7). The aim in this situation is not to heal but to keep wounds clean and free of infection, to control pain and provide maximum comfort. Dressings must be cosmetically acceptable. Antibiotics effective against anaerobes, e.g. metronidazole, given either systemically or topically, can relieve malodour. Tranexamic acid can also be given topically to prevent bleeding. Superficial radiotherapy will prevent ulceration of a subcutaneous lesion and can provide local control over limited areas.

Constipation

Although trivial to the well, constipation is a common and most distressing symptom to those with advanced disease and, as with pain, treatment should be continuous and anticipatory. It can lead to considerable abdominal discomfort and is a common cause of nausea and vomiting. Unfortunately, almost all strong analgesics cause constipation and the situation is often exacerbated by inactivity, poor diet, dehydration and hypercalcaemia. This condition should be taken seriously and treated aggressively with regular oral laxatives along with enema and suppositories as indicated (Table 12.8). Opioid-induced constipation is best treated with compound preparations such as codanthramer which contains both a faecal softener (poloxamer) and a

Table 12.7 *Wound dressings*

Type of wound	Deep		Shallow	
	Low exudate	**High exudate**	**Low exudate**	**High exudate**
Necrotic Brown/black hard dead tissue must be removed to allow granulation	Require debridement by: Surgery Hydrogel Enzymes			
Sloughy Yellow dead tissue must be removed to allow granulation	Hydrogel Hydrocolloid paste	Alginate	Hydrogel Hydrocolloid sheet	Alginate
	(Enzymes can be used if above methods fail)			
Infected Identified by clinical signs: pain, heat, swelling, redness. Dressing needs changing daily. May require *systemic* antibiotics. Irrigate with sodium chloride 0.9% only; do not use topical antiseptic/antibiotics	Hydrogel	Alginate Foam cavity dressing	Hydrogel Hydrocolloid	Alginate
Malodorous Need to eradicate organisms causing odour. Can use dressing to absorb odour. Consider systemic antibiotics	Metronidazole gel + primary dressing of choice + secondary dressing if required + charcoal dressing			
Granulating Pink/red appearance. Bleeds easily. Do not change dressing frequently. Requires protection	Hydrogel Hydrocolloid	Alginate Foam cavity dressing	Hydrogel sheet Hydrocolloid	Alginate Foam sheet
Epithelialising Pink/white tissue, still fragile. Requires protection.	Thin hydrocolloid sheet Hydrogel sheet Semi-permeable film			

From: Royal Marsden Hospital Wound Care Guidelines.

Table 12.8 *Aperients*

Drug	Indication/mechanism of action	Comments
Bran Ispaghula husk (Fybogel®) Sterculia (Normacol®)	Bulking agents increase stool by absorbing water	Avoid in patients with bowel obstruction Maintain adequate fluid intake
Liquid paraffin	Faecal softeners Lubricates and softens impacted faeces	Should not be used in patients with swallowing difficulties (danger of aspiration lipoid pneumonia)
Docusate sodium Arachis oil enema	For 'per rectum intervention'	Added stimulant properties
Magnesium sulphate	Osmotic laxatives, retain fluid in bowel	Useful when rapid bowel evacuation is required; use with caution in the elderly and debilitated
Lactulose		Semisynthetic disaccharide, not absorbed from bowel, added antimicrobial effect may take up to 48 h to act
Phosphate suppositories	For clearance of rectal impaction	
Senna Bisacodyl	Bowel stimulants, increase colonic motility	May increase colicky pain
Danthron		Colours urine red, skin contact can cause irritation and excoriation
Glycerol suppositories	Rectal stimulant because of irritant action of glycerol	

stimulant (danthron) or co-danthrusate (danthron 50 mg, docusate 60 mg). Care must be taken in those patients who are incontinent or catheterised as the danthron can cause skin staining, irritation and occasionally excoriation. The combination of bisacodyl and docusate is a logical alternative in this situation.

Confusion Common causes of confusion are drug toxicity, infection, hypoxia, hypercalcaemia and direct cancer involvement of the central nervous system. The cause should be actively sought and treated accordingly.

Hypercalcaemia presents with polyuria, poldypsia, dehydration, nausea and vomiting, confusion and somnolence that can progress to coma and death if not treated. Tumour-induced hypercalcaemia (TIH) is a particularly common complication of advanced metastatic bone disease. Intravenous bisphosphonates remain the treatment of choice for TIH as they are easy to deliver and relatively devoid of side effects.[15] Patients should be re-hydrated with at least two litres of normal saline prior to intravenous bisphosphonates (either pamidronate 90 mg or sodium clodronate 1500 mg in 500 ml normal saline over 4–6 h). The serum calcium should return to normal within three to four days, associated with an improvement in symptoms. The hypercalcaemia will almost certainly recur after two to four weeks if no further specific systemic anticancer therapy is available. It can be re-treated but will eventually become resistant. Maintenance therapy with oral bisphosphonates does not generally delay the recurrence of hypercalcaemia. TIH is a preterminal event and the median survival following an initial episode of TIH is two months, except in those patients in whom further systemic anticancer therapy is available.[16] Although the symptoms associated with hypercalcaemia are distressing and should be treated, the benefit of treating TIH in a patient in whom no further anti-cancer therapy is possible and who presents with no symptoms must be questioned.

The brain is frequently a site of metastases and patients may present with a localised weakness, convulsions or personality change as well as confusion. If one suspects cerebral secondaries, the patient should be commenced on high dose steroids (e.g. dexamethasone 8 mg bd) while awaiting confirmation of the diagnosis. An improvement on steroids bodes well for subsequent response to radiotherapy. Short courses of radiotherapy (up to five fractions) are as effective as prolonged courses. The median survival following the diagnosis of cerebral metastases is about three months although some patients live longer.

Weakness

Weakness, lethargy and fatigue are common but rarely reported symptoms of advanced disease. General debility, poor nutrition, depression, electrolyte disturbance (e.g. hyponatraemia or hypomagnesaemia) and treatment can all contribute.

If a patient suddenly 'goes off her legs', especially if this is associated with bowel or bladder disturbance and sensory loss, malignant cord compression should be considered and investigated immediately. Vertebral disease is common in metastatic breast cancer and is often unsuspected until imaged by a magnetic resonance scan[17] (Fig. 12.5). Cord compression is not uncommon and must be treated with urgency. The success of treatment is often dependent on early detection. High dose steroids should be commenced at first suspicion and continued until treatment is complete. Surgical decompression may be appropriate for single lesions or early in the disease course, but as this condition is often associated with widespread metastatic disease, radiotherapy is normally the treatment of choice.

Figure 12.5
Malignant cord compression as demonstrated by MRI scanning

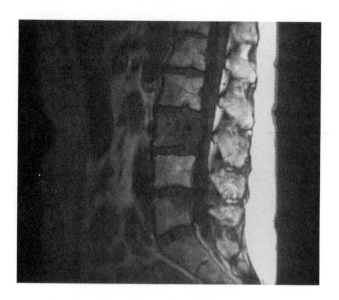

The dying patient

The ability to deliver drugs subcutaneously has in some ways revolutionised the dying process, although some believe that this has resulted in the institutionalisation of death and a further loss of the ability to die naturally.[18] Drugs that can be delivered subcutaneously via a syringe-driver in this situation are listed in Table 12.9. Recommended sites for the placement of subcutaneous needles are shown in Fig. 12.6 and some guidelines for the use of a syringe driver are given in Table 12.10.

It is crucial to continue to deliver analgesia to dying patients. Those that can no longer take oral medications can be given drugs per rectum, transdermally or via a subcutaneous infusion. Diamorphine is the strong opioid of choice when delivered subcutaneously. It is much more soluble than morphine allowing for larger doses to be delivered in a smaller volume. The appropriate dose of subcutaneous diamorphine is one-third the total daily dose of oral morphine although this often needs to be increased during the terminal phase.

A common problem encountered when managing the dying patient is terminal restlessness. The former may result from uncontrolled pain although recent work suggests that it may be exacerbated by dehydration and consequent accumulation of toxic metabolites of strong opioids.[19] Midazolam, a benzodiazepine derivative, is the drug most commonly used to combat terminal restlessness. When nausea and vomiting has been a major problem, a more appropriate agent to use in this situation may be methotrimeprazine which has both antipsychotic sedative and antiemetic properties.[20] Both drugs can be delivered subcutaneously. Rectal diazepam provides an alternative choice if the subcutaneous route is not being used.

Figure 12.6
*Recommended sites
for the placement of
subcutaneous
needles.*

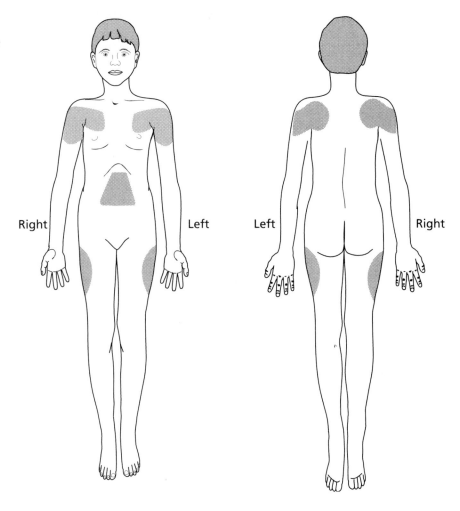

Right   Left   Left   Right

In terminal dyspnoea the primary aim is to depress respiratory drive, control anxiety and calm the patient. This can be achieved pharmacologically with small doses of morphine or diamorphine given regularly in conjunction with benzodiazepines. Retained bronchial secretions can result in alarming sounds of laboured breathing in the dying patient. This can be alarming to relatives and carers but can be lessened with the judicious use of hyoscine hydrobromide which dries secretions in large airways.

Many relatives and carers find it difficult to cope with loved ones dying and not receiving fluid or nourishment when intravenous lines are taken down or removed. Up to 2 litres/day normal saline can be delivered via the subcutaneous route, but in a patient who is obviously dying of an incurable disease, a death without lines or tubes seems more dignified and can break down barriers between carers and dying patient.

Table 12.9 *Drugs suitable for subcutaneous administration to the dying patient*

Drug	Indication	Comments
Diamorphine	Analgesia	The 24 h dose of diamorphine is one-third the 24 h oral morphine dose
Midazolam	Terminal restlessness and agitation Convulsions	Can be mixed with diamorphine in syringe driver Usual dose 20–60 mg 24 hourly
Methotrimeprazine	Terminal restlessness Vomiting/nausea	Antipsychotic effect can help terminal confusion, usual starting dose 25 mg 24 hourly
Hyoscine hydrobromide	Retained bronchial secretions	Should be given prophylactically, can result in profound dryness Maximum 24 h dose 2–4 mg
Dexamethasone	Chronic steroid use	Sudden discontinuation can exacerbate terminal distress
Haloperidol	Nausea and vomiting	Commonly used with diamorphine to combat opioid-induced vomiting Sedative at high doses (> 3 mg/day)
Cyclizine	Bowel obstruction	Does not exacerbate colicky pain, may precipitate at concentrations > 10 mg/ml

Conclusion Although metastatic breast cancer is an incurable malignancy, it is possible to live with advanced disease for many years. With the provision of good palliative measures it is possible to achieve good quality of life for many women. This care encompasses not only the patient but their relatives and carers. Palliative care should be considered early in the course of the disease and should continue throughout the illness trajectory.

Many thousands of women die of breast cancer each year. In the UK women can usually have the choice of place of death (hospice, hospital or home), because of the well-developed hospice and palliative care services. Similarly there is a large number of support services available in the community for breast cancer sufferers (e.g. Macmillan nurses, Marie Curie Cancer Care, The Sue Ryder Foundation and the British Association of Cancer United Patients) to provide counselling and general support to women with breast cancer and to their friends and carers.

Table 12.10 *Guidelines for the use of subcutaneous infusions in palliative care*

1. Use of a simple battery-operated portable syringe driver with a butterfly infusion set to deliver drugs at a predetermined site.

2. The best sites to place the subcutaneous needle are the lateral aspects of the upper arms and thigh, the abdomen, the anterior chest and below the clavicle, avoiding any bony prominence (Fig. 12.6).

3. Provided there is evidence of compatibility, selected injections can be mixed in syringe drivers; e.g. the following can be used with diamorphine: midazolam, methotrimeprazine, hyoscine, haloperidol, cyclizine[a] and dexamethasone[a] – where possible avoid more than two drugs in one combination.

4. Some medications are *not* suitable for subcutaneous infusion, e.g. chlorpromazine, prochlorperazine and diazepam, all of which cause skin reactions at the injection site.

5. Small volumes of water for injection are usually used to dissolve drugs as normal saline increases the likelihood of precipitation when more than one drug is used.

6. The infusion site should be checked regularly. Swelling at the site of injection is not an indication for site change whereas pain or obvious inflammation is.

7. Cover the infusion site with a semi-occlusive dressing, e.g. Tegaderm®, to allow observation of needle site.

8. The infusion can be programmed to run over 6, 12 or 24 h, and drug doses should be reviewed regularly.

9. Check syringe driver frequently to ensure correct administration rate.

[a] May precipitate at higher dose levels.

References

1. Ventafridda V, Tamburini M, Caraceni A, de Conno F, Naldi F. A validation study of the WHO method for cancer pain relief. Cancer 1987; 59: 850–6.

2. Hanks GW, de Conno F, Hanna M, *et al.* Morphine in cancer pain: modes of administration. Br Med J 1996; 312: 823–6.

3. Gorman DJ. Opioid analgesics in the management of pain in patients with cancer: an update. Palliat Med 1991; 5: 277–94.

4. Walsh TD, Baxter R, Bowman K, Leban B. High dose morphine and respiratory function in chronic pain. Pain 1981; Supp 1: 539.

5. Vainio A, Ollila J, Matikainen E, Rosenberg P, Kalso E. Driving ability in cancer patients receiving long-term morphine analgesia. Lancet 1995; 346: 667–70.

6. Zech DFJ, Lehmann KA, Grond S. A new treatment option for chronic cancer pain. Eur J Palliat Care 1995; 1: 26–30.

7. de Stoutz ND, Bruera E, Suarez-Almazor M. Opioid rotation for toxicity reduction in terminal care patients. J. Pain Symptom Manage. 1995; 10: 378–84.

8. Twycross R. Corticosteroids in advanced cancer. Br Med J 1992; 305: 969–70.

9. Price P, Hoskin P, Easton D, Austin D, Palmer S, Yarnold J. Prospective randomised trial of single and multifraction radiotherapy schedules in the treatment of painful bony metastases. Radiother Oncol 1986; 6: 247–55.

10. Pace V. Use of nonsteroidal anti-inflammatory drugs in cancer. Palliat Med 1995; 9: 273–86.

11. Holten-Verzantvoort AT, Kroon HM, Bijvoet OI, Cleton FJ, *et al.* Palliative pamidronate treatment in patients with bone metastases from breast cancer. J. Clin. Oncol 1993; 11: 491–8.

12. Miles DW, Knight RK. Diagnosis and management of malignant pleural effusion. Cancer Treat Rev 1993; 19: 151–68.

13. Loprinzi CL, Goldberg M, Burnham NL. Cancer associated anorexia and cachexia; implications for therapy. Drugs 1992; 43: 499–506.

14. Tchekmedyian NS, Hickman M, Sian J, *et al.* Megesterol acetatate in cancer anorexia and weight loss. Cancer 1992; 69: 1268–74.

15. Ralston SH, Gardner MD, Dryburgh FJ, Jenkins AS, Cowan RA, Boyle IT. Comparison of aminohydroxypropylidene diphosphonate mithramycin and corticosteroids/calcitonin in the treatment of cancer associated hypercalcaemia. Lancet 1985; ii: 907–16.

16. Ling PJ, A'Hern RP, Hardy JR. Analysis of survival following treatment of tumour-induced hypercalcaemia with intravenous pamidronate (APD). Br J Cancer 1995; 72: 206–9.

17. Jones AL, Williams MP, Powles TJ, *et al.* Magnetic resonance imaging in the detection of skeletal metastases in patients with breast cancer. Br J Cancer 1990; 62: 296–8.

18. O'Neil WM. Subcutaneous infusions – a medical last rite. Palliat Med 1994; 8: 91–3.

19. Bruera E, Franco JJ, Maltoni M, Watanabe S, Suarez-Almazor M. Changing pattern of agitated impaired mental status in patients with advanced cancer: association with cognitive monitoring, hydration and opioid rotation. J. Pain and Sympt Manage. 1995; 10: 287–91.

20. Oliver DJ. The use of methotrimeprazine in terminal care. Br J Clin Pract 1985; 39: 9.

Index

Page numbers in *italic* refer to illustrations and tables; **bold** page numbers indicate a main discussion.